Client Teaching Guides for Home Health Care

Third Edition

Linda H. Gorman, BSN, RN

JONES AND BARTLETT PUBLISHERS

Sudbury, Massachusetts

BOSTON   TORONTO   LONDON   SINGAPORE

World Headquarters
Jones and Bartlett Publishers
40 Tall Pine Drive
Sudbury, MA 01776
978-443-5000
info@jbpub.com
www.jbpub.com

Jones and Bartlett Publishers Canada
6339 Ormindale Way
Mississauga, Ontario L5V 1J2
Canada

Jones and Bartlett Publishers International
Barb House, Barb Mews
London W6 7PA
United Kingdom

Jones and Bartlett's books and products are available through most bookstores and online booksellers. To contact Jones and Bartlett Publishers directly, call 800-832-0034, fax 978-443-8000, or visit our website www.jbpub.com.

Substantial discounts on bulk quantities of Jones and Bartlett's publications are available to corporations, professional associations, and other qualified organizations. For details and specific discount information, contact the special sales department at Jones and Bartlett via the above contact information or send an email to specialsales@jbpub.com.

The authors, editor, and publisher have made every effort to provide accurate information. However, they are not responsible for errors, omissions, or for any outcomes related to the use of the contents of this book and take no responsibility for the use of the products and procedures described. Treatments and side effects described in this book may not be applicable to all people; likewise, some people may require a dose or experience a side effect that is not described herein. Drugs and medical devices are discussed that may have limited availability controlled by the Food and Drug Administration (FDA) for use only in a research study or clinical trial. Research, clinical practice, and government regulations often change the accepted standard in this field. When consideration is being given to use of any drug in the clinical setting, the health care provider or reader is responsible for determining FDA status of the drug, reading the package insert, and reviewing prescribing information for the most up-to-date recommendations on dose, precautions, and contraindications, and determining the appropriate usage for the product. This is especially important in the case of drugs that are new or seldom used.

Production Credits
Executive Editor: Kevin Sullivan
Acquisition Editor: Emily Ekle
Associate Editor: Amy Sibley
Editorial Assistant: Patricia Donnelly
Senior Production Editor: Susan Schultz
Associate Marketing Manager: Rebecca Wasley
Associate Project Manager: Courtney Robin Fleishman

Manufacturing and Inventory Control
  Supervisor: Amy Bacus
Interactive Technology Manager: Dawn Mahon Priest
Text Design and Composition: Cape Cod Compositors
Cover Design: Anne Spencer
Cover Image: © Robert Saroseik/Shutterstock, Inc.
Printing and Binding: Courier Corporation
Cover Printing: Courier Corporation

ISBN-13: 978-0-7637-4934-7
ISBN-10: 0-7637-4934-6

6048
Printed in the United States of America
14 13 12 11   10 9 8 7 6 5 4 3

Contents

Contents

Contents

Contents

Introduction

Time is money. We as health care providers now have a shorter amount of time to provide the same quality of care and teaching to our clients. Shorter hospital stays, more outpatient procedures, and rising medical costs have increased the need for teaching a client and/or caregiver about his or her disease process and procedures required. What was once done only under the umbrella of home health care is now considered under community-based nursing. Health care and health education are given in many settings in addition to the acute-care setting. Community-based nursing is needed in clinics, workplaces, outpatient facilities, schools, physician's offices, and so forth.

An important, cost-effective way to deal with providing health care is to stress the need for prevention. Understanding the basic disease process and treatment should also include ways to prevent additional problems or complications. Having this knowledge can promote faster recovery and more personal independence or responsibility and save money. Most of the teaching guides in this book include information about how to prevent complications or when to seek additional help.

Client Teaching Guides for Home Health Care covers a variety of health concerns: medical disorders/diseases, procedures and surgeries, diseases that affect specific age groups, and numerous specialty disorders such as psychiatric, maternal and neonatal, pediatric, and neurological (including dementia), as well as hospice care. The medication section was expanded with new information to meet the needs of clients, many of whom have polypharmacy issues. Also expanded was the nutrition section, which can be used by all clients to improve or maintain a healthy lifestyle. Additions that cover safety issues for specific age groups can be used to promote health and prevent injury or illness.

Each teaching guide is designed to provide a large amount of information in a condensed, easily understood way. The teaching guides and information that they provide are to be used by a nurse or professional health care provider. Teaching the client and/or caregiver is best achieved by providing verbal and written instructions for care. These guides can be photocopied or printed from the CD-ROM included in the back of this book as needed and given to the client and/or caregiver to provide continuity of care and promote his or her independence with self-care.

No book can cover all health care issues. Included with this book are many resources for further research or to reinforce the current health care treatments. Basic information to aid the professional nurse in making his or her nursing diagnosis and care plan is included with the discussion of the North American Nursing Diagnosis Association.

Part I

Nursing Diagnoses

Teaching Guides

Nursing Care Plans and the Use of Teaching Guides

1

Patient name: _____ Admission: _____

NRS
DATE INITIAL

I. **The nurse plays a major role in two important concepts of healthcare.**

A. Health promotion
B. Disease prevention
C. Reasons to adopt these two concepts are
   • More cost-effective
   • Increased client satisfaction
   • Faster recovery
D. The prevention focus is addressed at three levels:
   1. Primary prevention is the prevention of the initial occurrence of disease or injury.
   2. Secondary prevention is the early identification and treatment of disease or injury.
   3. Tertiary prevention maximizes the recovery after an illness or injury.

II. **The nurse is frequently responsible to initiate a client's plan of care. It is important to understand the components of a care plan. They are as follows:**

A. Assessment
B. Diagnosis (nursing)
C. Determine outcomes (set goals or desired outcomes for client)
D. Plan interventions (actions to be taken)
E. Give nursing care (interventions in action)
F. Evaluate nursing care (evaluate effectiveness of intervention and/or need to change plan).
G. Document (this tracks the client's condition and response, care provided, and effectiveness of any teaching given)

III. **The nursing responsibility in plan of care is as follows:**

A. The use of a nursing diagnosis provides the base on which to select and builds nursing interventions or nursing care.
B. Components of the nursing diagnosis are as follows:
   • Diagnostic label—problem
   • Etiology—cause or risk factor

NRS
DATE INITIAL

   • Signs and symptoms—defining characteristics

IV. **Explain the use of nursing diagnoses.**

A. A nursing diagnosis describes a client's response to disease or injury.
B. The most used list has been created by NANDA.
C. The medical diagnosis and nursing diagnosis are not the same.
D. The medical diagnosis describes the actual disease or injury and can be found in the ICD-9-CM codes.
E. The three types of nursing diagnosis are as follows:
   1. Actual problem
   2. Risk for problem
   3. Wellness issues

RESOURCES

2005-2006 NANDA-I-Approved Nursing Diagnosis

North American Nursing Diagnosis Association
NANDA International
100 N. 20th Street, 4th floor
Philadelphia, PA 19103
800-647-9002
E-mail: info@nanda.org
www.nanda.org/

REFERENCES

Ackley, B. J., & Ladwig, G. B. (2006). *Nursing diagnosis handbook: A guide to planning care.* St. Louis: Mosby Inc.

Canobbio, M. M. (2006). *Mosby's handbook of patient teaching.* St. Louis: Mosby Inc.

Cohen, B. J., & Taylor, J. J. (2005). *Memmler's the human body in health and disease* (10th ed.). Philadelphia: Lippincott Williams & Wilkins.

Hunt, R. (2005). *Introduction to community based nursing.* Philadelphia: Lippincott Williams & Wilkins.

Perry, A., & Potter, P. (2006). *Clinical nursing skills & technique.* St. Louis: Mosby Inc.

Part II

Diseases

Teaching Guides

1 Latex Allergy

Patient name: _____ **Admission:** _____

NRS
DATE INITIAL

I. **The client/caregiver can define latex allergy.**

A. Latex sensitivity is an allergic response to the protein in latex.

B. Latex gloves are often coated with powder that gives the latex particles the ability to become airborne.

C. Latex allergy symptoms can range from mild to severe.

II. **The client/caregiver can define the two types of allergic reaction to latex.**

A. Contact dermatitis is usually a delayed localized skin reaction that occurs within 6 to 8 hours of contact and can last several days. The most common place of reaction is the hands.

B. Immediate hypersensitivity is an instant system reaction of swelling, itching, respiratory distress, hypotension, and even death.

C. General symptoms of latex allergy can be as follows:
- Itchy, red, or watery eyes
- Sneezing or runny nose
- Coughing
- Rash or hives
- Chest tightness and shortness of breath
- Shock

III. **The client/caregiver can list common items containing latex found in the health care facility.**

- Medical gloves
- Medication vial stoppers
- Band-aids
- Stethoscope tubing
- Urinary catheters
- Tourniquets
- Blood pressure cuff and tubing
- Intravenous injection ports

IV. **The client/caregiver can list common items containing latex in the home or work areas.**

- Balloons
- Rubber toys

NRS
DATE INITIAL

- Pacifiers and baby bottle nipples
- Rubber bands
- Adhesive tape
- Diapers and sanitary pads
- Condoms
- Dental bands

V. **The client/caregiver can list ways to deal with latex allergy.**

A. Avoid direct exposure to latex.

B. Educate yourself to which products contain latex.

C. Wear a medical alert bracelet or identification.

D. Inform any employer of your allergy.

E. Discuss with your physician the severity of your allergy and whether you could benefit from use of epinephrine self-injection pen.

RESOURCES

American Academy of Allergy, Asthma and Immunology
www.aaaai.org

CDC National Institute for Occupational Health and Safety
www.cdc.gov/niosh

REFERENCES

Cohen, B. J., & Taylor, J. J. (2005). *Memmler's the human body in health and disease* (10th ed.). Philadelphia: Lippincott Williams & Wilkins.

Hitchcock, J. E., Schubert, P. E., & Thomas, S. A. (2003). *Community health nursing: Caring in action.* Clifton Park, NY: Thomson Delmar Learning.

Latex allergy: A prevention guide (NIOSH Publication No. 98-113). (1999). National Institute for Occupational Safety and Health. Centers for Disease Control and Prevention. Washington DC.

Timby, B. K., & Smith, N. C. (2003). *Introductory medical-surgical nursing* (8th ed.). Philadelphia: J. B. Lippincott Williams & Wilkins.

2 Rheumatoid Arthritis

Patient name: _____   Admission: _____

NRS
DATE INITIAL

I. **The client/caregiver can define rheumatoid arthritis (RA).**

A. It is a systemic inflammatory disorder of connective tissue and joints.
B. It is a chronic disease characterized by remissions and exacerbations.
C. The cause of this disease is unknown, but it is considered an autoimmune disease.
D. RA affects small joints early and progresses to involve large joints.
E. RA strikes most often between the ages of 20 to 40 years of age, but it can also be found in children and older adults.

II. **The client/caregiver can recognize signs and symptoms of rheumatoid arthritis.**

A. Localized symptoms are joint pain, swelling, warmth, redness (erythema), stiffness, limited mobility of affected joints, and fluid on joints.
B. The swelling and pain can come and go.
C. Stiffness can occur, particularly in the morning and when sitting for long periods of time.
D. Joints are usually affected bilaterally and symmetrically.
E. Fatigue, weakness, loss of appetite, depression, and weight loss can occur.
F. Flu-like symptoms are possible, including a low-grade fever.
G. Anemia is possible.
H. Decreased tolerance to stress can occur.

III. **The client/caregiver can list measures to manage rheumatoid arthritis.**

A. Adequate exercise
  1. Always get physician's approval for level of exercise.
  2. Regular exercise includes
    • Flexibility (stretching, range of motion)
    • Strengthening (resistance)
    • Cardiovascular (aerobic)
  3. Exercise at a slow steady pace.

NRS
DATE INITIAL

  4. Perform active or passive range of motion exercises.
  5. Never exercise a hot, inflamed joint.
  6. Balance exercise with rest.
  7. Set realistic goals.
  8. Stop exercise or activity if pain occurs.
B. Proper diet
  1. Maintain healthy weight to decrease pressure on joints.
  2. Eat well-balanced meals that are high in protein, vitamins, zinc, and iron to promote tissue building and repair.
C. Stress management skills
D. Pain control
  1. Apply heat or cold as ordered.
  2. Apply splints as ordered.
  3. Use transcutaneous electrical nerve stimulation as ordered.
  4. Take pain medications as ordered.
  5. Consider other alternatives, such as biofeedback, relaxation techniques, Tai Chi exercise, and pain clinics.
  6. Avoid extremes in temperature and damp, moist environments.
E. Physical or occupational therapy referrals
F. Assistive, adaptive, or protective devices (braces, splints, etc.)
G. Joint protection principles.
H. Medications as ordered (report any side effects to physician)
I. Reporting of exacerbation of symptoms to physician
J. Surgery as recommended
K. Keep follow-up appointments with physician, laboratory tests, or therapies

IV. **The client/caregiver is aware of possible complications.**

A. Deformity and disability
B. Infections
C. Neuropathy
D. Chronic renal failure
E. Cardiac complications
F. Sjogren's syndrome (dry eyes and mucous membranes)

RESOURCES

Arthritis Foundation
www.arthritis.org

National Institute of Arthritis and Musculoskeletal and Skin
   Diseases
www.niams.nih.gov

American College of Rheumatology
www.rheumatology.org

Exercise program (i.e., YMCA and health clubs)

Support Groups

REFERENCES

Ackley, B. J., & Ladwig, G. B. (2006). *Nursing diagnosis handbook: A guide to planning care.* Philadelphia: Mosby Inc.

Cohen, B. J., & Taylor, J. J. (2005). *Memmler's the human body in health and disease* (10th ed.). Philadelphia: Lippincott Williams & Wilkins.

Diet and your arthritis. (2007). Arthritis Foundation. *ww2.arthritis.org/default.asp.*

Hitchcock, J. E., Schubert, P. E., & Thomas, S. A. (2003). *Community health nursing: Caring in action.* Clifton Park, NY: Thomson Delmar Learning.

Timby, B. K., & Smith, N. C. (2003). *Introductory medical-surgical nursing* (8th ed.). Philadelphia: J. B. Lippincott Williams & Wilkins.

3   Sjogren's Syndrome

Patient name: _____   **Admission:** _____

NRS
DATE INITIAL

I. **The client/caregiver can describe Sjogren's syndrome.**

A. The white blood cells incorrectly produce antibodies which attack, inflame, and damage moisture producing glands.

B. Damage is most common to the tear and saliva glands.

C. Risk factors
- Greater for women
- Greater over the age of 40 years
- Higher for people who have rheumatoid arthritis, lupus, polymyositis, Raynaud's, and scleroderma or those who have family history of rheumatic disease

D. The more serious form is called primary Sjogren's. Damage is done to the moisture-producing tissue in the skin, muscle, joints, thyroid, blood vessels, liver, or pancreas.

II. **The client/caregiver can list symptoms of Sjogren's syndrome.**

A. Three or more month history of a dry or gritty eye sensation, blurred vision, or bright-light sensitivity.

B. Chronic complaints of dry or "cotton" mouth often combined with thickened saliva that becomes sticky.

C. Decreased saliva will
1. Increase the risk of cavities
2. Cause lips to crack and bleed
3. Cause mouth sores and fungal infections
4. Make taste and smell abilities fade

D. Damaged moisture production in other areas can cause
- Dry and itchy skin with rashes
- Joint pain
- Gastrointestinal problems
- Heartburn
- Weight loss
- Thyroid problems
- Lung and respiratory problems

III. **The client/caregiver can describe treatment for Sjogren's syndrome.**

A. The goal is to moisturize and protect any problem areas.

NRS
DATE INITIAL

B. Treatment for the mouth
- Regular dental care
- Sugar-free hard candy or gum
- Good oral care using fluoride gel, floss, and rinses
- Over-the-counter artificial saliva products
- No smoking
- Use of humidifiers in home

C. Treatment for the eyes
1. Avoid wind, sand, and smoke.
2. Goggles can be used as protection.
3. Artificial tears can be helpful.

D. Treatment for skin
- Moisturizing soaps
- Oil-based ointments
- Protection against sunlight
- Vaginal lubricants

E. Use medication only as directed by physician.

F. Because various medical specialist and health providers are involved, coordinate and inform all care providers to maximize treatment.

RESOURCES

Sjogren's Syndrome Foundation
www.sjogrens.org

National Institute of Arthritis and Musculoskeletal and Skin Diseases (NIAMS)
www.niams.nih.gov

REFERENCES

Ackley, B. J., & Ladwig, G. B. (2006). *Nursing diagnosis handbook: A guide to planning care.* Philadelphia: Mosby Inc.

Cohen, B. J., & Taylor, J. J. (2005). *Memmler's the human body in health and disease* (10th ed.). Philadelphia: Lippincott Williams & Wilkins.

Timby, B. K., & Smith, N. C. (2003). *Introductory medical-surgical nursing* (8th ed.). Philadelphia: J. B. Lippincott Williams & Wilkins.

4 Systemic Lupus Erythematosus

Patient name: _____

Admission: _____

I. **The client/caregiver can define systemic lupus erythematosus (SLP).**

   A. With SLP the body's immune system does not function as it should. It produces antibodies that fight against the body's healthy cells and tissue.
   B. It is a chronic disorder with exacerbations and remissions.
   C. It is an inflammatory disorder that causes structural changes in connective tissue affecting the skin, joints, muscles, and other organs.
   D. Symptoms may range from mild to severe.
   E. Symptoms may vary during the course of the disease.

II. **The client/caregiver can list signs and symptoms.**

   A. Painful or swollen joints and muscle pain
   B. Unexplained fever
   C. Red rashes, most commonly on the face (butterfly rash over nose and checks)
   D. Chest pain upon deep breathing
   E. Unusual loss of hair
   F. Pale or purple fingers or toes from cold or stress
   G. Sensitivity to the sun
   H. Swelling in legs/ankles or around eyes
   I. Mouth ulcers
   J. Swollen glands
   K. Extreme fatigue
   L. Headache

III. **The client/caregiver can list body systems that can be affected by lupus.**

   A. Kidneys—inflammation and renal disease
   B. Lungs—pleuritis and pneumonia
   C. Central nervous system—dizziness, vision problems, memory and personality changes, seizure, or stroke

   D. Blood vessels—mild to severe vasculitis
   E. Blood—anemia, leukopenia (decreased white blood cells), or increased risk for blood clots
   F. Heart—inflammation of heart and surrounding membrane or increased risk for atherosclerosis

IV. **The client/caregiver can list measures to manage this disease.**

   A. Take medications as ordered.
   B. Be alert to specific medication treatments. Have education about the use of corticosteroids, and follow physician instructions for dosage and discontinuation.
   C. Plan regular exercise and rest. Pace activities to allow for rest.
   D. Avoid sunlight or ultraviolet radiation. Never use tanning booths. When outdoors use sunscreen and wear clothing to protect arms, legs, and face.
   E. Eat a diet high in protein, vitamins, and iron to prevent anemia.
   F. Maintain adequate fluid intake.
   G. Avoid crowds or people with known infections.
   H. Provide meticulous mouth care.
   I. Apply hot packs or cold packs to lessen pain and stiffness.
   J. Bathe in cool water to decrease itchiness and rash.
   K. Keep follow-up appointments with physician. Report any signs of flare-up promptly.
   L. Wear a Medic Alert bracelet.
   M. Use any adaptive equipment to maintain activity of daily living, such as cooking or dressing.
   N. For fever over 100 degrees, call your doctor.

(Continued)

RESOURCES

Local lupus support groups

S.L.E. Lupus Foundation
www.lupusny.org/

National Institute of Arthritis and Musculoskeletal and Skin
Diseases Information Clearinghouse NIAMS/National
Institutes of Health
www.niams.nih.gov/

American College of Rheumatology/Association of
Rheumatology Health Professionals
www.rheumatology.org

Arthritis Foundation
www.arthritis.org

REFERENCES

Ackley, B. J., & Ladwig, G. B. (2006). *Nursing diagnosis
handbook: A guide to planning care.* Philadelphia: Mosby Inc.

Cohen, B. J., & Taylor, J. J. (2005). *Memmler's the human body
in health and disease* (10th ed.). Philadelphia: Lippincott
Williams & Wilkins.

Hitchcock, J. E., Schubert, P. E., & Thomas, S. A. (2003).
Community health nursing: Caring in action. Clifton Park, NY:
Thomson Delmar Learning.

Lutz, C., & Przytulski, K. (2001). *Nutrition and diet therapy.*
Philadelphia: F. A. Davis Company.

Nutrition made incredibly easy. (2003). Philadelphia: Lippincott
Williams & Wilkins.

Timby, B. K., & Smith, N. C. (2003). *Introductory medical-
surgical nursing* (8th ed.). Philadelphia: J. B. Lippincott
Williams & Wilkins.

5 AIDS

Patient name: _____

Admission: _____

I. The client/caregiver can define AIDS.

A. AIDS is caused by HIV.
B. HIV kills or damages cells of the body's immune system.
C. This damage destroys the body's ability to fight infections and certain cancers.
D. Viruses or bacteria that are not a threat to healthy people become opportunistic and life-threatening infections for the person diagnosed with AIDS.
E. The term AIDS usually applies to the most advanced stages of HIV infection.

II. The client/caregiver can list methods of transmission.

A. HIV is spread through contact with contaminated blood. Because of blood screening and heat treatment to donated blood, the risk of getting HIV from transfusions is extremely small.
B. HIV is spread most often by having unprotected sex with an infected partner.
C. The virus can enter the body through the lining of the vagina, vulva, penis, rectum, or mouth during sex.
D. HIV can spread among injection drug users by sharing of needles or syringes that are contaminated with infected blood.
E. Women can transmit HIV to their babies during pregnancy or time of birth.

III. The client/caregiver can list risky behavior practices to be avoided in prevention of the spread of the HIV.

A. Sharing of drug needles or syringes
B. Having sexual contact, including oral, with an infected person without using a condom
C. Having sexual contact with someone whose HIV status is unknown

IV. The client/caregiver can recognize early signs and symptoms of HIV.

A. Flu-like symptoms within a month or two after exposure to the virus

B. Fever
C. Headache
D. Swollen glands
E. Fatigue

V. The client/caregiver can recognize symptoms experienced later in the course of the disease.

A. "Swollen glands" for more than 3 months
B. Weight loss
C. Frequent fevers and sweats
D. Persistent or frequent yeast infections of mouth or vagina
E. Persistent skin rashes
F. Pelvic inflammatory disease in women that does not respond to treatment
G. Short-term memory loss
H. Frequent or severe herpes infections that cause mouth, genital, or anal sores or the painful nerve disease called shingles

VI. The client/caregiver can list tests common for diagnosis of AIDS.

A. Enzyme-linked immunosorbent assay (ELISA)
B. Western blot, which is used to confirm the results of the ELISA test

VII. The client/caregiver can list measures to prevent AIDS.

A. Avoid sex with multiple partners.
B. Avoid intravenous drug abuse.
C. Avoid sharing needles or syringes.
D. Use condoms correctly.

VIII. The client/caregiver can list measures to manage AIDS and prevent opportunistic infections.

A. Avoid infections with good handwashing and personal hygiene.
B. Avoid exposure to infection, such as people with respiratory infections, shingles, and tuberculosis or children with chicken pox.

(Continued)

C. Report any signs and symptoms of infection.

D. Use stress-management techniques.

E. Set up an emotional support network with family, friends, or support groups.

F. Eat a nutritious diet. Check high-calorie diet in therapeutic diets. Check food safety and prevention of food-borne illness in nutrition education.

G. Maintain a balance of rest and exercise.

H. Avoid donating blood or semen.

I. Inform health care providers of diagnosis.

J. Inform sex partners of diagnosis.

K. Keep follow-up appointments with physician and laboratory.

L. Avoid alcohol and tobacco product use.

M. Avoid exposure to infection, such as people with respiratory infections, shingles, and tuberculosis or children with chicken pox.

N. Use extra care when dealing with pets. Do not touch pet litter boxes, feces, bird droppings, or water in fish tanks.

O. Use extra care with gardening activities. Germs live in garden and potting soil. Wear gloves while handling dirt, and use good hand hygiene.

IX. **The client/caregiver can list measures to maintain body requirements for nutrition.**

A. Provide good oral hygiene.

B. Eat small, more frequent meals.

C. Rest one-half hour after meals.

D. Take vitamin and mineral supplements as ordered.

E. Take medication (antiemetics) for nausea and vomiting as needed.

X. **The client/caregiver can list precautions to prevent transmission of the virus.**

A. Personal care
  1. Hands and other parts of the body should be washed immediately after contact with blood or other body fluids. Surfaces soiled with blood should be disinfected appropriately.
  2. Gloves should be worn during contact with blood or other body fluids that could possibly contain visible blood, such as urine, feces, or vomit.

  3. Cuts, sores, or breaks on both the caregiver and client's exposed skin should be covered with bandages.

B. Equipment
  1. Needles and other sharp instruments should be used only when medically necessary.
  2. Do not put caps back on needles by hand. Do not remove needles from syringes. Dispose of needles in puncture-proof containers out of the reach of children and visitors.
  3. Infected persons should not share razors, toothbrushes, tweezers, nail or cuticle items, pierced earrings, or other pierced jewelry.
  4. Disposable gloves should only be used once and then discarded.

C. Household items and linens
  1. Clothes and bed sheets used by someone with AIDS can be washed the same way as other laundry.
  2. If clothes or sheets have blood, vomit, semen, vaginal fluids, urine, or feces on them, use disposable gloves and handle the clothes or sheets as little as possible.
  3. Put soiled linens in plastic bags until you can wash them. You can but do not need to add bleach to kill HIV; a normal wash cycle will kill the virus.
  4. Fabrics and furniture can be cleaned with soap and water or cleansers that you can buy in a store; follow the directions on the box. Wear gloves while cleaning.
  5. About one-quarter cup of bleach mixed with 1 gallon of water makes a good disinfectant for floors, showers, tubs, sinks, mops, sponges, and so forth.
  6. Soiled disposable items such as gloves, soiled underpads, or dressings should be secured in heavy-duty plastic garbage bags.
  7. Clean food preparation area and bathroom area with hot, soapy water and then with a solution that is one part bleach to nine parts water.

D. Personal
  1. The proper and consistent use of latex or polyurethane (a type of plastic) condoms

(Continued)

NRS
DATE INITIAL

when engaging in sexual intercourse—vaginal, anal, or oral—can greatly reduce a person's risk of acquiring or transmitting sexually transmitted diseases, including HIV infection.

2. If a person with AIDS has a cough that lasts longer than a week, the doctor should check for tuberculosis.
3. If the person with AIDS has fever blisters or cold sores (herpes simplex) around the mouth or nose, do not kiss or touch the sores.
4. If you have to touch the sores to help the person, wear gloves and wash your hands carefully as soon as you take the gloves off.

E. Proper condom use
1. Use latex or polyurethane condoms. Never reuse a condom.
2. Store condoms in cool, dry place. Do not store in car or wallet.
3. Check expiration date.
4. Place condom on an erect (hard) penis before any contact with partner's genital area.
5. Use water-based lubricant with latex condoms to help prevent the condom from tearing. Do not use oil-based products, such as baby or cooking oils, hand lotion or petroleum jelly as lubricants.
6. Hold condom in place at the base of penis before withdrawing after sex.
7. Properly dispose of condom.
8. Avoid use of lubricants with spermicide called nonoxynol-9 (N-9). It may cause skin irritation or abrasions that can make the area more susceptible to sexually transmitted diseases.

RESOURCES

Centers for Disease Control and Prevention
www.aidsinf.nih.gov/guidelines/
www.cdc.gov/hiv/
www.cdc.gov/hiv/resources/factsheets/index.htm

National Institute of Allergy and Infectious Diseases (NIAID)
www.niaid.nih.gov/

National Institutes of Health (NIH)
www.nih.gov/

Department of Health and Human Services (HHS)
www.hhs.gov/

AIDSinfo
800-HIV-0440 (800-448-0440) or 301-519-0459
888-480-3739 (TTY/TDD)
http://aidsinfo.nih.gov

CDC National Prevention Information Network (NPIN)
800-458-5231
www.cdcnpin.org

Caring for Someone with AIDS at Home
www.cdc.gov/hiv/pubs/BROCHURE/careathome.htm

CDC-INFO 24 Hours/Day for more information about sex
800-CDC-INFO (232-4636)
888-232-6348 (TTY), in English, en Español

American Social Health Organization
www.ashastd.org/condom/condom

REFERENCES

Ackley, B. J., & Ladwig, G. B. (2006). *Nursing diagnosis handbook: A guide to planning care.* Philadelphia: Mosby Inc.

Caring for someone with AIDS at home. Retrieved from *www.cdc.gov/hiv/pubs/BROCHURE/careathome.htm.*

Cohen, B. J., & Taylor, J. J. (2005). *Memmler's the human body in health and disease* (10th ed.). Philadelphia: Lippincott Williams & Wilkins.

Hitchcock, J. E., Schubert, P. E., & Thomas, S. A. (2003). *Community health nursing: Caring in action.* Clifton Park, NY: Thomson Delmar Learning.

How to use a condom. (1999–2007). American Social Health Organization. Research Triangle Park, NC.

Hunt, R. (2005). *Introduction to community based nursing.* Philadelphia: Lippincott Williams & Wilkins.

Lutz, C., & Przytulski, K. (2001). *Nutrition and diet therapy.* Philadelphia: F. A. Davis Company.

Nutrition made incredibly easy. (2003). Philadelphia: Lippincott Williams & Wilkins.

Timby, B. K., & Smith, N. C. (2003). *Introductory medical-surgical nursing* (8th ed.). Philadelphia: J. B. Lippincott Williams & Wilkins.

Cardiomyopathy

Patient name: _____ **Admission:** _____

NRS
DATE INITIAL

I. **The client/caregiver can define cardiomyopathy.**

   A. There is a chronic condition with structural changes in the heart muscle.
   B. The heart muscle loses its ability to pump blood efficiently and is a chronic condition often resulting in heart failure.
   C. There are three major types of cardiomyopathy: dilated, hypertrophic, and restrictive.

II. **The client/caregiver can recognize signs and symptoms of cardiomyopathy.**

   A. Shortness of breath (dyspnea) on exertion and when lying down
   B. Fatigue leading to decreased activity tolerance
   C. Swelling of the legs
   D. Palpitations
   E. Chest pain
   F. Fainting, lightheadedness, or passing out after activity
   G. Low amount of urine during day but need to urinate at night
   H. Possible cough

III. **The client/caregiver can list factors that will help manage the disease.**

   A. Encourage healthy weight
   B. Follow dietary instructions such as fluid restriction and low-sodium diet
   C. Avoid the use of tobacco, alcohol, and caffeine-containing products
   D. Receive pneumonia and influenza vaccinations
   E. Monitor the level of activity/exercise for signs of dyspnea or chest pain
   F. Restrict driving if syncope is common symptom
   G. Monitor for irregular pulse or rapid heart rate

   H. Take medication as ordered by physician
   I. Use of oxygen as needed and ordered
   J. Relaxation and positive-thinking techniques
   K. Monitor for depression or social isolation

IV. **The client/caregiver can list complications of cardiomyopathy.**

   A. Pulmonary diseases that compromise cardiac function
   B. Need for various cardiac surgeries, pacemaker insertion, implanted automatic defibrillator, dynamic cardiomyoplasty surgery, or even heart transplant.
   C. Formation of blood clots

RESOURCES

National Heart, Lung, and Blood Institute (NHLBI)
www.nhlbi.nih.gov

Support groups such as Mended Hearts
www.mendedhearts.org

American Heart Association
www.americanheart.org

Advance directives (American Medical Association)
www.medem.com/index.cfm

Hospice

REFERENCES

Advance care planning: Guidance for patients. (2001). American Medical Association.

Hitchcock, J. E., Schubert, P. E., & Thomas, S. A. (2003). *Community health nursing: Caring in action.* Clifton Park, NY: Thomson Delmar Learning.

Timby, B. K., & Smith, N. C. (2003). *Introductory medical-surgical nursing* (8th ed.). Philadelphia: J. B. Lippincott Williams & Wilkins.

2 Cardiac Arrhythmias

Patient name: _____ Admission: _____

<table>
<tr><td>DATE</td><td>NRS INITIAL</td></tr>
</table>

I. **The client/caregiver can define cardiac arrhythmia (dysrhythmia).**

A. The heart has its own conduction system that produces the rate and rhythm of each heart beat.
B. When this conduction system is not working properly, the result is an abnormally slow or rapid heart rate that does not function in the usual manner.
C. Some arrhythmias do not need treatment, whereas other can quickly lead to life-threatening situations.

II. **The client/caregiver can define normal cardiac rhythm.**

A. A normal heart rate is between 60 and 100 beats per minute.
B. Each impulse or beat occurs in an even, regular rate.

III. **The client/caregiver can discuss possible predisposing factors for arrhythmias.**

A. Myocardial ischemia related to coronary artery disease
B. Congestive heart failure
C. Pain
D. Anxiety and stress
E. Endocrine disorders
F. Electrolyte imbalances
G. Valvular heart disease
H. Side effects of medications

IV. **The client/caregiver can be knowledgeable of methods of treatment for dysrhythmias.**

A. Drug therapy
B. Elective electrical cardioversion is used with non–life-threatening dysrhythmias. It is a nonemergency procedure done by a physician usually as an outpatient status.
C. Defibrillation. This treatment is used only in a life-threatening situation.
D. Automatic implanted cardiac defibrillator (AICD) is an internal electrical device used

for clients with life-threatening dysrhythmias. This client has had previous episodes of cardiac arrest and survived but is still at risk for sudden cardiac death.
E. Pacemaker. They treat clients with abnormally slow heart rhythms and can be temporarily used or surgically implanted for permanent use. Permanent pacemakers function either on demand or at a fixed-rate pacer. The demand pacer will activate if pulse rate falls below a set rate per minute. The fixed-rate is preset when inserted to a specific rate (use the pacemaker teaching guide).

V. **The client/caregiver can list educational topics and skills needed for post-hospital care.**

A. Knowledge of how to monitor blood pressure and the rate and rhythm of pulse.
B. Awareness of how to secure emergency help. Call 911. Have telephone numbers of physician and brief history including medication available for first responders.
C. Have home emergency alert system for client who lives alone.
D. Be able to evaluate for symptoms of distress other than change in pulse rate:
   • Shortness of breath
   • Lightheadedness
   • Sweating
   • Chest pain
   • Palpitations
   • Skin becomes pale and cool
   • Disoriented or confused mental state
E. Ensure understanding and compliance of medication prescribed.
F. Understanding of need for follow-up care by physician and/or any appointments for testing.
G. Wear medical alert identification for disease and any use of pacemaker or AICD.

(Continued)

NRS
DATE INITIAL

H. Ensure understanding of any implanted pacemaker or AICD maintenance (use the pacemaker teaching guide).

VI. **The client/caregiver can list possible complications of dysrhythmias.**

A. Myocardial infarction.
B. Cardiac arrest leading to sudden death.

RESOURCES

National Heart, Lung, and Blood Institute (NHLBI)
www.nhlbi.nih.gov

Support groups such as Mended Hearts
www.mendedhearts.org

American Heart Association
www.americanheart.org

Advance directives (American Medical Association)
www.medem.com/index.cfm

REFERENCES

Ackley, B. J., & Ladwig, G. B. (2006). *Nursing diagnosis handbook: A guide to planning care.* Philadelphia: Mosby Inc.

Cohen, B. J., & Wood, D. L. (2000). *Memmler's the human body in health and disease* (9th ed.). Philadelphia: Lippincott Williams & Wilkins.

Hitchcock, J. E., Schubert, P. E., & Thomas, S. A. (2003). *Community health nursing: Caring in action.* Clifton Park, NY: Thomson Delmar Learning.

Timby, B. K., & Smith, N. C. (2003). *Introductory medical-surgical nursing* (8th ed.). Philadelphia: J. B. Lippincott Williams & Wilkins.

3 Angina Pectoris

Patient name: _____   **Admission:** _____

I. **The client/caregiver can define "angina pectoris."**

A. Chest pain is caused by insufficient oxygen to meet demands of the heart.

B. A lack of oxygen occurs when insufficient blood flows through the coronary arteries.

C. Stable angina usually has a precipitating cause while unstable angina can occur at rest.

II. **The client/caregiver can recognize signs and symptoms of angina pectoris.**

A. Chest pain (may range from very mild to very severe)

B. Anxiety

C. Indigestion

D. Sweating

E. Shortness of breath

III. **The client/caregiver can list locations where chest pain can occur.**

A. Midanterior chest

B. Neck and jaw

C. Inner aspects of arms (left arm is more common)

D. Upper abdomen

E. Shoulders and between shoulder blades

IV. **The client/caregiver can list possible precipitating factors and appropriate measures to decrease risk.**

A. Factors: sudden physical exertion
Measures:
1. Exercise regularly.
2. Take regular rest periods, and avoid strenuous activities.
3. Have nitroglycerin available to take as directed if chest pain presents (use nitroglycerin/nitrates medication teaching guide).

B. Factors: emotional stress
Measures:
1. Learn relaxation and stress management.

C. Factors: consumption of a heavy meal
Measures:
1. Eat small, frequent meals.
2. Rest after meals.

D. Factors: temperature extremes
Measures:
1. Dress warmly in cold weather.
2. Avoid sleeping in cold rooms.
3 Avoid becoming overheated.
4. Monitor reaction to hot shower in morning and sitting near fireplace.

E. Factors: nicotine
Measures:
1. Avoid smoking and other people's smoke

F. Factors: hypertension
Measures:
1. Take medications as prescribed.
2. Monitor blood pressure closely.
3. Monitor cholesterol levels.

G. Factors: obesity
Measures:
1. Achieve and maintain ideal weight (use weight-reduction teaching guide).
2. Eat healthy meal low in saturated fat, cholesterol and sodium (use cardiovascular related nutrition teaching guide).

H. Factors: constipation accompanied by excessive straining.
Measures:
1. Eat a diet high in fiber (use the high-fiber diet teaching guide).
2. Exercise regularly.
3. Take stool softeners as needed. Discuss use with physician.

(Continued)

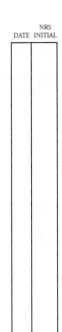

NRS
DATE INITIAL

V.   **The client/caregiver can list what to do if an angina attack occurs.**

 A. Take nitroglycerin at the first sign of angina.
 B. Rest in a lying or sitting position.
 C. Maintain a quiet environment.
 D. If the client feels no relief 5 minutes after taking nitroglycerin, take nitroglycerin again. If another 5 minutes pass and the client feels no relief, take nitroglycerin a third time.
 E. If the client feels no relief 5 minutes after the third nitroglycerin, get medical attention.

VI.   **The client/caregiver can list possible complications.**

 A. Dysrhythmias of the heart
 B. Myocardial infarction
 C. Cardiac arrest leading to sudden death

RESOURCES

American Heart Association
www.americanheart.org

National Institutes of Health
www.nih.gov

American Dietetic Association
www.eatright.org

REFERENCES

Ackley, B. J., & Ladwig, G. B. (2006). *Nursing diagnosis handbook: A guide to planning care.* Philadelphia: Mosby Inc.

Cohen, B. J., & Wood, D. L. (2000). *Memmler's the human body in health and disease* (9th ed.). Philadelphia: Lippincott Williams & Wilkins.

Nutrition made incredibly easy. (2003). Springhouse: Lippincott, Williams & Wilkins.

Portable RN: The all-in-one nursing reference. (2002). Springhouse: Lippincott, Williams & Wilkins.

Taylor, C., Lillis, D., & LeMone, P. (2005). *Fundamentals of nursing.* Philadelphia: Lippincott Williams & Wilkins.

Timby, B. K., & Smith, N. C. (2003). *Introductory medical-surgical nursing* (8th ed.). Philadelphia: J. B. Lippincott Williams & Wilkins.

4   Congestive Heart Failure

■ Patient name: _____ Admission: _____

<table>
<tr><td>NRS
DATE INITIAL</td><td></td></tr>
</table>

I. **The client/caregiver can define congestive heart failure.**

   A. The heart is unable to pump sufficient blood to meet the body's metabolic needs.

   B. Heart failure describes the accumulation of blood and fluids in organs and tissues as a result impaired heart function.

   C. Heart failure is classified as acute or chronic and right sided or left sided.

II. **The client/caregiver can briefly describe the anatomy and physiology of the heart.**

   A. The heart consists of four chambers: the right and left ventricles and the right and left atria.

   B. The upper chambers, the atria, receive the blood from various parts of the body and pump it into the ventricles.

   C. The right ventricle pumps blood into the lungs, and the left ventricle pumps blood into all parts of the body.

   D. The primary reason for heart failure or decreased cardiac output is damage to muscular wall of the heart.

III. **The client/caregiver can list factors that may increase risk.**

   A. Myocardial infarction
   B. Coronary artery disease
   C. Hypertension
   D. Congenital heart defects
   E. Obesity
   F. Aging
   G. Diabetes mellitus

IV. **The client/caregiver can recognize the signs and symptoms.**

   A. Left-sided failure produces hypoxemia and respiratory symptoms
     1. Fatigue with activity
     2. Effort at breathing when active (exertional dyspnea)
     3. Inability to breathe unless sitting upright (orthopnea)
     4. Awakening at night by breathlessness (paroxysmal nocturnal dyspnea)
     5. Elevated blood pressure
     6. Productive cough with pink, frothy sputum
     7. Decreased urine output
     8. In acute situation, pulmonary edema develops demonstrated by sudden hypoxic, restlessness, and confusion
     9. Elevated blood pressure

   B. Right-sided failure
     1. Gradual unexplained weight gain from fluid retention
     2. Dependent pitting edema in feet and ankles
     3. Fluids retention in sacral area or abdomen (ascites)
     4. Loss of appetite and/or nausea
     5. Dyspnea as a result of enlarged abdomen

V. **The client/caregiver can report measures to prevent congestive heart failure.**

   A. Lifestyle changes include stress reduction and energy conservation.

   B. Schedule rest periods to reduce fatigue and dyspnea.

   C. Follow the diet or any fluid restrictions prescribed by physician.

   D. Take medication exactly as prescribed.

   E. Avoid tobacco and alcohol.

   F. Weigh daily at the same time of day using the same scale. Notify physician if a more than 2-pound gain in 24 hours is identified.

   G. Measure pulse rate and blood pressure daily. Report a heart rate that is less than 60 beats per minute or more than 120 beats per minute.

   H. Elevate legs while sitting.

   I. Avoid extreme heat, cold, or humidity.

   J. Keep follow-up appointments with physician and have laboratory work obtained as ordered.

(Continued)

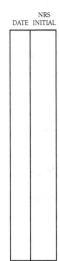

NRS
DATE INITIAL

VI. The client/caregiver can demonstrate understanding of nutritional issues related to congestive heart disease (refer to Nutrition and Cardiovascular Disease).

VII. The client/caregiver can list possible complications of congestive heart disease.

A. Acute pulmonary edema
B. Damage to organs such as liver, kidney, or brain
C. Pneumonia
D. Electrolyte imbalance related to diuretic therapy
E. Need for oxygen therapy

RESOURCES

American Heart Association
www.americanheart.org

National Heart, Lung, and Blood Institute (NHLBI)
www.nhlbi.nih.gov

REFERENCES

Ackley, B. J., & Ladwig, G. B. (2006). *Nursing diagnosis handbook: A guide to planning care*. Philadelphia: Mosby Inc.

Cohen, B. J., & Wood, D. L. (2000). *Memmler's the human body in health and disease* (9th ed.). Philadelphia: Lippincott Williams & Wilkins.

Nutrition made incredibly easy. (2003). Springhouse: Lippincott, Williams & Wilkins.

Portable RN: The all-in-one nursing reference. (2002). Springhouse: Lippincott, Williams & Wilkins.

Taylor, C., Lillis, D., & LeMone, P. (2005). *Fundamentals of nursing*. Philadelphia: Lippincott Williams & Wilkins

Timby, B. K., & Smith, N. C. (2003). *Introductory medical-surgical nursing* (8th ed.). Philadelphia: J. B. Lippincott Williams & Wilkins.

5 Coronary Artery Disease

Patient name: _____ Admission: _____

NRS
DATE INITIAL

I. **The client/caregiver can define coronary artery disease.**

   A. It is a progressive disease characterized by a narrowing or blockage of one or both of the coronary arteries causing a decreased blood supply to the heart.
   B. The decreased blood supply creates a lack of oxygen and nutrients to the heart and can cause tissue damage.
   C. The disease develops slowly and may be very advanced before symptoms occur.
   D. The primary cause is atherosclerosis, which is the buildup of fatty, fibrous plaque on the inner wall of the artery, causing it to become narrowed and hardened.
   E. Another cause is arteriosclerosis, produced by loss of elasticity of arteries.

II. **The client/caregiver can list factors that may increase risk of coronary heart disease.**

   A. Controllable factors
      1. Cigarette smoking
      2. Elevated blood pressure
      3. Stress
      4. High-cholesterol diet
      5. Obesity
      6. Sedentary lifestyle
      7. Diabetes mellitus
      8. The use of estrogen oral contraceptives
   B. Noncontrollable factors
      1. Age (risk increases with age)
      2. Sex (incidence rate in men is three times that of women)
      3. Race (incidence rate is higher in blacks than in whites)
      4. Family history

III. **The client/caregiver can list measures to prevent or manage coronary heart disease.**

   A. Limit cholesterol, sodium, and saturated fat intake (diets related to cardiovascular disease).
   B. Take medication as prescribed.
   C. Establish exercise program approved by physician.

NRS
DATE INITIAL

IV. **The client/caregiver can list possible complications of coronary heart disease.**

   A. Myocardial infarction
   B. Angina pectoris
   C. Heart failure
   D. Dysrhythmias
   E. Cardiac arrest

RESOURCES

American Heart Association
www.americanheart.org

National Institutes of Health
www.nih.gov

American Dietetic Association
www.eatright.org

National Cholesterol Education Program—National Institutes of Health
www.nhlbi.nih.gov/chd/

CDC: Tobacco Information and Prevention Source (TIPS)
www.cdc.gov/tobacco/how2quit

United States Department of Health and Human Resources: Tobacco Cessation
www.surgeongeneral.gov/tobacco/

REFERENCES

Ackley, B. J., & Ladwig, G. B. (2006). *Nursing diagnosis handbook: A guide to planning care.* Philadelphia: Mosby Inc.

Cohen, B. J., & Wood, D. L. (2000). *Memmler's the human body in health and disease* (9th ed.). Philadelphia: Lippincott Williams & Wilkins.

Nutrition made incredibly easy. (2003). Springhouse: Lippincott, Williams & Wilkins.

Portable RN: The all-in-one nursing reference. (2002). Springhouse: Lippincott, Williams & Wilkins.

Taylor, C., Lillis, D., & LeMone, P. (2005). *Fundamentals of nursing.* Philadelphia: Lippincott Williams & Wilkins.

Timby, B. K., & Smith, N. C. (2003). *Introductory medical-surgical nursing* (8th ed.). Philadelphia: J. B. Lippincott Williams & Wilkins.

6 | Hypertension

Patient name: _____ Admission: _____

NRS
DATE INITIAL

I. **The client/caregiver can define hypertension.**

   A. It is the occasional or continued elevation of diastolic or systolic pressure.
   B. The systolic reading (the top number) represents the pressure exerted on the blood vessel wall when the heart is contracting.
   C. The diastolic reading (the bottom number) represents the pressure on the blood vessel while the heart is at rest.

II. **The client/caregiver can state normal blood pressure values. (No absolute dividing line exists between normal and high blood pressure, but the American Heart Association and National Heart, Lung, and Blood Institute gives the following guidelines.)**

   A. Normal blood pressure readings should be 120/80 or below.
   B. If your systolic reading is 120 to 139 or diastolic is 80 to 89 (or both), then this is considered "prehypertension."
   C. High blood pressure is a pressure of 140 systolic or higher and/or 90 diastolic or higher that stays elevated over time.

III. **The client/caregiver can recognize signs and symptoms of high blood pressure, although it is frequently asymptomatic and is considered the "silent killer."**

   A. Dizziness
   B. Headaches, often described as throbbing or pounding
   C. Palpitations
   D. Blurring of vision
   E. Fatigue
   F. Nosebleeds
   G. Insomnia
   H. Nervousness
   I. Chest pain (angina)
   J. Shortness of breath (dyspnea)

NRS
DATE INITIAL

IV. **The client/caregiver can list factors that increase risk.**

   A. Age (persons older than 35 years)
   B. Black
   C. Close blood relative with hypertension
   D. Overweight
   E. Stress
   F. High sodium intake
   G. High cholesterol intake
   H. Oral contraceptives
   I. Cigarette smoking
   J. Excessive alcohol use
   K. History of diabetes, gout, or kidney disease
   L. Sedentary lifestyle

V. **The client/caregiver can list measures to control hypertension.**

   A. Monitor blood pressure at home, and know what it should be.
   B. Take medication exactly as prescribed.
   C. Lifestyle changes to reduce stress.
   D. Eat balanced meals low in saturated fat, cholesterol, and sodium.
   E. Stop smoking (use tobacco-cessation teaching guide).
   F. Lose weight if overweight (use weight-reduction teaching guide).
   G. Avoid oral contraceptives.
   H. Avoid alcohol.
   I. Have regular medical checkups.
   J. Avoid over-the-counter medications unless recommended by physician.
   K. Exercise regularly.
   L. Use Medic Alert cards/bracelet.

VI. **The client/caregiver is aware of possible complications.**

   A. Myocardial infarction
   B. Heart failure
   C. Stroke
   D. Kidney failure
   E. Malignant hypertension

(Continued)

RESOURCES

American Heart Association
www.americanheart.org

National Institutes of Health
www.nih.gov

American Dietetic Association
www.eatright.org

Cardiac Rehab Programs offered at many hospital centers

Support groups for weight control and smoking cessation

REFERENCES

Ackley, B. J., & Ladwig, G. B. (2006). *Nursing diagnosis handbook: A guide to planning care.* Philadelphia: Mosby Inc.

Cohen, B. J., & Wood, D. L. (2000). *Memmler's the human body in health and disease* (9th ed.). Philadelphia: Lippincott Williams & Wilkins.

Nutrition made incredibly easy. (2003). Springhouse: Lippincott, Williams & Wilkins.

Portable RN: The all-in-one nursing reference. (2002). Springhouse: Lippincott, Williams & Wilkins.

Taylor, C., Lillis, D., & LeMone, P. (2005). *Fundamentals of nursing.* Philadelphia: Lippincott Williams & Wilkins.

Timby, B. K., & Smith, N. C. (2003). *Introductory medical-surgical nursing* (8th ed.). Philadelphia: J. B. Lippincott Williams & Wilkins.

7   Myocardial Infarction

Patient name: _____   Admission: _____

NRS
DATE INITIAL

I. The client/caregiver can define myocardial infarction.

 A. A myocardial infarction results from reduced or blocked blood flow through one of the coronary arteries to the myocardial tissue.

 B. This blockage causes death of the heart tissue.

II. The client/caregiver can list factors that may increase risk of myocardial infarction but cannot be changed.

 A. Increasing age

 B. Gender (men are at greater risk)

 C. Heredity, which includes individual family history and race

III. The client/caregiver can list major risk factors that can be modified to decrease risk for heart disease.

 A. Use of tobacco products

 B. High blood cholesterol

 C. High blood pressure

 D. Physical inactivity

 E. Obesity

 F. Diabetes mellitus

 G. Stress

 H. Alcohol abuse

IV. The client/caregiver can recognize signs and symptoms of a myocardial infarction.

 A. Chest discomfort or pain often described as an uncomfortable pressure, crushing or squeezing pain, or substernal pain. Pain usually occurs in the middle of chest.

 B. Discomfort or pain in one or both arms, back, neck, jaw or stomach

 C. Shortness of breath

 D. Complaints of nausea, lightheadedness, or sweating

 E. Anxiety or feeling of dread

NRS
DATE INITIAL

V. The client/caregiver will know what to do if signs of myocardial infarction occur.

 A. Remain calm and assist client into comfortable position.

 B. Call 911.

 C. Follow any previous instructions from physician regarding medication to be used in this type of emergency.

 D. If the client loses consciousness and no pulse is found, cardiopulmonary resuscitation should begin and continue until trained help arrives.

VI. The client/caregiver can list measures to prevent a reoccurrence of myocardial infarction.

 A. Explain the medication treatment plan ordered by physician. Understanding the medication regimen will promote compliance.

 B. Lose weight if overweight (weight-loss diet guide).

 C. Follow the cardiac disease dietary recommendation of low-fat, low-cholesterol, and low-sodium diet (give related teaching guides).

 D. Encourage client to participate in a cardiac rehabilitation program.

 E. Understand physical limitations as dictated by physician and cardiac rehabilitation program. Clarify when and how to resume sexual activity.

 F. Monitor blood pressure and pulse.

 G. Avoid alcohol.

 H. Avoid use of tobacco products (tobacco-cessation guide).

 I. Learn and use stress-management techniques (stress-management guide).

 J. Learn what symptoms to report to physician immediately, such as chest pain, shortness of breath, or changes in blood pressure or pulse.

(Continued)

NRS
DATE INITIAL

K. Monitor and report symptoms of depression to physician.
L. Use Medic Alert cards or bracelets indicating health history and medications.

VII. The client/caregiver is aware of possible complications.

A. Dysrhythmias
B. Cardiogenic shock
C. Arterial or pulmonary embolism
D. Pericarditis
E. Mitral insufficiency

Cardiac rehabilitation programs offered at many hospital centers

Support groups for weight control and smoking cessation

United States Department of Health and Human Services
www.surgeongeneral.gov/tobacco/

U.S. Food and Drug Administration
www.fda.gov/hearthealth

RESOURCES

American Heart Association
www.americanheart.org

National Institutes of Health
www.nih.gov

American Red Cross Services—CPR
www.redcross.org/services

American Dietetic Association
www.eatright.org

REFERENCES

Ackley, B. J., & Ladwig, G. B. (2006). *Nursing diagnosis handbook: A guide to planning care.* Philadelphia: Mosby Inc.

Cohen, B. J., & Wood, D. L. (2000). *Memmler's the human body in health and disease* (9th ed.). Philadelphia: Lippincott Williams & Wilkins.

Nutrition made incredibly easy. (2003). Springhouse: Lippincott, Williams & Wilkins.

Portable RN: The all-in-one nursing reference. (2002). Springhouse: Lippincott, Williams & Wilkins.

Taylor, C., Lillis, D., & LeMone, P. (2005). *Fundamentals of nursing.* Philadelphia: Lippincott Williams & Wilkins.

Timby, B. K., & Smith, N. C. (2003). *Introductory medical-surgical nursing* (8th ed.). Philadelphia: J. B. Lippincott Williams & Wilkins.

8 Peripheral Vascular Disease

Patient name: _____   Admission: _____

I.   **The client/caregiver can define peripheral vascular disease.**

   A. It is diminished blood supply to or from the lower extremities.
   B. It can involve either the veins or the arteries.

II. **The client/caregiver can recognize the signs and symptoms.**

   A. Arterial insufficiency
      1. Sharp pain that increases after exercise
      2. Cool, pale skin
      3. Absent or diminished pulse in legs and feet
      4. Reddish-blue color of skin
      5. Delayed healing
      6. Decreased capillary filling time
   B. Venous insufficiency
      1. Aching, cramping-type pain
      2. Edema
      3. Mottled and pigmented skin
      4. Ulcers close to the ankle

III. **Client/caregiver can list measures for management of disease.**

   A. Prevent decreased circulation
      1. Avoid smoking.
      2. Avoid constrictive clothing.
      3. Never cross legs.
      4. Avoid letting lower extremities to be exposed to extreme temperatures.
      5. Avoid long periods of sitting or standing.
      6. Eat a diet low in cholesterol, fats, and sodium (nutrition guides for specific diets).
   B. Promote increased circulation
      1. Walking as ordered by physician.
      2. Wear support hose.
      3. Perform Buerger-Allen exercises.
         a. Prop legs in elevated position; hold legs at approximately 45 degrees for 1 minute to drain blood.

         b. Sit with legs dangled on side of bed. Stretch feet downward holding for 30 seconds, and then stretch feet inward, outward, and upward, holding each position for 30 seconds.
         c. Lie flat on back with legs straight for 1 minute.
   C. Prevent injury to lower extremities
      1. Never go barefooted.
      2. Cut toenails carefully straight across after soaking them for 10 minutes.
      3. Wear well-fitting shoes with hose or stockings.
      4. Avoid scratching lower extremities.
      5. See a podiatrist for corns, calluses, ingrown toenails, and so forth.
      6. Avoid use of hot water bottles or heating pad.
      7. Wash feet carefully and pat dry. Observe for any redness or open areas.
      8. Wear clean cotton socks.
   D. Take medications as ordered.
   E. Obtain laboratory tests as ordered, and attend follow-up appointments with physician.

IV. **The client/caregiver is aware of possible complications.**

   A. Ulcers
   B. Cellulitis
   C. Gangrene
   D. Thrombophlebitis
   E. Embolism

RESOURCES

American Heart Association
www.americanheart.org

National Institutes of Health
www.nih.gov

(Continued)

American Dietetic Association
www.eatright.org

Support groups for weight reduction or cessation of smoking

Stress management

Exercise classes at local YMCA

REFERENCES

Ackley, B. J., & Ladwig, G. B. (2006). *Nursing diagnosis handbook: A guide to planning care.* Philadelphia: Mosby Inc.

Cohen, B. J., & Wood, D. L. (2000). *Memmler's the human body in health and disease* (9th ed.). Philadelphia: Lippincott Williams & Wilkins.

Nutrition made incredibly easy. (2003). Springhouse: Lippincott, Williams & Wilkins.

Portable RN: The all-in-one nursing reference. (2002). Springhouse: Lippincott, Williams & Wilkins.

Taylor, C., Lillis, D., & LeMone, P. (2005). *Fundamentals of nursing.* Philadelphia: Lippincott Williams & Wilkins.

Timby, B. K., & Smith, N. C. (2003). *Introductory medical-surgical nursing* (8th ed.). Philadelphia: J. B. Lippincott Williams & Wilkins.

9 Thrombophlebitis

Patient name: _____ Admission: _____

NRS
DATE INITIAL

I. **The client/caregiver can define thrombophlebitis.**

   A. It is an inflammation of the vein with a clot or thrombus formation.
   B. It usually occurs deep in the lower extremities but may occur in other areas of the body.
   C. Clots forming in the deep veins are deep-vein thrombosis (DVT).

II. **The client/caregiver can list factors that increase the risk of thrombophlebitis.**

   A. Immobility or inactivity
   B. Reduced cardiac output
   C. Oral contraceptives
   D. Trauma or injury that creates compression of the veins of the pelvis or legs
   E. Varicose veins
   F. Intravenous therapy
   G. Advancing age
   H. Cardiac and blood vessel disease
   I. Cigarette smoking
   J. Obesity
   K. Surgery
   L. History of thrombophlebitis
   M. Gender (more common in women)

III. **The client/caregiver can list signs and symptoms; often no signs or symptoms are present.**

   A. Heat, redness, and swelling along the affected vein
   B. Fever, malaise, fatigue, and possibly anorexia
   C. Positive Homan's sign (pain upon extending or straightening toes)

IV. **The client/caregiver can list measures for prevention.**

   A. Avoid constrictive clothing.
   B. Avoid smoking, alcohol, and caffeine.
   C. Lose weight if overweight.
   D. Avoid oral contraceptives. Discuss other methods of birth control with physician.

NRS
DATE INITIAL

   E. Avoid prolonged sitting and crossing the legs at the knee.
   F. Avoid standing for long periods and shift weight frequently when standing.
   G. Exercise daily.

V. **The client/caregiver can list measures for treatment.**

   A. Maintain bed rest until the physician removes activity restrictions. Elevate the affected extremity in a straight line using pillows without bending the knee.
   B. Complete rest of the affected extremity as ordered by physician.
   C. Apply warm moist compresses or apply an aquathermia pad to protected skin over affected area as ordered. Remove and reapply compresses after 20 minutes or sooner if cooling occurs. Remove the aquathermia pad every 2 hours for 20 minutes to do skin assessment.
   D. Wear knee or thigh-high antiembolism hose if prescribed by the physician. (Remove every 8 hours to assess extremity and condition of skin.) Launder hose if soiled and have extra pair for continual use.
   E. Use pneumatic compression device to the affected area if prescribed by the physician.
   F. Take nonnarcotic analgesics and anti-inflammatory agents as ordered.
   G. Take anticoagulants therapy or drugs that prevent platelet aggregation may be ordered. Obtain ordered laboratory tests to help physician determine the effectiveness of medication.
   H. Observe for symptoms of impaired clotting such as nosebleeds, bleeding gums, or easy bruising.
   I. Avoid massaging extremity to prevent emboli.
   J. Eat a well-balanced diet.
   K. Increase fluid intake to at least six to eight glasses per day.

(Continued)

NRS
DATE INITIAL

L. Keep follow-up appointments with physician.
M. Avoid over-the-counter medications or supplements unless approved by physician.
N. Measure the size of affected extremity daily.
O. Report increase in size of extremity, skin breakdown, redness, pain, warmth, and numbness.
P. Keep follow-up appointments with physician.
Q. Use Medic Alert bracelet or card to identify coagulation therapy if used.

VI. **The client/caregiver is aware of possible complications.**

A. Pulmonary embolism
B. Venous insufficiency
C. Stroke

RESOURCES

Support groups for cessation of smoking and weight loss.

REFERENCES

Ackley, B. J., & Ladwig, G. B. (2006). *Nursing diagnosis handbook: A guide to planning care.* Philadelphia: Mosby Inc.

Cohen, B. J., & Wood, D. L. (2000). *Memmler's the human body in health and disease* (9th ed.). Philadelphia: Lippincott Williams & Wilkins.

Nutrition made incredibly easy. (2003). Springhouse: Lippincott, Williams & Wilkins.

Portable RN: The all-in-one nursing reference. (2002). Springhouse: Lippincott, Williams & Wilkins.

Taylor, C., Lillis, D., & LeMone, P. (2005). *Fundamentals of nursing.* Philadelphia: Lippincott Williams & Wilkins.

Timby, B. K., & Smith, N. C. (2003). *Introductory medical-surgical nursing* (8th ed.). Philadelphia: J. B. Lippincott Williams & Wilkins.

10 | Varicose Veins

Patient name: _____   **Admission:** _____

NRS
DATE INITIAL

I.   **The client/caregiver has a basic knowledge of the anatomy and physiology of the vascular system.**

   A. Arteries carry blood away from the heart while veins carry blood to the heart.
   B. Veins have a series of valves that allow blood to be carried against gravity and prevent a backflow of blood.

II. **The client/caregiver can define varicose veins.**

   A. Varicose veins are abnormally dilated veins that may twist and turn.
   B. They are caused by valves in the veins that stretch and weaken, causing blood to pool in the lower extremities.
   C. Varicose veins can occur in legs, esophagus, or rectal area.

III. **The client/caregiver can list factors that may increase risk.**

   A. Congenital weakness of vein structure
   B. Obesity
   C. Pregnancy
   D. Constrictive clothing
   E. Prolonged periods of sitting
   F. Venous obstruction (blood clots, tumors, etc.)
   G. Advanced age

IV. **The client/caregiver can recognize signs and symptoms.**

   A. Enlarged, twisted veins that appear under the skin as dark blue or purple
   B. Leg pain, especially after long periods of sitting
   C. Swelling of feet, ankles, and legs
   D. Complaint of legs feeling heavy or tired
   E. Area with impaired circulation may appear darker than surrounding skin

NRS
DATE INITIAL

V.   **The client/caregiver can list measures to prevent or manage varicose veins.**

   A. Avoid sitting or standing for long periods of time. Do not cross legs at the knee.
   B. Avoid injury to extremities.
   C. Avoid constrictive clothing.
   D. Have frequent rest periods with feet elevated.
   E. Exercise regularly such as swimming or walking.
   F. Wear elastic support hose. Demonstrate how to apply and remove support hose.
   G. Proper foot and nail care. Report any open areas.
   H. Lose weight if overweight (refer to weight-reduction diet teaching guide).
   I. Avoid smoking (refer to tobacco abuse teaching guide).

VI. **The client/caregiver can list treatments available if the above measures are not sufficient.**

   A. Surgery includes vein ligation or vein stripping.
   B. Sclerotherapy uses a clotting solution, which is injected into vein, which closes it off.
   C. Endovenous ablation therapy uses laser energy to cauterize the vein.

VII. **The client/caregiver is aware of possible complications.**

   A. Superficial thrombophlebitis
   B. Rupture
   C. Venous stasis ulcers
   D. Cellulitis

RESOURCES
Vein clinics

Registered dietician for weight loss

(Continued)

REFERENCES

Ackley, B. J., & Ladwig, G. B. (2006). *Nursing diagnosis handbook: A guide to planning care.* Philadelphia: Mosby Inc.

Cohen, B. J., & Wood, D. L. (2000). *Memmler's the human body in health and disease* (9th ed.). Philadelphia: Lippincott Williams & Wilkins.

MedlinePlus *Varicose Vein Therapy.* Updated December 2006, by Janet L. Albright, MD, General Vascular Associates, Reno, NV.

Nutrition made incredibly easy. (2003). Springhouse: Lippincott, Williams & Wilkins.

Portable RN: The all-in-one nursing reference. (2002). Springhouse: Lippincott, Williams & Wilkins.

Taylor, C., Lillis, D., & LeMone, P. (2005). *Fundamentals of nursing.* Philadelphia: Lippincott Williams & Wilkins.

Timby, B. K., & Smith, N. C. (2003). *Introductory medical-surgical nursing* (8th ed.). Philadelphia: J. B. Lippincott Williams & Wilkins.

11 Venous Stasis Ulcer

Patient name: _____

NRS
DATE INITIAL

I. **The client/caregiver can define venous stasis ulcer.**

   A. It is the breakdown of the skin caused by incompetent valves in the veins.
   B. Incompetent valves cause excessive venous pressure that cause small skin veins and venules to rupture.
   C. Venous ulcers frequently occur on front of lower legs or around the ankle.
   D. They are slow to heal, prone to trauma, and may lead to secondary infections.

II. **The client/caregiver can list factors that increase risk of venous stasis ulcers.**

   A. Thrombophlebitis
   B. Varicose veins
   C. Poor hygiene
   D. Poor nutritional status
   E. General debilitation

III. **The client/caregiver can recognize signs and symptoms of venous insufficiency.**

   A. Thickened leathery skin
   B. Reddish brown skin discoloration
   C. Swelling of extremity
   D. Pain (relieved with elevation of foot)

IV. **The client/caregiver can list measures to prevent or treat venous stasis ulcers.**

   A. Use elastic compression stockings. Have more than one pair of stockings so that one pair can be worn while the other pair is laundered.
   B. Apply stockings each morning before legs are lowered to floor.
   C. Promote weight loss if necessary.
   D. Eat a well-balanced diet high in protein, vitamin C, zinc, and iron.
   E. Avoid heating pads, hot water bottles, and so forth.

   F. Elevate legs at regular periods for 15 to 20 minutes.
   G. Walk or do isometric calf muscle pumps frequently.
   H. Raise the foot of the bed to promote venous drainage during sleep.
   I. Wear shoes with laces to reduce pooling of blood in the feet.
   J. Avoid poorly fitting shoes and sandals to avoid injury.
   K. Avoid morning showers or sitting in front of a fire because the heat dilates the blood vessels and may add to congestion and swelling.
   L. Avoid extreme temperatures.
   M. Avoid nicotine and caffeine.

V. **The client/caregiver can provide treatment as ordered by physician.**

   A. Provide dressing changes of wound as ordered by physician using aseptic technique. Avoid tape directly on skin.
   B. Application of Unna boots.
   C. Chronic nonhealing ulcers may be treated with topical hyperbaric oxygen therapy.
   D. Vascular surgery for repair or debridement of wound.
   E. Pain medication as directed.

VI. **The client/caregiver is aware of possible complications.**

   A. Infection
   B. Reoccurrence of venous stasis ulcer
   C. Amputation of extremity
   D. Cellulitis

RESOURCES

Registered dietician

Certified nurse wound specialist

Podiatrist

(Continued)

REFERENCES

Ackley, B. J., & Ladwig, G. B. (2006). *Nursing diagnosis handbook: A guide to planning care.* Philadelphia: Mosby Inc.

Cohen, B. J., & Wood, D. L. (2000). *Memmler's the human body in health and disease* (9th ed.). Philadelphia: Lippincott Williams & Wilkins.

Nutrition made incredibly easy. (2003). Springhouse: Lippincott, Williams & Wilkins.

Portable RN: The all-in-one nursing reference. (2002). Springhouse: Lippincott, Williams & Wilkins.

Taylor, C., Lillis, D., & LeMone, P. (2005). *Fundamentals of nursing.* Philadelphia: Lippincott Williams & Wilkins.

Timby, B. K., & Smith, N. C. (2003). *Introductory medical-surgical nursing* (8th ed.). Philadelphia: J. B. Lippincott Williams & Wilkins.

12 Metabolic Syndrome

Patient name: _____ Admission: _____

NRS
DATE INITIAL

I. **The client/caregiver can define metabolic syndrome.**

A. Metabolic syndrome is the cluster of metabolic risk factors that increase the risk of coronary artery disease.

B. The American Heart Association and the National Heart, Lung, and Blood Institute suggest the following perimeters for the diagnosis of metabolic syndrome. They include the following:
   1. Obesity, including a waist circumference more than 40 inches for men and 35 inches for women.
   2. Blood pressure of 130/85 mm Hg or higher.
   3. Triglyceride level of 150 mg/dl or higher.
   4. HDL level below 40 mg/dl in men and 50 mg/dl in women.
   5. Fasting serum glucose level of 100 mg/dl.

II. **The client/caregiver can list objective methods used to evaluate for this syndrome during a physical examination.**

A. BMI is the body mass index, which compares a person's weight to their height to give an estimate of body fat.

B. Waist circumference is a reflection of body fat distribution. Fat that is distributed in large amounts around the waist is often called an apple-shaped body type. This body type is at the greatest risk for cardiovascular disease.

C. Skinfold measurements are usually taken at the triceps, and biceps areas. This also helps to establish the body fat percentage of an individual.

D. Measure blood pressure and pulse.

E. Assess for shortness of breath and/or edema.

NRS
DATE INITIAL

III. **The client/caregiver can discuss laboratory diagnostic tests the physician may use to evaluate for the presence of metabolic syndrome.**

A. Total cholesterol and LDL and HDL levels
B. Serum triglycerides
C. Blood glucose level

IV. **The client/caregiver can list additional testing the physician may use to evaluate for damage to the cardiovascular system by the metabolic syndrome.**

A. Electrocardiogram (ECG)
B. Stress test
C. Echocardiography
D. Cardiac catherization
E. Chest x-ray

V. **The client/caregiver can list resources included in this book for the metabolic syndrome.**

A. Diabetes mellitus teaching guide
B. The hypertension teaching guide
C. Coronary artery disease teaching guide
D. Nutrition teaching guides
E. Weight-loss diet
F. Cardiovascular-related diets: low-fat, low-cholesterol, and low-sodium diets
G. Diabetes mellitus diet

RESOURCES

National Cholesterol Education Program (NCEP)
www.nhibi.nih.gov/about/ncep

National Heart, Lung, and Blood Institute
www.nhlbi.nih

American Heart Association
www.americanheart.org

National Institutes of Health
www.nih.gov

(Continued)

American Dietetic Association
www.eatright.org

American Diabetes Association
www.diabetes.org

REFERENCES

Ackley, B. J., & Ladwig, G. B. (2006). *Nursing diagnosis handbook: A guide to planning care.* Philadelphia: Mosby Inc.

Cohen, B. J., & Wood, D. L. (2000). *Memmler's the human body in health and disease* (9th ed.). Philadelphia: Lippincott Williams & Wilkins.

Nutrition made incredibly easy. (2003). Springhouse: Lippincott, Williams & Wilkins.

Portable RN: The all-in-one nursing reference. (2002). Springhouse: Lippincott, Williams & Wilkins.

Taylor, C., Lillis, D., & LeMone, P. (2005). *Fundamentals of nursing.* Philadelphia: Lippincott Williams & Wilkins.

Timby, B. K., & Smith, N. C. (2003). *Introductory medical-surgical nursing* (8th ed.). Philadelphia: J. B. Lippincott Williams & Wilkins.

1 Cushing's Syndrome

Patient name: _____   **Admission:** _____

I. **The client/caregiver can define Cushing's syndrome.**

   A. It is a hormonal disorder caused by prolonged exposure to high levels of cortisol.
   B. The adrenal glands release cortisol into the blood stream.
   C. Cushing's syndrome is caused by an overproduction of cortisol.
   D. It most commonly affects adults who are 20 to 50 years old.

II. **The client/caregiver can explain what causes the high levels of cortisol.**

   A. Use of glucocorticoid hormones like prednisone for chronic health conditions.
   B. The body overproduces the amount of cortisol because
      1. Benign pituitary tumors, benign adrenal tumors cause a chain reaction that results in increased cortisol levels.
      2. Other benign or malignant tumors that grow outside the pituitary can cause the same reaction. The most common is malignant lung tumors.

III. **The client/caregiver can list symptoms of Cushing's syndrome.**

   A. General physical features or change in appearance are as follows:
      1. A tendency to gain weight, especially around abdomen, face (moon face), and neck and upper back (buffalo hump)
      2. Thinning and weakness of the muscle of the upper arms and legs
      3. Thinning of skin with easy bruising and pink or purple stretch marks on the abdomen, thighs, breasts, and shoulders
      4. Increased acne
      5. Growth of facial hair
      6. Scalp hair loss for women
      7. Reddening complexion on the face and neck
      8. Skin darkening (acathosis) on the neck

   B. Other symptoms may be as follows:
      • Elevated blood pressure
      • Fatigue and weakness
      • Depression or mood swings
      • Increased thirst and urination
   C. Common laboratory finding changes are as follows:
      • Elevated white blood count
      • Elevated blood sugar
      • Low serum potassium

IV. **The client/caregiver can list complications of untreated disease.**

   A. Increased weakness and fatigue
   B. Poor skin healing
   C. Osteoporosis of the spine
   D. Increased susceptibility to infections such as pneumonia or tuberculosis
   E. Increased risk of peptic ulcers

V. **The client/caregiver can list treatments for Cushing's syndrome.**

   A. If the cause is long-term use of glucocorticoid hormones to treat another disorder, the physician will reduce it to the lowest adequate dose and monitor the use carefully.
   B. Other treatments may include the following:
      • Surgery
      • Radiation
      • Chemotherapy
      • The use of cortisol-inhibiting drugs

VI. **The client/caregiver can discuss important measures to manage disease.**

   A. Monitor
      • Blood glucose (sugar) levels
      • Blood pressure
      • Weight (weekly)
      • Signs of edema
      • Stools for change in color or that test positive for blood
      • Mood changes or increasing depression

(Continued)

NRS
DATE INITIAL

B. Teach
   1. Safety precautions to prevent falls or injury
   2. The use of medications such as diuretic (fluid pills) or changes in medications
   3. Rest periods between activities
   4. Exercise with rest periods
   5. Avoidance of exposure to infections
   6. No nonprescription drugs without physician's approval
   7. Recommended diet, usually sodium-restricted diet
   8. Good skin care and hygiene
   9. Expression of feelings over any physical changes
   10. Ways to modify appearance to improve self-esteem
C. Report
   1. Any epigastric pain or discomfort
   2. Any sores or cuts that do not heal
   3. Any changes in glucose levels, weight, and blood pressure or evidence of blood in stool
   4. Any mood changes or depression

RESOURCES

Counseling

Support groups

National Institutes of Health
www.nih.gov

Cushing's Support and Research Foundation, Inc.
www.CSRF.net

REFERENCES

Ackley, B. J., & Ladwig, G. B. (2006). *Nursing diagnosis handbook: A guide to planning care.* St. Louis: Mosby Inc.

Cohen, B. J., & Taylor, J. J. (2005). *Memmler's the human body in health and disease* (10th ed.). Philadelphia: Lippincott Williams & Wilkins.

Lutz, C., & Przytulski, K. (2001). *Nutrition and diet therapy.* Philadelphia: F. A. Davis Company.

Nursing 2006 drug handbook. (2006). Philadelphia: Lippincott Williams and Wilkins.

Perry, A., & Potter, P. (2006). *Clinical nursing skills & technique.* St. Louis, Missouri: Mosby Inc.

Timby, B. K., & Smith, N. C. (2003). *Introductory medical-surgical nursing* (8th ed.). Philadelphia: J. B. Lippincott Williams & Wilkins.

2 | Diabetes Mellitus

Patient name: _____   **Admission:** _____

NRS
DATE INITIAL

I. **The client/caregiver can define diabetes mellitus.**

   A. It is a disease in which the body does not produce or properly use insulin.
   B. Insulin is a hormone produced in the pancreas and is necessary for the body to turn sugar and other foods into energy.
   C. A lack of insulin leads sugars to build up to unsafe levels in the blood.

II. **The client/caregiver can explain current diabetes definitions.**

   A. Diabetes mellitus is defined as a fasting blood sugar level of 126 mg/dl or more.
   B. "Prediabetes" is when blood glucose (sugars) are higher than normal, but not yet diabetic.
      1. Prediabetics have an increased risk for developing type 2 diabetes, heart disease, and stroke.
      2. They have impaired fasting glucose levels (100 to 125 mg/dl).
      3. They have impaired glucose tolerance (fasting glucose less than 126 mg/dl and a glucose level between 140 and 199 mg/dl 2 hours after taking an oral glucose tolerance test).

III. **The client/caregiver can list the three major types of diabetes.**

   A. Types of diabetes:
      1. Type 1 diabetes is usually diagnosed in childhood. Daily injections of insulin are required to sustain life.
      2. Type 2 diabetes usually occurs in adulthood. The pancreas does not make enough insulin to keep blood glucose (sugar) levels normal. Many people do not know they have this type. This type is becoming more common because of age, obesity, and a lack of exercise.
      3. Gestational diabetes is high blood glucose levels that develop at any time

during pregnancy in a person who does not have diabetes.

IV. **The client/caregiver can list risk factors for diabetes.**

   A. A parent, brother, or sister with diabetes
   B. Obesity
   C. Age greater than 45 years
   D. Member of some ethnic groups (particularly African American and Hispanics)
   E. Gestational diabetes or delivering a baby weighing more than 9 pounds
   F. High blood pressure
   G. High triglyceride or cholesterol levels

The American Diabetes Association recommends that all adults be screened for diabetes at least every 3 years. A person at high risk should be screened more often.

V. **The client/caregiver can recognize signs and symptoms.**

   A. Symptoms of type 1 diabetes
      • Increased thirst
      • Increased urination
      • Weight loss in spite of increased appetite
      • Fatigue
      • Nausea
      • Vomiting
   B. Symptoms of type 2 diabetes
      • Increased thirst
      • Increased urination
      • Increased appetite
      • Fatigue
      • Blurred vision
      • Slow-healing infections
      • Impotence in men

VI. **The client/caregiver can list ways the diabetic can test glucose levels.**

   A. Urine analysis to check for glucose and ketones
   B. Fasting blood glucose level
   C. Random (nonfasting) blood glucose level

(Continued)

NRS
DATE INITIAL

D. Oral glucose tolerance test
E. Hemoglobin A1c to measure the average blood glucose during the previous 2 to 3 months. A nondiabetic person has a value of 5%. The diabetic client should try to keep it below 7%.

VII. **The client/caregiver can list necessary skills to deal with diabetes.**

A. Know when and what to eat
B. Know how to test and record blood glucose
C. Know how to test urine for ketones (type 1 diabetics)
D. Know how to recognize and treat low blood sugar (hypoglycemia) and high blood sugar (hyperglycemia)
E. Know how to take insulin and/or oral medication
F. Know how to adjust insulin and/or food intake when changing exercise and eating habits

VIII. **The client/caregiver can list measures important in management of diabetes mellitus.**

A. Achieve and maintain ideal weight. Some people with type 2 diabetes find that they no longer need oral medication if they lose weight and increase daily activity.
B. The diet should be
 1. Consistent in carbohydrates during three meals and three snacks daily (check consistent carbohydrate therapeutic diets—Chapter 25).
 2. A registered dietician can help in learning glycemic index of foods.
 3. MyPyramid is a great source for information.
C. Exercise
 1. Do daily.
 2. Perform at the level appropriate for current fitness level.
 3. Monitor blood glucose levels before and after exercise.
 4. Drink extra fluids (without sugar) before, during, and after exercise.
 5. Carry a diabetic identification card.
 6. Carry cell phone in case of emergency.
 7. Carry food that contains a fast-acting carbohydrate in case you experience hypoglycemic reaction.

NRS
DATE INITIAL

D. Oral medications (see Medication Classifications—Chapter 27)
 1. Oral medications that perform an increase in insulin production by the pancreas, increase sensitivity to insulin, or delay absorption of glucose.
 2. Different types of oral medications may be combined.
E. Foot care
 1. Check feet daily. Report any sores or changes with signs of infection.
 2. Wash feet daily with lukewarm water and mild soap. Dry completely.
 3. Soften dry skin with lotion or prescribed creams.
 4. Exercise daily to promote good circulation.
 5. Wear comfortable, well-fitting shoes.
 6. See a podiatrist for foot problems, such as corns or calluses.
 7. Remind health care provider to examine feet without shoes and socks during your routine visits.
 8. Stop smoking.
 9. Avoid going without shoes.
 10. Clip nails straight across, and gently file with an emery board.
F. Eye care
 1. Have a complete dilated eye examination every year.
 2. Have a comprehensive eye exam that includes visual acuity testing that measures how well you see at various distances and a dilated eye exam that can reveal any damage to retina or optic nerve. Tonometry uses an instrument to measure pressure inside the eye.
G. Skin care
 1. Bathe every day with mild soap and lukewarm water. Use lotion as needed.
 2. Avoid scratches or bruises. Wash cuts and scrapes with soap and water, and cover with bandage.
 3. Wear gloves when you work.
 4. Use sunscreen.
 5. Dress appropriate to weather.
 6. Call physician if skin injury does not heal.

(Continued)

H. Dental care
1. Brush and floss every day.
2. Visit the dentist every 6 months.

IX. **The client/caregiver can recognize signs, symptoms, and possible causes of hyperglycemia (high blood sugar).**

A. Signs and symptoms
- Polyuria (frequent or excessive urination)
- Polydipsia (extreme thirst)
- Polyphagia (excessive hunger)

B. Possible causes of hyperglycemia
- One of the first signs of diabetes
- Excess food
- Insufficient insulin production
- Lack of exercise
- Infection
- Obesity

X. **The client/caregiver can recognize signs, symptoms, and possible causes of hypoglycemia (low blood sugar). This usually occurs when the blood sugar is below 50 mg/dl.**

A. Signs and symptoms include the following:
- Sweating
- Tremors
- Anxiety
- Hunger
- Dizziness
- Headache
- Cloudy vision
- Confusion
- Abnormal behavior
- Convulsions
- Loss of consciousness

B. Possible causes of hypoglycemia (low blood sugar) include the following:
- An excessive amount of insulin
- Inadequate amount of food
- Excessive exercise

XI. **The client/caregiver will know what to do if symptoms of high or low blood sugar occurs.**

A. High blood sugar
1. Go to the emergency room.
B. Low blood sugar
1. Eat some form of simple carbohydrate as soon as possible.

2. Sources of concentrated simple carbohydrates are sweetened fruit juice, candy, cake frosting, or glucose tablets.
3. The following on the list each contain about 15 grams of carbohydrate:
- Three glucose tablets
- One-half cup of fruit juice or regular soda
- Six or seven hard candies (not sugar free)
- One tablespoon of honey or sugar
4. Go to the emergency room if symptoms persist.

XII. **The client/caregiver can state management of diabetes during illnesses.**

A. Take your insulin or oral medications.
B. Test your blood sugar before each meal and at bedtime.
C. Follow your meal plan, if you can eat. If you are not eating, take in at least 4 ounces of sugar-containing beverage every hour. Encourage fluids to maintain hydration.
D. Contact your physician if
1. You are unable to keep down food, liquids or medications.
2. Your illness lasts more than 24 hours.
3. You have blood sugars higher than 240 mg/ml for more than 1 day.

XIII. **The client/caregiver is aware of possible emergency complications.**

A. Diabetic hyperglycemic hyperosmolar coma
1. It is caused by complications of type 2 diabetes and extremely high blood glucose (sugar) levels without presence of ketones.
2. The symptoms are decreased consciousness, extreme dehydration, and very high blood glucose (sugar) levels (600 to 2400 mg/dl).
3. It can be triggered by infection or increased fluid loss.
4. Symptoms are elevated pulse, low blood pressure, speech impairment, confusion, convulsions, and coma.

(Continued)

NRS
DATE INITIAL

B. Diabetic ketoacidosis results from extremely high blood sugar levels causing metabolic acidosis. Symptoms are as follows:
- Increased thirst and urination
- Nausea
- Deep and rapid breathing
- Abdominal pain
- Sweet-smelling breath
- Loss of consciousness

C. Hypoglycemic coma or severe insulin reaction. Symptoms are as follows:
- Weakness and drowsiness
- Headache
- Confusion
- Dizziness
- Double vision
- Lack of coordination
- Convulsions
- Unconsciousness

XIV. **The client/caregiver is aware of possible long-term complications.**

- Diabetic retinopathy—damage to retina possibly leading to blindness
- Diabetic nephropathy—kidney damage
- Diabetic neuropathy—loss of sensation in extremities, loss of bladder control, and impotence
- Hyperlipidemia
- Hypertension—strokes
- Coronary artery disease, peripheral vascular disease, atherosclerosis
- Amputation of extremities

RESOURCES

American Diabetes Association
www.diabetes.org

Diabetes Risk Test
www.diabetes.org/risk-test

Community support group

Dietician or nutritionist

MyPyramid from the United States Department of Agriculture
www.mypyramid.gov/

National Institute of Diabetes and Digestive and Kidney Diseases
www2.niddk.nih.gov/

REFERENCES

American College of Endocrinology and American Diabetes Association consensus statement on inpatient diabetes and glycemic control. (2006). *Diabetes Care, 29,* 1955–1962 (this article is based on a consensus conference held in Washington, DC, January 30 and 31, 2006).

Ackley, B. J., & Ladwig, G. B. (2006). *Nursing diagnosis handbook: A guide to planning care.* St. Louis: Mosby Inc.

Cohen, B. J., & Taylor, J. J. (2005). *Memmler's the human body in health and disease* (10th ed.). Philadelphia: Lippincott Williams & Wilkins.

Hitchcock, J. E., Schubert, P. E., & Thomas, S. A. (2003). *Community health nursing: Caring in action.* Clifton Park, NY: Thomson Delmar Learning.

Lutz, C., & Przytulski, K. (2001). *Nutrition and diet therapy.* Philadelphia: F. A. Davis Company.

Nursing 2006 drug handbook. (2006). Philadelphia: Lippincott Williams and Wilkins.

Perry, A., & Potter, P. (2006). *Clinical nursing skills & technique.* St. Louis: Mosby Inc.

Timby, B. K., & Smith, N. C. (2003). *Introductory medical-surgical nursing* (8th ed.). Philadelphia: J. B. Lippincott Williams & Wilkins.

3 Insulin Teaching Guide

Patient name: _____

Admission: _____

I. The client/caregiver can state action of insulin.

A. Helps to control blood-sugar levels in clients with type 1 diabetes mellitus.
B. It is administered by insulin subcutaneous injection or insulin pump.
C. Types of insulin are
  1. Humalog, Novolog (very short acting). The onset of action is 5 to 15 minutes, and the peak effect is after 30 to 60 minutes.
  2. Regular (short acting). The onset of action is 30 minutes. The peak effect is after 2 to 5 hours.
  3. NPH (intermediate acting). The onset of action in 1 to 2.5 hours. The peak effect is after 8 to 14 hours.
  4. Lente (intermediate acting). The onset of action is 1 to 2.5 hours. The peak effect is after 8 to 12 hours.
  5. Ultra Lente (long acting). The onset of action is 4 to 6 hours. The peak effect is after 10 to 18 hours.
  6. Premixed combinations have the onset of action in 30 minutes. The peak effect is after 7 to 12 hours. Examples of combinations are 70/30 (70 intermediate/30 rapid acting), 50/50 (50 intermediate/50 rapid acting), and 75/25 (75 intermediate/25 rapid acting).
  7. Lantus (insulin glargine). It has a constant long duration with no defined peak of action. It is usually given once a day and usually at bedtime.

II. The client/caregiver can list possible adverse reactions to insulin.

A. Hypoglycemia or low blood sugar
  • Headache
  • Sweating
  • Hunger
  • Nervousness
  • Weakness
  • Restlessness or sweating during sleep

B. Hyperglycemia or high blood sugar
  • Flushed
  • Dry skin
  • Nausea
  • Fatigue
  • Headache
  • Dizziness
C. Allergic reaction (seek emergency treatment)

III. The client/caregiver can list precautions when storing, preparing, and administering insulin.

A. Keep insulin vials that are currently in use at room temperature. When not needed, store in refrigerator. Never freeze insulin.
B. Take insulin exactly as prescribed, and never adjust dose without orders from physician.
C. Do not interchange beef, pork, or human insulins.
D. Lantus insulin should never be mixed with other insulins.
E. Never use insulin that has changed color or consistency.
F. Rotate sites to prevent skin complications using abdomen, upper and outer thighs, upper arms, and buttocks.
G. Administer insulin promptly (within 5 minutes) after mixing insulins.
H. Use only insulin syringes to administer insulin.
I. Press—do not massage injection site after administration of insulin.
J. Dispose of syringes in an impermeable container.

IV. The client/caregiver can list other precautions when taking insulin.

A. Limit cigarette smoking because it decreases the amount of insulin absorbed when given subcutaneously.
B. Avoid alcohol and aspirin, which may increase effect of insulin.
C. Never omit meals.

(Continued)

D. Carry a snack (source of simple sugar) at all times in case of low blood sugar.

E. Wear a medical identification bracelet.

F. Monitor and record blood or urine glucose levels.

G. Monitor factors that affect amount of insulin required:

1. Follow diet closely as instructed.
2. Exercise daily in constant amounts.
3. Use stress management techniques.
4. Obtain prompt treatment for any infections.
5. Test blood sugar more frequently if a change in diet, activity, stress, illness, or infection occurs, and notify the physician.

H. Keep follow-up appointments with the physician and laboratory.

I. Report any signs of hypoglycemia, that is, headache, sweating, hunger, nervousness, and weakness.

J. Report any signs of hyperglycemia, that is, flushed, dry skin; nausea; fatigue; headache; and dizziness.

V. **The client/caregiver can list measures to safely use insulin pump.**

A. The insulin pump is used for continuous (24 hour) insulin delivery.

B. The insulin pump has a pump reservoir and a computer chip that allows the user to control the exact amount of insulin being delivered and is battery operated.

C. They are approximately the size of a beeper. It is attached to a thin plastic tube that has a soft cannula or needle at the end to deliver insulin.

D. The cannula (needle) is inserted under the skin, usually on the abdomen. It needs to be changed every 3 days.

E. The tubing can be disconnected when showering or swimming.

VI. **The client/caregiver can demonstrate syringe preparation.**

A. Wash hands thoroughly.

B. Assemble equipment: syringe, insulin, alcohol swab.

C. Check that you are using appropriate type of insulin and that it has not expired.

D. Verify that you are using appropriate type of syringe (only insulin syringe).

E. Roll the insulin bottle gently to mix it.

F. Cleanse top of bottle with alcohol.

G. Pull plunger of syringe back the number of units of insulin to be injected, not allowing the needle to touch anything.

H. Insert the needle into the bottle and inject air.

I. Invert the bottle and syringe, and slowly withdraw prescribed amount of insulin, being sure that the needle is under the fluid level.

J. Check the syringe for air bubbles, and remove by tapping the syringe. Draw up more insulin, and discard excess if necessary for accurate amount.

VII. **The client/caregiver can demonstrate procedure for insulin injection.**

A. Wash hands. Check previous rotation site and select new site.

B. Prepare the injection site by swabbing the center of the area with alcohol and moving outward in a circular manner about 2 inches. Allow the area to air dry.

C. Pinch the skin approximately 2 inches with thumb and forefinger at the injection site, not touching the area that was cleaned.

D. Inject the needle into the skin using a quick, firm motion at a 45-degree (normal weight) or 90-degree angle (obese patient).

E. Inject insulin slowly into the tissue. Remove the needle, and hold swab over site briefly.

F. Place the manufacturer's needle guard to cover needle and dispose syringe/needle in safety container.

VIII. **The client/caregiver can list sites of body for insulin injections.**

A. Upper arms
B. Abdomen
C. Thighs
D. Buttocks

(Continued)

RESOURCES

American Diabetes Association

800-232-3472

www.diabetes.org

Medical supply company

Pharmacist

REFERENCES

Adams, M. P., Josephson, D. L., & Holland, L. N. Jr. (2005). *Pharmacology for nurses: A pathophysiologic approach*. Upper Saddle River, NJ: Pearson Education, Inc.

Canobbio, M. M. (2006). *Mosby's handbook of patient teaching*. St. Louis: Mosby Inc.

Nursing 2006 drug handbook. (2006). Philadelphia: Lippincott Williams and Wilkins.

Standards of medical care in diabetes—2007. *Diabetes Care, 30*(Suppl 1), S4–S41.

Perry, A., & Potter, P. (2006). *Clinical nursing skills & technique*. St. Louis: Mosby Inc.

4 Hyperthyroidism

Patient name: _____

Admission: _____

DATE | NRS INITIAL

I. The client/caregiver has a basic understanding of the anatomy and physiology of the thyroid gland.

A. The thyroid gland is located in the lower neck and in front of the trachea.
B. It is divided into two lobes and is joined by a band of tissue called the isthmus, making it resemble a butterfly.
C. It concentrates iodine from food and uses it to synthesize two hormones.
D. These two hormones regulate the body's metabolic rate.

II. The client/caregiver can define hyperthyroidism and possible causes.

A. It is a syndrome that occurs when the thyroid gland produces an excess of thyroid hormones.
B. Excess thyroid hormones cause an increased rate at which the body uses energy.
C. Noncancerous lumps growing in the thyroid gland can also increase the production of hormones and cause hyperthyroidism.
D. Graves' disease (an autoimmune disorder) can attack the thyroid gland and cause overproduction of hormones.

III. The client/caregiver can recognize signs and symptoms of hyperthyroidism.

- Heat intolerance, sweating
- Sudden weight loss
- Alterations in appetite
- Frequent bowel movements
- Changes in vision
- Fatigue and muscle weakness
- Menstrual disturbance
- Impaired fertility
- Mental disturbances possibly depression
- Sleep disturbances
- Tremors
- Thyroid enlargement
- Rapid heartbeat

DATE | NRS INITIAL

- Wider, swollen or red eyes
- In severe cases exophthalmos, in which eyes appear to protrude because of enlarged muscle and fatty tissue surrounding the eyes

IV. Client/caregiver can list measures to alleviate symptoms of hyperthyroidism.

A. Restlessness
 1. Avoid emotional or physical stimulation until metabolism returns to normal
 2. Avoid excessive exercise and plan for rest periods
 3. Avoid caffeine, yellow and red food dyes, and artificial preservatives
 4. Avoid aspirin and aspirin products
B. Weight loss
 1. Eat a high-carbohydrate, high-protein diet
 2. Monitor weight on a regular basis
C. Diarrhea
 1. Avoid highly seasoned foods
 2. Use BRAT (bananas, rice, apples, tea) during acute episode
 3. Increase fluids to maintain hydration
D. Eyeball protrusion and eye irritation
 1. Apply cool moist compresses
 2. Shield eyes with eye patches or sunglasses
 3. Cover or tape eyelids shut at night
 4. Sleep with head of bed elevated
 5. Limit fluids and sodium to decrease fluid retention in eyes
 6. Notify physician of visual disturbances
 7. Use artificial tears or eye lubricants as ordered
E. Heat intolerance
 1. Provide cool environment
 2. Dress appropriately
 3. Encourage good hygiene
F. Depression
 1. Obtain emotional support or counseling as needed
 2. Dress attractively to increase self-esteem

(Continued)

NRS
DATE INITIAL

V.   **The client/caregiver is aware of possible medical treatment.**

   A. Suppression of hormone production with medication (check medication classification for thyroid medication)
   B. Destruction of thyroid tissue with radioactive iodine
   C. Surgical removal of part of the thyroid gland

VI.   **The client/caregiver is aware of signs and symptoms of possible complications.**

   A. Thyroid storm or thyrotoxic crisis has a sudden onset with symptoms of high fever, very rapid heart rate, delirium, dehydration, and extreme irritability. Prompt treatment is necessary because it can be life threatening.
   B. If untreated, thyroid disease can cause elevated cholesterol levels, heart disease, infertility, and osteoporosis.

RESOURCES

National Institute of Diabetes and Digestive and Kidney Diseases
www2.niddk.nih.gov/

American Thyroid Association
www.thyroid.org/

National Institutes of Health/Thyroid Disease
www.nlm.nih.gov/medlineplus/thyroiddiseases

Community support group

Dietician or nutritionist

REFERENCES

Ackley, B. J., & Ladwig, G. B. (2006). *Nursing diagnosis handbook: A guide to planning care.* St. Louis: Mosby Inc.

Cohen, B. J., & Taylor, J. J. (2005). *Memmler's the human body in health and disease* (10th ed.). Philadelphia: Lippincott Williams & Wilkins.

Lutz, C., & Przytulski, K. (2001). *Nutrition and diet therapy.* Philadelphia: F. A. Davis Company.

Nursing 2006 drug handbook. (2006). Philadelphia: Lippincott Williams and Wilkins.

Nutrition made incredibly easy. (2003). Philadelphia: Lippincott Williams & Wilkins.

Portable RN: The all-in-one nursing reference. (2002). Springhouse: Lippincott, Williams & Wilkins.

Timby, B. K., & Smith, N. C. (2003). *Introductory medical-surgical nursing* (8th ed.). Philadelphia: J. B. Lippincott Williams & Wilkins.

5 Hypothyroidism

Patient name: _____

Admission: _____

I. **The client/caregiver has a basic understanding of the anatomy and physiology of the thyroid gland.**

A. The thyroid gland is located in the lower neck and in front of the trachea.
B. It is divided into two lobes and is joined by a band of tissue called isthmus.
C. It concentrates iodine from food and uses it to synthesize two hormones.
D. These two hormones regulate the body's metabolic rate.

II. **The client/caregiver can define hypothyroidism.**

A. Hypothyroidism is a disease resulting from a deficiency of thyroid hormones.
B. Hypothyroidism can affect infants, children, and adults.
C. Severe hypothyroidism is myxedema.

III. **The client/caregiver can state possible causes of hypothyroidism.**

A. Congenital deficiency
B. Tumors
C. Inflammation of the thyroid
D. Pituitary disease
E. Surgical removal of thyroid
F. Iodine deficiency
G. Radioactive iodine treatment

IV. **The client/caregiver can recognize signs and symptoms of hypothyroidism.**

A. Adults
  • Lethargy and fatigue
  • Forgetfulness
  • Weight gain
  • Dry, scaly skin
  • Puffy face and swollen around the eyes
  • Thinning and loss of hair
  • Hoarse voice
  • Constipation
  • Irregular menstrual periods or heavy flow

  • Increased sensitivity to cold
  • Hypersensitivity to drugs such as barbiturates and sedatives and to anesthesia
B. Congenital hypothyroidism
  • Excessive sleeping and lack of energy
  • Greater risk for delayed mental development
  • Constipation or bloated abdomen
  • Puffy face and swollen tongue
  • Hoarse cry
  • Low muscle tone
  • Cold extremities
  • Increased birth weight, but little to no growth later

V. **The client/caregiver can list measures for management symptoms of the disease.**

A. Exercise regularly with planned rest periods.
B. Set realistic goals to increase activity as tolerated.
C. Eat a diet that is low in sodium, cholesterol, fat, and calories.
D. Avoid constipation with a diet high in fiber, adequate fluids, stool softeners, and so forth.
E. Take thyroid medication as instructed at the same time each day (thyroid medication and laboratory testing must be taken lifelong).
F. Contact physician before taking any over-the-counter medication (sedatives or hypnotics can cause respiratory depression).
G. Keep follow-up appointments with physician.
H. Provide a warm environment to promote comfort.
I. Avoid pressure or irritation to the skin to prevent skin breakdown.
J. Avoid excess stress, which increases metabolic rate.
K. Use a Medic Alert bracelet or card.

(Continued)

NRS
DATE INITIAL

VI. **The client/caregiver can list what signs and symptoms to report to physician.**

  A. Signs/symptoms of hyperthyroidism are weight loss, restlessness, fast heart rate, fatigue, loose bowel movements, or heat intolerance (hyperthyroidism can be caused by hormone therapy).
  B. Signs/symptoms of hypothyroidism are a puffy, mask-like face and swelling around the eyes.
  C. Signs/symptoms of respiratory infections are fever, cough, and cold symptoms.
  D. Signs/symptoms of urinary infections are burning, frequency, and urgency.

VII. **The client/caregiver is aware of signs and symptoms of possible complications.**

  A. Enlarged heart and/or heart failure
  B. Organic psychosis
  C. Myxedema coma
  D. Intestinal obstruction
  E. Anemia

RESOURCES

National Institute of Diabetes and Digestive and Kidney Diseases
www2.niddk.nih.gov/

American Thyroid Association
www.thyroid.org/

National Institutes of Health/Thyroid Disease
www.nlm.nih.gov/medlineplus/thyroiddiseases

Community support group

Dietician or nutritionist

REFERENCES

Ackley, B. J., & Ladwig, G. B. (2006). *Nursing diagnosis handbook: A guide to planning care.* St. Louis: Mosby Inc.

Cohen, B. J., & Taylor, J. J. (2005). *Memmler's the human body in health and disease* (10th ed.). Philadelphia: Lippincott Williams & Wilkins.

Lutz, C., & Przytulski, K. (2001). *Nutrition and diet therapy.* Philadelphia: F. A. Davis Company.

Nursing 2006 drug handbook. (2006). Philadelphia: Lippincott Williams and Wilkins.

Perry, A., & Potter, P. (2006). *Clinical nursing skills & technique.* St. Louis, Missouri: Mosby Inc.

Portable RN: The all-in-one nursing reference. (2002). Springhouse: Lippincott, Williams & Wilkins.

Timby, B. K., & Smith, N. C. (2003). *Introductory medical-surgical nursing* (8th ed.). Philadelphia: J. B. Lippincott Williams & Wilkins.

1 Bowel Obstruction

Patient name: _____ Admission: _____

NRS
DATE INITIAL

I. The client/caregiver has a basic understanding of the anatomy and physiology of the intestines.

   A. The small intestine is approximately 18 feet long and extends from the stomach to the large intestine.
   B. The large intestine, which is much shorter and wider, ascends up the right side of the abdomen, is horizontal across the abdomen, and descends on the left side of the abdomen.
   C. Digestion and absorption occur in the intestines.

II. The client/caregiver can define contents obstruction.

   A. A blockage prevents the contents from passing normally through the intestines, and it can occur in either the large or small intestine.
   B. There are two basic types of obstructions:
      1. Mechanical obstruction occurs when something physically stops the passage of fecal contents (may be caused by tumors, adhesions, hernias, etc.).
      2. Paralytic obstruction is the cessation of peristalsis caused by trauma, infection, toxins, surgery, and so forth.
   C. When obstruction occurs, intestinal contents, fluids, and gas accumulate.

III. The client/caregiver can list factors that increase the risk of bowel obstruction.

   A. Inflammatory disease
   B. Tumor
   C. Hernia
   D. Fecal impaction
   E. Postoperative scar tissue (adhesions)
   F. Foreign bodies (ingested materials that obstruct the intestines)
   G. Congenital strictures
   H. Strictures or scars from radiation therapy

NRS
DATE INITIAL

IV. The client/caregiver can recognize signs and symptoms.

   A. Paralytic ileus is marked by
      • Abdominal distention
      • Absent bowel sounds
      • Relatively little pain
   B. Mechanical obstruction
      • Abdominal fullness and distention
      • Abdominal pain and cramping
      • Vomiting
      • Failure to pass gas or stool
      • Breath odor

V. The client/caregiver can state possible treatment.

   A. Intravenous fluids to replace fluids
   B. Nasogastric tube to drain fluids and gas
   C. Surgery

VI. The client/caregiver can list possible complications.

   A. A lack of blood supply to the bowel, which can cause gangrene and death of the bowel tissue
   B. Perforation (hole) in the intestine

REFERENCES

Ackley, B. J., & Ladwig, G. B. (2006). *Nursing diagnosis handbook: A guide to planning care.* St. Louis: Mosby Elsevier.

Cohen, B. J., & Taylor, J. J. (2005). *Memmler's the human body in health and disease* (10th ed.). Philadelphia: Lippincott Williams & Wilkins.

Perry, A., & Potter, P. (2006). *Clinical nursing skills & technique.* St. Louis: Mosby Inc.

Taylor, C., Lillis, C., & LeMone, P. (2005). *Fundamentals of nursing.* Philadelphia: Lippincott, Williams & Wilkins.

Timby, B. K., & Smith, N. C. (2003). *Introductory medical-surgical nursing* (8th ed.). Philadelphia: J. B. Lippincott Williams & Wilkins.

2   Diverticular Disease

Patient name: _____ **Admission:** _____

DATE / NRS INITIAL

I. **The client/caregiver can define two types of diverticular disease.**

   A. Diverticulosis is a condition in which there are multiple diverticula that are outpouchings of mucosa through a weakened area in the intestinal wall in the lower bowel.

   B. Diverticulitis is the inflammation of diverticula that results when undigested food particles and bacteria become trapped in the diverticula.

II. **The client/caregiver can identify factors that may increase risk of diverticular disease.**

   A. Low-fiber diet

   B. Advancing age

   C. Chronic constipation

   D. Obesity

   E. History of ulcerative colitis or Crohn's disease

III. **The client/caregiver can recognize signs and symptoms of diverticular disease.**

   A. Symptoms of diverticulosis include
- Mild cramps, bloating, and constipation

   B. Symptoms of diverticulitis
- Abdominal pain
- Tenderness around the left side of the lower abdomen
- Fever and chills
- Nausea and vomiting
- Cramping
- Constipation

IV. **The client/caregiver can list measures to prevent or manage diverticular disease.**

   A. Avoid constipation.
1. Eat a diet high in fiber to prevent constipation after inflammation has subsided (high-fiber diet in therapeutic diet).
2. Use stool softeners or bulk laxatives as ordered by the physician.
3. Avoid harsh laxatives and enemas.
4. Drink at least eight glasses of water per day.
5. Establish a regular time for bowel evacuation.
6. Exercise regularly.

   B. Lose weight if necessary (weight-reduction diet).

   C. Report any fever, nausea or vomiting, cloudy or foul odor of urine, constipation, or diarrhea to physician.

   D. Ask the physician about recommendations for colon cancer screening.

V. **The client/caregiver can list possible complications.**

   A. Intestinal obstruction

   B. Peritonitis

   C. Hemorrhage

   D. Perforations

   E. Abscess or fistula formation

   F. Peritonitis and sepsis

RESOURCE

National Digestive Diseases Information Clearinghouse
E-mail: nddic@info.niddk.nih.gov

REFERENCES

Ackley, B. J., & Ladwig, G. B. (2006). *Nursing diagnosis handbook: A guide to planning care.* St. Louis: Mosby Elsevier.

Cohen, B. J., & Taylor, J. J. (2005). *Memmler's the human body in health and disease* (10th ed.). Philadelphia: Lippincott Williams & Wilkins.

Lutz, C., & Przytulski, K. (2001). *Nutrition and diet therapy.* Philadelphia: F. A. Davis Company.

Perry, A., & Potter, P. (2006). *Clinical nursing skills & technique.* St. Louis: Mosby Inc.

Taylor, C., Lillis, C., & LeMone, P. (2005). *Fundamentals of nursing.* Philadelphia: Lippincott, Williams & Wilkins.

Timby, B. K., & Smith, N. C. (2003). *Introductory medical-surgical nursing* (8th ed.). Philadelphia: J. B. Lippincott Williams & Wilkins.

3 Hemorrhoids

Patient name: _____ Admission: _____

NRS DATE INITIAL		

I. The client/caregiver can define hemorrhoids.

  A. They are dilated veins in swollen tissue around the anus.

  B. Hemorrhoids can be internal or external.

  C. Prolapsed hemorrhoids may come out during defecation.

II. The client/caregiver can identify factors that may increase the risk of hemorrhoids.

  A. Straining at stool because of constipation

  B. Pregnancy and constipation

  C. Heavy lifting

  D. Prolonged sitting and standing

  E. Cirrhosis of the liver

III. The client/caregiver can recognize signs and symptoms.

  A. External hemorrhoids
    1. Enlarged mass at the anus
    2. Inflammation
    3. Pain
    4. Bleeding with bowel movement

  B. Internal hemorrhoids
    1. Pain
    2. Bleeding with bowel movements
    3. Itching in perianal area
    4. Constipation

IV. The client/caregiver can list measures to prevent or manage hemorrhoids.

  A. Relieve pressure and straining of constipation.
    1. Increase fluids to at least six to eight glasses per day. Avoid alcohol.
    2. Use stool softeners or laxatives as needed.
    3. Increase fiber in diet.

NRS DATE INITIAL		

    4. Never delay urges to evacuate stool.

    5. Do moderate exercise daily such as walking.

  B. Use warm compresses or tub baths several times a day in plain, warm water for about 10 minutes.

  C. Apply hemorrhoidal cream or suppository as ordered.

  D. Gently wash and dry perianal area after each bowel movement.

  E. Avoid prolonged sitting, squatting, or standing.

  F. Contact the physician for evaluation.

  G. Surgical intervention may be necessary.

V. The client/caregiver is aware of possible complications.

  A. Iron-deficiency anemia

  B. Anal fissures (cracks in mucosa)

  C. Bleeding

  D. Blood clots within hemorrhoids

  E. Strangulated hemorrhoids

REFERENCES

Ackley, B. J., & Ladwig, G. B. (2006). *Nursing diagnosis handbook: A guide to planning care.* St. Louis: Mosby Elsevier.

Cohen, B. J., & Taylor, J. J. (2005). *Memmler's the human body in health and disease* (10th ed.). Philadelphia: Lippincott Williams & Wilkins.

Lutz, C., & Przytulski, K. (2001). *Nutrition and diet therapy.* Philadelphia: F. A. Davis Company.

Perry, A., & Potter, P. (2006). *Clinical nursing skills & technique.* St. Louis: Mosby Inc.

Taylor, C., Lillis, C., & LeMone, P. (2005). *Fundamentals of nursing.* Philadelphia: Lippincott, Williams & Wilkins.

Timby, B. K., & Smith, N. C. (2003). *Introductory medical-surgical nursing* (8th ed.). Philadelphia: J. B. Lippincott Williams & Wilkins.

Hiatal Hernia

Patient name: _____ **Admission:** _____

I. **The client/caregiver has a basic under-standing of the anatomy of the esophagus, stomach, and diaphragm.**

  A. The diaphragm is a large sheet of muscle that separates the abdomen from the chest cavity.

  B. The esophagus (the food tube) extends down through a small opening in the diaphragm to connect to the stomach.

  C. The stomach lies just below the diaphragm.

II. **The client/caregiver can define a hiatal hernia.**

  A. Hernias occur when one part of the body protrudes through a gap or opening into another part.

  B. Hiatal hernia occurs when the muscle tissue surrounding this opening becomes weak and the upper part of the stomach bulges through the diaphragm into the chest cavity.

III. **The client/caregiver can list factors that may increase the risk of hiatal hernia.**

  A. Congenital weakness

  B. Advanced age

  C. Smoking

  D. Prolonged illness

  E. Obesity

  F. Pregnancy

  G. Tumors

  H. Restrictive clothing

  I. Heavy lifting

IV. **The client/caregiver can recognize the signs and symptoms of hiatal hernia, although the condition frequently exists without symptoms.**

  A. Heartburn (burning sensation in the esophagus)

  B. Belching

  C. Regurgitation of sour tasting liquid in the mouth

  D. Difficulty swallowing because of muscle spasms

  E. Chest pain

  F. Symptoms become worse when leaning forward, straining, lifting heavy objects, lying down, and during pregnancy.

V. **The client/caregiver can list measures to manage or prevent symptoms.**

  A. Nutritional measures

    1. Avoid caffeine, coffee, soda, chocolate, and so forth.

    2. Avoid onions, spicy foods, spearmint, and peppermint.

    3. Limit citrus fruits and tomato-based foods.

    4. Limit fatty foods.

    5. Eat small, frequent meals.

    6. Increase fluids.

    7. Increase fiber to prevent constipation.

  B. Drink water after meals to cleanse the esophagus.

  C. Wait at least 3 hours after eating before going to bed or lying down.

  D. Avoid eating before going to bed at night.

  E. Do not exercise immediately after eating.

  F. Avoid smoking.

  G. Lose weight if you are overweight.

  H. Elevate the head of your bed. Raise the head of the bed 6 to 9 inches. Use blocks to raise the bed or a foam wedge to raise the mattress. Do not use pillows because they will increase pressure on your abdomen.

  I. Avoid wearing tight clothing.

  J. Discuss medications with physician for possible causes of heartburn. Do not use over the counter medications without physician approval.

  K. Reduce stress by relaxation techniques such as deep breathing, meditation, tai chi, or yoga.

(Continued)

NRS
DATE INITIAL

L. Avoid heavy lifting.
M. Take medications as ordered.
N. Keep follow-up appointments with physician.

VI. **The client/caregiver can list possible complications.**

A. Gastroesophageal reflux disease
B. Ulceration of the herniated portion of the stomach
C. Gastritis
D. Lung aspiration
E. Slow bleeding and iron-deficiency anemia

REFERENCES

Ackley, B. J., & Ladwig, G. B. (2006). *Nursing diagnosis handbook: A guide to planning care.* St. Louis: Mosby Elsevier.

Cohen, B. J., & Taylor, J. J. (2005). *Memmler's the human body in health and disease* (10th ed.). Philadelphia: Lippincott Williams & Wilkins.

Lutz, C., & Przytulski, K. (2001). *Nutrition and diet therapy.* Philadelphia: F. A. Davis Company.

Perry, A., & Potter, P. (2006). *Clinical nursing skills & technique.* St. Louis: Mosby Inc.

Taylor, C., Lillis, C., & LeMone, P. (2005). *Fundamentals of nursing.* Philadelphia: Lippincott, Williams & Wilkins.

Timby, B. K., & Smith, N. C. (2003). *Introductory medical-surgical nursing* (8th ed.). Philadelphia: J. B. Lippincott Williams & Wilkins.

5 Pancreatitis

Patient name: _____ Admission: _____

I. The client/caregiver has a basic understanding of anatomy and physiology of the pancreas.

A. It is located behind the stomach in a horizontal position, with the head attached to the small intestine and the tail reaching to the spleen.

B. The pancreas excretes a digestive juice that is emptied into the small intestine.

C. The pancreas also produces two hormones: insulin and glucagon.

II. The client/caregiver can define pancreatitis.

A. It is an inflammation of the pancreas that may be acute or chronic.

B. Damage to the pancreas is caused by premature activation of enzymes.

C. Chronic pancreatitis is progressive destruction of pancreatic tissue replaced by fibrotic tissue.

III. The client/caregiver can list factors that increase risk of pancreatitis.

A. Alcohol abuse (accounts for most chronic pancreatitis)

B. Gallbladder disease

C. Drug toxicity

D. A higher risk in African Americans

E. A higher risk in men than women

F. Cystic fibrosis

IV. The client/caregiver can recognize signs and symptoms of acute pancreatitis.

A. Pain
   1. Pain usually has a sudden, severe onset after ingestion of a heavy meal or alcohol.
   2. Pain is located in left upper quadrant of abdomen or mid to upper abdomen and may radiate to the back.

B. Nausea or vomiting

C. Abdominal rigidity and tenderness

D. Fever and/or chills

E. Sweating and clammy skin

F. Low blood pressure

G. Fast heart rate

H. Respiratory distress

I. Mild jaundice

J. Weight loss

V. The client/caregiver can recognize symptoms of chronic pancreatitis.

A. Dull, aching chronic epigastric pain

B. Jaundice

C. Impaired glucose tolerance

D. Frothy, foul-smelling stools

E. Weight loss

F. Nausea and vomiting

G. Symptoms of diabetes mellitus

VI. The client/caregiver can list measures to prevent or manage pancreatitis.

A. Avoid alcohol and tobacco products.

B. Limit the fat in your diet.

C. Use a high-carbohydrate diet. Stress complex carbohydrates found in grains, vegetables, and legumes.

D. Take fat-soluble vitamin supplements (vitamins A, D, and E) and calcium as ordered.

E. Avoid stimulants such as nicotine and caffeine (coffee, tea, and colas) to decrease pancreatic secretions.

F. Eat small, frequent meals to minimize the secretion of pancreatic enzymes.

G. Take analgesics for pain control as ordered. Be aware of the potential for drug abuse with uncontrolled pain.

H. Take medications as ordered.

I. Use lotions or creams to decrease itchy dry skin.

J. Report any symptoms of severe epigastric pain, nausea and vomiting, foul-smelling, clay-colored stools, weight loss, and dark urine.

K. Surgical intervention may be necessary.

(Continued)

NRS
DATE INITIAL

VII. The client/caregiver is aware of signs and symptoms of possible complications.

   A. Respiratory distress
   B. Jaundice
   C. Abscess
   D. Circulatory or renal failure
   E. Hemorrhage/shock
   F. Diabetes
   G. Peptic ulcer
   H. Infection
   I. Drug addiction
   J. Depression

RESOURCES

National Pancreas Foundation
www.pancreasfoundation.org/

Pain-control clinic

Dietician

Mental health counseling

Support groups

REFERENCES

Ackley, B. J., & Ladwig, G. B. (2006). *Nursing diagnosis handbook: A guide to planning care.* St. Louis: Mosby Elsevier.

Cohen, B. J., & Taylor, J. J. (2005). *Memmler's the human body in health and disease* (10th ed.). Philadelphia: Lippincott Williams & Wilkins.

Lutz, C., & Przytulski, K. (2001). *Nutrition and diet therapy.* Philadelphia: F. A. Davis Company.

Perry, A., & Potter, P. (2006). *Clinical nursing skills & technique.* St. Louis: Mosby Inc.

Taylor, C., Lillis, C., & LeMone, P. (2005). *Fundamentals of nursing.* Philadelphia: Lippincott, Williams & Wilkins.

Timby, B. K., & Smith, N. C. (2003). *Introductory medical-surgical nursing* (8th ed.). Philadelphia: J. B. Lippincott Williams & Wilkins.

6

Celiac Disease

Patient name: _____ Admission: _____

I. **The client/caregiver can define celiac disease and risk factors.**

A. It is a disease that makes the body not able to tolerate a protein called gluten.

B. Gluten is found in wheat, rye, and barley. Gluten can also be found in the products we use, such as stamps, envelopes, some medicines, and some vitamins.

C. This disease creates damage to the small intestines and interferes with absorption of nutrients from food when gluten is ingested or touched.

D. It is considered a digestion disease and an autoimmune disorder.

E. Celiac disease is a genetic disease.

F. It can be triggered or activated for the first time after
   • Surgery
   • Pregnancy
   • Childbirth
   • Viral infection
   • Severe emotional stress

II. **The client/caregiver can list symptoms of celiac disease.**

A. Celiac disease may exist without symptoms. There is still a risk for complications, such as malnutrition.

B. It affects people differently. Symptoms may include one or more of the following:
   • Recurring gas, abdominal bloating, and pain
   • Chronic diarrhea
   • Pale, foul-smelling, or fatty stool
   • Weight loss or gain
   • Fatigue
   • Anemia
   • Bone or joint pain, osteoporosis
   • Behavioral changes (irritability is most common in children)
   • Tingling or numbness in legs
   • Muscle cramps
   • Seizures

   • Missed menstrual periods, infertility, and recurrent miscarriage
   • Delayed growth (failure to thrive in infants)
   • Mouth ulcers and tooth discoloration
   • Itchy skin rash

III. **The client/caregiver can list measures to manage celiac disease.**

A. The only treatment for celiac disease is to follow a gluten-free diet. It is a lifetime requirement.
   1. Avoid wheat, rye, or barley products.
   2. Use corn, rice, soy, arrowroot, tapioca, or potato flours in recipes.
   3. Buy plain, frozen, or canned vegetables and season with herbs or spices.
   4. When eating out, select meat, poultry, or fish made without breading, gravies, or sauces.
   5. Store all gluten-free products in the refrigerator or freezer because they do not contain preservatives.
   6. Read labels carefully. Buy "gluten-free" products. Contact a food manufacturer for product information if in doubt.

B. Family members of a person with celiac disease may want to be tested.

C. Seek others with celiac disease for information and support.

IV. **The client/caregiver can list possible complications.**

A. Malnutrition and anemia
B. Lymphoma and adenocarcinoma
C. Osteoporosis
D. Miscarriage or congenital malformation
E. Short stature
F. Increased risk for other autoimmune diseases

(Continued)

RESOURCES

Dietician

Support groups

Celiac Disease Foundation
www.celiac.org

National Foundation for Celiac Awareness
www.celiacawareness.org

American Dietetic Association
www.eatright.org

REFERENCES

Ackley, B. J., & Ladwig, G. B. (2006). *Nursing diagnosis handbook: A guide to planning care.* St. Louis: Mosby Elsevier.

Cohen, B. J., & Taylor, J. J. (2005). *Memmler's the human body in health and disease* (10th ed.). Philadelphia: Lippincott Williams & Wilkins.

Lutz, C., & Przytulski, K. (2001). *Nutrition and diet therapy.* Philadelphia: F. A. Davis Company.

Perry, A., & Potter, P. (2006). *Clinical nursing skills & technique.* St. Louis: Mosby Inc.

Taylor, C., Lillis, C., & LeMone, P. (2005). *Fundamentals of nursing.* Philadelphia: Lippincott, Williams & Wilkins.

Timby, B. K., & Smith, N. C. (2003). *Introductory medical-surgical nursing* (8th ed.). Philadelphia: J. B. Lippincott Williams & Wilkins.

7 Peptic Ulcer

Patient name: _____ **Admission:** _____

I. **The client/caregiver can describe anatomy and cause of a peptic ulcer.**

A. A peptic ulcer is a sore in the lining of the stomach or duodenum (the first part of the small intestine).
B. It is also called duodenal or gastric ulcer.
C. Causes of peptic ulcers
1. Acids that help digest foods can also damage the walls of the stomach or duodenum
2. Most commonly an infection with a bacterium called *Helicobacter pylori*
3. Long-term use of nonsteroidal anti-inflammatory medicines (NSAIDs), which includes prescription medicine and nonprescription NSAIDs such as aspirin, ibuprofen, and naproxen
4. Excessive alcohol consumption
5. Smoking

II. **The client/caregiver can list symptoms of a peptic ulcer.**

A. Burning stomach pain
B. Pain that may come and go for a few days or weeks
C. Pain that may be noticed more when stomach is empty
D. Pain that usually goes away after you eat
E. Pain that may be worse when under stress
F. Pain that may start after eating spicy foods

III. **The client/caregiver can list possible complications.**

A. Internal bleeding
B. Ulceration through the wall of stomach or small intestine
C. Peritonitis (serious infection in abdominal cavity)
D. The formation of scar tissue leading to stricture to the passage of food

IV. **The client/caregiver can list measures to treat and manage this condition.**

A. Medications that may be used in treatment are
1. Antibiotic medications are used to treat *Helicobacter pylori*.
2. Acid blockers reduce amount of acid.
3. Proton pump inhibitors reduce stomach acids.
4. Antacids can neutralize existing stomach acid and provide pain relief. They can also be taken with acid blockers. Cytoprotective agents help to protect stomach lining.
B. Abstain from smoking.
C. Limit or avoid alcohol.
D. Avoid spicy or acidic foods.
E. Control stress.
F. Review use of NSAIDs with physician.

RESOURCE
Dietician

REFERENCES
Ackley, B. J., & Ladwig, G. B. (2006). *Nursing diagnosis handbook: A guide to planning care*. St. Louis: Mosby Elsevier.

Cohen, B. J., & Taylor, J. J. (2005). *Memmler's the human body in health and disease* (10th ed.). Philadelphia: Lippincott Williams & Wilkins.

Lutz, C., & Przytulski, K. (2001). *Nutrition and diet therapy*. Philadelphia: F. A. Davis Company.

Perry, A., & Potter, P. (2006). *Clinical nursing skills & technique*. St. Louis: Mosby Inc.

Taylor, C., Lillis, C., & LeMone, P. (2005). *Fundamentals of nursing*. Philadelphia: Lippincott, Williams & Wilkins.

Timby, B. K., & Smith, N. C. (2003). *Introductory medical-surgical nursing* (8th ed.). Philadelphia: J. B. Lippincott Williams & Wilkins.

8 Inflammatory Bowel Diseases (Ulcerative Colitis/Crohn's)

Patient name: _____ Admission: _____

NRS
DATE INITIAL

I. The client/caregiver can explain the disease process of ulcerative colitis and Crohn's disease.

A. Both are inflammatory bowel diseases.
B. Both are chronic disorders.
C. The damage created in both diseases is the result of inflammation of the lining of the digestive tract.
D. When damaged, the intestine secretes large amounts of water and sodium. This results in the inability to absorb excess fluid and diarrhea occurs.
E. Crohn's disease can occur anywhere in the digestive tract. It causes damage deep in the layers of tissue.
F. Ulcerative colitis usually affects only the inner lining of the large intestine (colon) and rectum.

II. The client/caregiver can list risk factors for inflammatory bowel diseases.

A. Age—most likely to develop between ages of 15 and 35 years
B. Race
  1. Whites have the highest risk.
  2. Jewish or of European descent have four to five times the risk of Crohn's disease.
C. Family history of this disease
D. Where you live, as living in urban areas of an industrialized country or in Northern climates increases risk
E. Stress, which will increase the risk

III. The client/caregiver can list symptoms of inflammatory disease.

A. Diarrhea, ranging from looser or more frequent stools to dozens of bowel movements a day
B. Abdominal pain and cramping (in more severe cases, pain can be severe and accompany nausea and vomiting)
C. Blood in the stool

NRS
DATE INITIAL

D. Ulcers of the intestine that may progress and penetrate the intestinal wall
E. Reduced appetite and weight loss
F. Fever and fatigue

IV. The client/caregiver can list possible complications.

A. Obstruction of the bowel
B. Ulcers of digestive tract
C. Fistulas in the wall of digestive tract
D. Anal fissure
E. Malnutrition
F. Colon cancer
G. Crohn's disease can even cause other problems:
  • Arthritis
  • Inflammation of eyes or skin
  • Kidney stones
  • Gallstones
  • Osteoporosis
H. Depression and social isolation

V. The client/caregiver can lists measures to manage and cope with these diseases.

A. Diet—certain foods and beverages will aggravate symptoms.
  1. Limit dairy products (lactose diet in therapeutic diets).
  2. Try low-fat foods. Avoid butter, margarine, peanut butter, nuts, mayonnaise, avocados, cream, ice cream, fried foods, and chocolate and limit red meat.
  3. Experiment with amount of fiber in diet to evaluate tolerance. Try various ways to prepare fruits and vegetables. They may be better tolerated steamed, baked, or stewed. Problem foods may be cabbage, broccoli, cauliflower, apples, or carrots.
  4. Avoid other foods that make symptoms worse, such as citrus fruits, spicy food, popcorn, caffeine, and chocolate.

(Continued)

NRS
DATE INITIAL

5. Eat smaller, more frequent meals.
6. Drink plenty of fluids. Avoid alcohol, caffeine, or carbonated drinks.
7. Consult with physician regarding use of multivitamins.
8. Consult with dietician.

B. Avoid stress when possible. To help cope with stress, try some relaxation techniques, including the following:
   - Mild exercise
   - Biofeedback
   - Yoga or massage
   - Deep breathing and relaxation exercises
   - Set aside time each day for relaxing activity

C. Be informed about disease. Any situation is easier to handle when the facts are known.

D. Make contacts with support groups.

E. Seek health care professionals for information and emotional support.

RESOURCES

Crohn's and Colitis Foundation of America
www.ccfa.org
National Institutes of Health
www.nih.gov
American Dietetic Association
www.eatright.org

REFERENCES

Ackley, B. J., & Ladwig, G. B. (2006). *Nursing diagnosis handbook: A guide to planning care.* St. Louis: Mosby Elsevier.

Cohen, B. J., & Taylor, J. J. (2005). *Memmler's the human body in health and disease* (10th ed.). Philadelphia: Lippincott Williams & Wilkins.

Lutz, C., & Przytulski, K. (2001). *Nutrition and diet therapy.* Philadelphia: F. A. Davis Company.

Perry, A., & Potter, P. (2006). *Clinical nursing skills & technique.* St. Louis: Mosby Inc.

Taylor, C., Lillis, C., & LeMone, P. (2005). *Fundamentals of nursing.* Philadelphia: Lippincott, Williams & Wilkins.

Timby, B. K., & Smith, N. C. (2003). *Introductory medical-surgical nursing* (8th ed.). Philadelphia: J. B. Lippincott Williams & Wilkins.

9 | Gastroesophageal Reflux

Patient name: _____ Admission: _____

I. The client/caregiver can define gastro-esophageal reflux (GERD).

A. The esophagus carries food from the mouth to the stomach.
B. A ring of muscle at the bottom of the esophagus acts like a valve between the esophagus and stomach.
C. When that ring or sphincter does not close properly, stomach contents may leak back into the esophagus.
D. Stomach contents contain acid, and when they touch the lining of the esophagus, they create a burning sensation called heartburn.

II. The client/caregiver can list symptoms of GERD and explain when to seek medical attention.

A. Symptoms for adults with GERD are
   • Heartburn, which is the most common symptom (GERD can be present without this symptom)
   • Excessive clearing of the throat
   • Problems swallowing
   • Feeling that food is stuck in your throat
   • Burning in the mouth
   • Chest pain
B. Symptoms for children with GERD may be
   • Repeated vomiting
   • Coughing
   • Respiratory problems
   • Most babies will outgrow GERD by the age of 1 year
C. Reasons to consult with physician are
   • Heartburn or other symptoms more than twice a week
   • The use of antacids for more than 2 weeks

III. The client/caregiver can list methods of treatment and measures to manage this condition.

A. Medication ordered by physician
   1. Take medicine as ordered.
   2. Consult the physician if medication is not effective.
B. Lifestyle changes recommended by physician
   1. Do not consume alcohol.
   2. Do not smoke.
   3. Lose weight if necessary.
   4. Eat smaller, more frequent meals.
   5. Wear loose-fitting clothing.
   6. Avoid lying down for 3 hours after eating.
   7. Raise the head of bed 6 to 8 inches by placing blocks of wood under the bedposts.
   8. Use foam wedge to elevate head, but avoid pillows. Pillows create more pressure on stomach.
C. Nutritional recommendations are to avoid the following:
   • Chocolate
   • Drinks with caffeine or carbonation
   • Fatty and fried food
   • Garlic and onions
   • Mint flavorings
   • Spicy foods
   • Tomato-based foods such as chili and pizza

IV. The client/caregiver can list possible complications.

A. Prolonged irritation can result in bleeding, ulceration, or scar formation of the esophagus.
B. Development of Barrett's esophagus that over time can lead to cancer.
C. GERD can aggravate condition such as asthma, chronic cough, and pulmonary fibrosis.
D. There may be a need for surgical repair.

(Continued)

RESOURCES

Dietician

American College of Gastroenterology
www.acg.gi.org

North American Society for Pediatric Gastroenterology,
Hepatology, and Nutrition
www.naspghan.org

Pediatric/Adolescent Gastroesophageal Reflux
Association, Inc.
www.reflux.org

REFERENCES

Ackley, B. J., & Ladwig, G. B. (2006). *Nursing diagnosis handbook: A guide to planning care.* St. Louis: Mosby Elsevier.

Cohen, B. J., & Taylor, J. J. (2005). *Memmler's the human body in health and disease* (10th ed.). Philadelphia: Lippincott Williams & Wilkins.

Lutz, C., & Przytulski, K. (2001). *Nutrition and diet therapy.* Philadelphia: F. A. Davis Company.

Perry, A., & Potter, P. (2006). *Clinical nursing skills & technique.* St. Louis: Mosby Inc.

Taylor, C., Lillis, C., & LeMone, P. (2005). *Fundamentals of nursing.* Philadelphia: Lippincott, Williams & Wilkins.

Timby, B. K., & Smith, N. C. (2003). *Introductory medical-surgical nursing* (8th ed.). Philadelphia: J. B. Lippincott Williams & Wilkins.

1 Liver Cirrhosis

Patient name: _____ **Admission:** _____

NRS
DATE INITIAL

I.   The client/caregiver has a basic under-standing of the anatomy and physiology of the liver.

A. The liver is the largest organ of the body and is located in the upper right part of the abdominal cavity.

B. The liver has multiple functions:
1. It produces bile, which aids digestion in the intestines.
2. It stores vitamins A, D, E, K, and B12.
3. It stores glycogen, releasing it as glucose when needed.
4. It metabolizes fats, carbohydrates, and protein.
5. It metabolizes estrogens.
6. It is very important in the coagulation (blood clotting) process.
7. It destroys old, red blood cells and removes bacteria and foreign bodies from the blood stream.

II.   The client/caregiver can define cirrhosis.

A. It is the result of chronic liver disease that causes death of liver cells.

B. The death of cells is replaced by scar tissue and results in liver dysfunction.

III.   The client/caregiver is aware of causes of chronic liver disease.

A. Long-term alcohol abuse (primary cause)
B. Drug and substance abuse
C. A history of biliary obstruction and infection
D. Viral hepatitis infections
E. Exposure to chemical and industrial toxins
F. Metabolic disorders such as hemochromatosis and Wilson's disease

IV.   The client/caregiver can recognize signs and symptoms of cirrhosis.

A. Early symptoms
• Swelling of legs
• Vomiting blood

NRS
DATE INITIAL

• Confusion
• Jaundice (yellow tinted skin)
• Small red spider-like blood vessels on the skin
• Weakness and fatigue
• Weight loss
• Nausea and vomiting
• Impotence and loss of interest in sex
• Itching
• Ascites (swelling of abdomen)
• Bleeding hemorrhoids
• Decreased urine output
• Pale or clay colored stools
• Nose bleeds or bleeding gums
• General bleeding disorders
• Gynecomastia (breast development in males)

V.   The client/caregiver can list measures that prevent or manage cirrhosis.

A. Abstain from all alcohol.
B. Avoid over-the-counter drugs.
C. Plan regular rest periods to decrease demands of the body and increase blood supply to the liver.
D. Provide adequate skin care to protect from injury and to relieve itching.
1. Prevent trauma to skin with frequent position changes, pressure-relief devices, and so forth.
2. Follow good hygiene measures, using soap very sparingly.
3. Keep fingernails short to prevent irritation from scratching.
4. Take medications or treatment as ordered to decrease itching.
5. Use lotions to moisturize skin.
6. Keep the room temperature cool.
E. Assess for early signs of fluid retention
1. Weigh daily.
2. Measure abdominal girth.
F. Promote adequate nutrition
1. Eat small, frequent meals.
2. Eat foods that are high in calories and carbohydrates.

(Continued)

3. Eat foods that are low in fats and sodium (check the therapeutic diets chapter).
4. Proteins may be limited. Monitor ammonia levels.
5. Adjust texture of foods if mouth or esophagus bleeding.
6. Take vitamin supplements (especially B vitamins) as ordered.
7. Sodium and fluids may be restricted by physician to control edema.

G. Avoid contact with people who are ill to avoid infections and report any early signs of infection.

H. Report signs of bleeding and minimize possibility of trauma. Avoid forceful nose blowing, avoid straining at stool, use soft toothbrush, and so forth.

I. Report changes to physician such as any increased edema, fever, rapid weight loss, bleeding of any kind, confusion, personality change, and increased abdominal girth.

J. Take medications as prescribed and assess for side effects (decreased metabolism increases the risk for toxicity).

K. Keep follow-up appointments with the physician.

L. Use a Medic Alert bracelet or card.

VI. **The client/caregiver is aware of possible complications.**

A. Bleeding esophageal varices
B. Portal hypertension
C. Hepatic encephalopathy
D. Kidney failure
E. Ascites
F. Hepatic coma
G. Mental confusion
H. Liver cancer
I. Sepsis

RESOURCES

American Liver Foundation
www.liverfoundation.org

Hepatitis B Foundation
www.hepb.org

Alcoholics Anonymous
www.alcoholics-anonymous.org/

Narcotics Anonymous
www.na.org/

Community support groups

Mental health counseling

REFERENCES

Ackley, B. J., & Ladwig, G. B. (2006). *Nursing diagnosis handbook: A guide to planning care.* St. Louis: Mosby Inc.

Cohen, B. J., & Taylor, J. J. (2005). *Memmler's the human body in health and disease* (10th ed.). Philadelphia: Lippincott Williams & Wilkins.

Lutz, C., & Przytulski, K. (2001). *Nutrition and diet therapy.* Philadelphia: F. A. Davis Company.

Nutrition made incredibly easy. (2003). Philadelphia: Lippincott Williams & Wilkins.

Perry, A., & Potter, P. (2006). *Clinical nursing skills & technique.* St. Louis: Mosby Inc.

Taylor, C., Lillis, C., & LeMone, P. (2005). *Fundamentals of nursing.* Philadelphia: Lippincott, Williams & Wilkins.

Timby, B. K., & Smith, N. C. (2003). *Introductory medical-surgical nursing* (8th ed.). Philadelphia: J. B. Lippincott Williams & Wilkins.

2 Hepatitis

Patient name: _____ Admission: _____

I. **The client/caregiver will be able to define hepatitis and the types of hepatitis.**

   A. Hepatitis is an inflammation of the liver that can result in malfunction and liver damage. It can be acute or chronic.
   B. The most common cause of hepatitis is a viral infection. Forms of viral hepatitis are
   - Hepatitis A (infectious hepatitis or HAV)
   - Hepatitis B (serum hepatitis or HBV)
   - Hepatitis C (HCV)
   - Hepatitis D (HDV)
   - Hepatitis E (HEV)
   C. Forms of non viral hepatitis are
   - Toxic hepatitis—develops after exposure to chemicals toxic to the liver.
   - Drug induced hepatitis—develops as a result of drug reaction.

II. **The client/caregiver can describe mode of transmission for each form of hepatitis.**

   A. Hepatitis A (incubation period of 3 to 5 weeks) is transmitted by
      1. Oral route from feces (stool) and saliva of infected person
      2. Contaminated water, food, and equipment
   B. Hepatitis B (incubation period of 2 to 5 months) is transmitted by
      1. Infected blood products, needles, and dental and surgical equipment
      2. Sexually through vagina secretions and semen of carriers or with active infection
   C. Hepatitis C (incubation period of 2 to 20 weeks) is transmitted by
      1. Infected blood or blood products
      2. Sexual contact
   D. Hepatitis D (incubation period of 2 to 5 months) is transmitted by
      1. The same way as hepatitis B and occurs as dual infection but not alone
   E. Hepatitis E (incubation period is 2–9 weeks) is transmitted by
      1. Fecal (stool) to oral method. There is a low risk of person-to-person contact but can be severe in pregnant women.

III. **The client/caregiver can recognize signs and symptoms of hepatitis.**

   A. Signs and symptoms are divided into three phases of hepatitis: preicteric, icteric, and posticteric.
   B. The preicteric phase has the following symptoms:
   - Nausea and vomiting
   - A loss of appetite and weight loss
   - Fever
   - Complaints of tiredness
   - Headaches and joint pain
   - Discomfort in the right upper quadrant of abdomen
   - Enlargement of the spleen, liver, and lymph nodes
   - Rash and urticaria (itching of skin)
   C. The icteric phase has the additional symptoms:
   - Jaundice (yellowing tint to skin and eyes)
   - Pruritus
   - Clay- or light-colored stools
   - Dark urine
   D. The posticteric phase has the following symptoms:
   - Ending of previous symptoms
   - Liver enlargement
   - Continued fatigue

IV. **The client/caregiver can list measures to prevent hepatitis infections.**

   A. Receive vaccinations against hepatitis A, B, and E.
   B. Perform thorough handwashing techniques, especially after using toilet.
   C. Perform good personal and environmental hygiene.
   D. Obtain adequate rest and eat well-balanced diet.
   E. Use safe sex practices.
   F. Report any known exposure. You may receive immune globulin.
   G. Use standard precautions:
      1. Wear gloves if hands come in contact with body fluids.

(Continued)

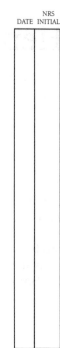

2. Wear gown and face shield if body fluids may be splashed.

H. Do not share razors, toothbrushes, or needles.

I. Use household bleach solution (10 parts water to one part bleach) to clean any surface contaminated with blood or feces (stool).

J. Avoid drinking or using any potentially contaminated water.

K. Screen food handlers. Screen public salad bars for presence of sneeze guards and hygienic devices and practices to prevent contamination.

L. Require child care providers to wear gloves during diaper changes and to use routine hand washing.

M. Do not share cigarettes, eating utensils, or beverage containers.

N. Use liquid soap dispensers and electric hand dryers in public restrooms.

O. Avoid placing fingers or hand held objects in mouth.

P. Avoid eating raw seafood.

V. **The client/caregiver is aware of measures to manage hepatitis.**

A. Assess and report any signs of bleeding, confusion, edema, lethargy, and weight changes.

B. Decrease itching.
  1. Take medications or apply lotions as prescribed.
  2. Take cool showers and avoid high temperatures.
  3. Keep fingernails short to prevent skin irritation if scratching.
  4. Wear cotton, loose-fitting clothing.

C. Provide general comfort measures.
  1. Quiet environment
  2. Good mouth care
  3. Good hygiene

D. Provide adequate nutrition.
  1. Offer small, frequent meals. Because of lack of appetite, try to offer foods that appeal to client and use some fat (in moderation) to make food appealing to the taste.
  2. Offer high-calorie, high-protein nutritious foods. Check with physician regarding protein content. High levels of ammonia can indicate a need to restrict protein intake.

3. Increase fluids to two liters per day unless contraindicated.
4. Weigh daily, weekly, or as ordered.
5. Avoid alcohol.

E. Rest as ordered. Avoid heavy lifting.

F. Use an electric razor and soft-bristled toothbrush to prevent bleeding.

G. Avoid alcohol and drugs that may cause further damage to liver.

H. Avoid over-the-counter medications unless recommended by physician, especially aspirin and aspirin products.

I. Keep follow-up appointments with physician and laboratory.

VI. **The client/caregiver is aware of possible complications.**

A. Need for liver transplant
B. Liver cirrhosis
C. Hepatitis coma and death

RESOURCES

Centers for Disease Control and Prevention
www.cdc.gov/ncidod/diseases/hepatitis/index.htm

Dietician

Community support groups

REFERENCES

Ackley, B. J., & Ladwig, G. B. (2006). *Nursing diagnosis handbook: A guide to planning care.* St. Louis: Mosby Inc.

Cohen, B. J., & Taylor, J. J. (2005). *Memmler's the human body in health and disease* (10th ed.). Philadelphia: Lippincott Williams & Wilkins.

Lutz, C., & Przytulski, K. (2001). *Nutrition and diet therapy.* Philadelphia: F. A. Davis Company.

Nutrition made incredibly easy. (2003). Philadelphia: Lippincott Williams & Wilkins.

Perry, A., & Potter, P. (2006). *Clinical nursing skills & technique.* St. Louis: Mosby Inc.

Taylor, C., Lillis, C., & LeMone, P. (2005). *Fundamentals of nursing.* Philadelphia: Lippincott, Williams & Wilkins.

Timby, B. K., & Smith, N. C. (2003). *Introductory medical-surgical nursing* (8th ed.). Philadelphia: J. B. Lippincott Williams & Wilkins.

Gallbladder and Gallbladder Diseases

3

Patient name: _____

Admission: _____

DATE | NRS INITIAL

I. The client/caregiver can define function of gallbladder and biliary system.

A. It is a muscular sac located under the liver.
B. It stores and concentrates the bile produced in the liver.
C. It has excess bile that is not immediately needed for digestion.
D. The bile is released into the small intestine in response to food.
E. The cystic duct drains the gallbladder. The common bile duct drains into the duodenum. These two ducts form the biliary system.

II. The client/caregiver can define diseases of the gallbladder.

A. Gallstones are formed in the gallbladder.
B. They are made up of water, salts, lecithin, cholesterol, and other substances.
C. They can be of various sizes, ranging from sand size particles to larger than 8 mm.
D. Biliary colic is when a stone is blocking the opening from the gallbladder.
E. If the stone blocks the cystic duct for a period of time, acute cholecystitis will occur.
F. If the blockage persists, bacteria can grow, resulting in cholangitis.
G. Stones that block the lower end of common bile duct may obstruct secretion from the pancreas and produce pancreatitis.

III. The client/caregiver can describe signs and symptoms of gallbladder disease.

A. Abdominal pain that
   • Is in the right upper abdomen or the middle of the upper abdomen
   • May be recurrent
   • May be sharp, cramping, or dull

DATE | NRS INITIAL

   • May radiate to the back or below the right should blade
   • May be made worse by eating fatty or greasy foods
   • Can occur within minutes of a meal
B. Jaundice
C. Fever
D. Clay-colored stools
E. Nausea and vomiting
F. Heartburn
G. Excess gas
H. Abdominal fullness

IV. The client/caregiver can list teaching needs for clients with gallbladder disease.

A. Nutrition instructions should include the following:
   1. Understand and follow diet as prescribed. High-fiber and low-fat diets are often recommended (check therapeutic diet chapter).
   2. Eat small, more frequent meals to prevent attacks.
   3. Replacement of water-soluble vitamins (vitamin A, D, E, and K) can sometimes be ordered by physician.
B. When to contact physician
   • Severe pain
   • Jaundice
   • Fever
   • Changes in color of stool or urine
C. Take medication as prescribed. Types of medication might include the following:
   1. Pain medication
   2. Medication to relax smooth muscles and spasm of gallbladder
   3. Medication to reduce nausea and vomiting
D. A follow-up appointment with physician and/or surgeon is given at time of discharge.

(Continued)

RESOURCE
Dietician

REFERENCES
Ackley, B. J., & Ladwig, G. B. (2006). *Nursing diagnosis handbook: A guide to planning care.* St. Louis: Mosby Inc.

Cohen, B. J., & Taylor, J. J. (2005). *Memmler's the human body in health and disease* (10th ed.). Philadelphia: Lippincott Williams & Wilkins.

Lutz, C., & Przytulski, K. (2001). *Nutrition and diet therapy.* Philadelphia: F. A. Davis Company.

Nutrition made incredibly easy. (2003). Philadelphia: Lippincott Williams & Wilkins.

Perry, A., & Potter, P. (2006). *Clinical nursing skills & technique.* St. Louis: Mosby Inc.

Taylor, C., Lillis, C., & LeMone, P. (2005). *Fundamentals of nursing.* Philadelphia: Lippincott, Williams & Wilkins.

Timby, B. K., & Smith, N. C. (2003). *Introductory medical-surgical nursing* (8th ed.). Philadelphia: J. B. Lippincott Williams & Wilkins.

Acute Renal Failure

1

Patient name: _____ **Admission:** _____

NRS
DATE INITIAL

NRS
DATE INITIAL

I. **The client/caregiver has a basic understanding of the anatomy and physiology of the renal system.**

A. The kidneys are two bean-shaped organs and are located on each side of the vertebral column at the 12th thoracic vertebrae at the posterior abdominal wall.

B. Each kidney has a ureter about 25 to 30 centimeters long that connects to the bladder.

C. The function of the kidneys is to remove waste materials from blood, balance body fluids, and form urine.

II. **The client/caregiver can define acute renal failure.**

A. Acute renal failure is the sudden inability of kidneys to remove metabolic waste and concentrate urine without losing electrolytes.

B. Renal cells are damaged by decreased renal blood flow and a lack of oxygen and other nutrients to the cells.

III. **The client/caregiver can list factors that may increase risk of renal failure.**

A. Low blood pressure caused by trauma, surgery, serious illness, septic shock, hemorrhagic shock, burns, or dehydration

B. Acute pyelonephritis or septicemia

C. Urinary tract obstruction

D. Blood transfusion reaction

E. Autoimmune kidney disease

IV. **The client/caregiver can recognize signs and symptoms.**

A. Nausea and vomiting

B. Urinary system changes
   • A decrease in the amount of urine
   • No urination
   • Excessive urination at night

C. Changes in mental status or mood
   • Drowsiness or lethargy
   • Agitation

   • Delirium or confusion
   • Coma
   • Mood changes
   • Trouble paying attention
   • Hallucinations

D. Generalized swelling and fluid retention

E. Flank pain between ribs and hips

F. Headache

G. Decreased sensation in hands and feet

H. Decreased appetite and metallic taste in mouth

I. Slow, sluggish movements, hand tremor, or seizures

J. Itchiness

K. Bruising and prolonged bleeding (nosebleeds, blood in stool)

V. **The client/caregiver can list measures to manage acute renal failure.**

A. Follow prescribed diet closely.
   • High in carbohydrates
   • Low in protein
   • Low in sodium
   • Low in potassium

B. Monitor fluid status closely.
   • Weigh daily using the same scale at the same time each day.
   • Measure intake and output.
   • Restrict fluids as instructed.

C. Take medication as ordered (possible use of antibiotics and/or diuretic).

D. Avoid infections, or get prompt treatment of infection.

E. Follow activity as ordered with regular rest periods.

F. Provide skin care and oral hygiene:
   1. Keep fingernails short and avoid scratching.
   2. Use lotions to moisturize skin and decrease itchiness.
   3. Use a soft-bristled toothbrush and mouthwash.

(Continued)

NRS
DATE INITIAL

    G. Keep follow-up appointments with physician and laboratory tests.

    H. Use Medic Alert card and bracelet.

VI. **The client/caregiver can list possible complications.**

    A. Fluid and electrolyte imbalance

    B. Chronic renal disease

    C. Anemia (loss of blood in the intestines)

    D. End-stage renal disease

    E. Damage to heart or nervous system

    F. Hypertension

    G. Need for dialysis

RESOURCES

National Kidney Foundation
www.kidney.org

National Kidney and Urologic Diseases Information Clearinghouse
http://kidney.niddk.nih.gov/about/index.htm

Support groups

REFERENCES

Ackley, B. J., & Ladwig, G. B. (2006). *Nursing diagnosis handbook: A guide to planning care.* St. Louis: Mosby Elsevier.

Cohen, B. J., & Taylor, J. J. (2005). *Memmler's the human body in health and disease* (10th ed.). Philadelphia: Lippincott Williams & Wilkins.

Lutz, C., & Przytulski, K. (2001). *Nutrition and diet therapy.* Philadelphia: F. A. Davis Company.

Perry, A., & Potter, P. (2006). *Clinical nursing skills & technique.* St. Louis: Mosby Inc.

Portable RN: The all-in-one nursing reference. (2002). Springhouse: Lippincott, Williams & Wilkins.

Timby, B. K., & Smith, N. C. (2003). *Introductory medical-surgical nursing* (8th ed.). Philadelphia: J. B. Lippincott Williams & Wilkins.

2

Chronic Renal Failure

Patient name: _____

Admission: _____

NRS
DATE INITIAL

NRS
DATE INITIAL

I. **The client/caregiver has a basic understanding of the anatomy and physiology of the renal system.**

   A. The kidneys are two bean-shaped organs. They are located on each side of the vertebral column at the 12th thoracic vertebrae at the posterior abdominal wall.

   B. Each kidney has a ureter about 25 to 30 centimeters long that connects to the bladder.

   C. The function of the kidneys is to remove waste materials from blood, balance body fluids, and form urine.

II. **The client/caregiver can define chronic renal failure.**

   A. It is the irreversible deterioration of renal function.

   B. Symptoms may occur very rapidly or very slowly over years.

   C. Uremia, an excess of urea and other nitrogenous wastes, occurs.

   D. Progression may continue to end-stage renal disease.

III. **The client/caregiver can list factors that increase risk of chronic renal failure.**

   A. Obstruction of the urinary tract

   B. Toxic agents

   C. Uncontrolled high blood pressure

   D. Diabetes mellitus

   E. Kidney diseases

   F. Recurrent infections

IV. **The client/caregiver can recognize signs and symptoms of chronic renal failure.**

   A. Initial symptoms of chronic renal failure are
- Loss of appetite
- Unintentional loss of weight
- Fatigue, apathy, and weakness
- Nausea or vomiting
- Frequent hiccups
- Generalized itching

   B. Later symptoms may include
- Increased or decreased urine output
- Easy bruising or prolonged bleeding
- Decreased alertness, confusion, and coma
- Muscle twitching or cramps
- Seizures
- Decreased sensation in hands and feet
- Uremic frost (deposits of white crystal in and on the skin)

   C. Late symptoms may be
- Excessive nighttime urination
- Excessive thirst
- Abnormally dark skin or paleness
- Nail abnormalities
- Breath odor
- High blood pressure
- Loss of appetite
- Agitation

V. **The client/caregiver can list measures to manage chronic renal failure.**

   A. Follow prescribed diet closely
- High in carbohydrates
- Low in protein
- Low in sodium
- Low in potassium

   B. Take vitamin and mineral supplements as ordered.

   C. Avoid infections or obtain prompt treatment for infections.

   D. Follow activity as instructed, with frequent rest periods.

   E. Avoid stress, which can aggravate symptoms.

   F. Monitor blood pressure closely.

   G. Monitor fluid status closely.
     1. Weigh daily (same time, same scale, and same amount of clothing).
     2. Measure intake and output.
     3. Restrict fluids as instructed.

   H. Provide skin care and oral hygiene.
     1. Keep fingernails short and avoid scratching.
     2. Use lotions to moisturize skin and decrease itchiness.

(Continued)

3. Use soft-bristled toothbrush and mouthwash.
4. Use medications and ointments as ordered to decrease itchiness.
5. Obtain regular dental checkups.

I. Prevent constipation with regular exercise and increased fiber.
J. Keep follow-up appointments with physician and for laboratory tests.
K. Take medications as ordered.
L. Monitor and report to physician signs of bleeding, mental status changes, edema, elevated blood pressure, loss of appetite, weight loss or rapid weight gain, and skin breakdown.
M. Wear Medic Alert bracelet.

VI. **The client/caregiver can list possible complications.**

A. End-stage renal disease
B. Congestive heart failure
C. Hypertension
D. A loss of blood from the gastrointestinal tract
E. Hemorrhage
F. Increased incidence of infection
G. Hepatitis B, hepatitis C, liver failure
H. Seizures
I. Dementia
J. Fractures and joint disorders
K. Changes in glucose metabolism
L. Electrolyte imbalance

M. Decreased libido, impotence
N. Menstrual problems and infertility
O. Dry, itchy skin with probable skin infections

RESOURCES

National Kidney Foundation
www.kidney.org

National Kidney and Urologic Diseases Information Clearinghouse
http://kidney.niddk.nih.gov/about/index.htm

Support groups

REFERENCES

Ackley, B. J., & Ladwig, G. B. (2006). *Nursing diagnosis handbook: A guide to planning care.* St. Louis: Mosby Elsevier.
Cohen, B. J., & Taylor, J. J. (2005). *Memmler's the human body in health and disease* (10th ed.). Philadelphia: Lippincott Williams & Wilkins.
Lutz, C., & Przytulski, K. (2001). *Nutrition and diet therapy.* Philadelphia: F. A. Davis Company.
Perry, A., & Potter, P. (2006). *Clinical nursing skills & technique.* St. Louis: Mosby Inc.
Portable RN: The all-in-one nursing reference. (2002). Springhouse: Lippincott, Williams & Wilkins.
Timby, B. K., & Smith, N. C. (2003). *Introductory medical-surgical nursing* (8th ed.). Philadelphia: J. B. Lippincott Williams & Wilkins.

3 Pyelonephritis

Patient name: _____   **Admission:** _____

NRS
DATE INITIAL

I. **The client/caregiver can define pyelonephritis.**

   A. It is the inflammation of kidney tissue and may be acute or chronic.
   B. Chronic pyelonephritis may destroy kidney tissue permanently.
   C. It is caused by bacterial infection of the lower urinary tract.

II. **The client/caregiver can list factors that may increase risk of pyelonephritis.**

   A. Pregnancy
   B. Testing or surgery of urinary tract or use of catheters to drain urine
   C. Trauma to the kidney
   D. Urinary stasis or back flow
   E. Bladder infections
   F. Conditions such as prostate enlargement, structural defects of ureters, or kidney stones
   G. Neurogenic bladder
   H. Chronic health problems (diabetes, kidney disease, etc.)

III. **The client/caregiver can recognize signs and symptoms.**

   A. Back, side, or groin pain
   B. Nausea or vomiting
   C. Fatigue
   D. Pain or burning on urination
   E. Urgent, frequent urination
   F. A loss of appetite
   G. Cloudy, foul-smelling urine
   H. Fever
   I. Decreased urine output
   J. Pus or blood in urine

NRS
DATE INITIAL

IV. **The client/caregiver can list measures to prevent or control pyelonephritis.**

   A. Females should follow practices to prevent urinary tract infections.
      1. Keep perineal area clean and dry.
      2. Wear cotton underpants and wear nonrestrictive clothing.
      3. Wipe from front to back after bowel movement.
      4. Urinate before and after sexual intercourse.
   B. Report early symptoms of urinary tract infection for early treatment (burning, frequency, cloudy urine, fever, and flank pain).
   C. Drink fluids, up to 3000 ml per day.
   D. Avoid caffeinated beverages and alcohol.
   E. Empty bladder routinely avoiding bladder distention.
   F. Use self-monitoring urine test for bacteria.
   G. Take antibiotics until completed.
   H. Consume acid-forming foods (such as meat, fish, poultry, eggs, grains, cranberries, prunes, and plum) to prevent stone formation.
   I. Keep follow-up physician and laboratory appointments.

V. **The client/caregiver is aware of possible complications.**

   A. Chronic pyelonephritis
   B. Scarring of the kidneys
   C. Hypertension
   D. General bacterial infection (shock or sepsis)

(Continued)

RESOURCES

American Foundation for Urologic Disease
www.afud.org

National Kidney and Urologic Diseases Information
  Clearinghouse
E-mail: nkudic@info.niddk.nih.gov

REFERENCES

Ackley, B. J., & Ladwig, G. B. (2006). *Nursing diagnosis
  handbook: A guide to planning care.* St. Louis: Mosby Elsevier.

Cohen, B. J., & Taylor, J. J. (2005). *Memmler's the human body
  in health and disease* (10th ed.). Philadelphia: Lippincott
  Williams & Wilkins.

Lutz, C., & Przytulski, K. (2001). *Nutrition and diet therapy.*
  Philadelphia: F. A. Davis Company.

Perry, A., & Potter, P. (2006). *Clinical nursing skills & technique.*
  St. Louis: Mosby Inc.

Portable RN: The all-in-one nursing reference. (2002).
  Springhouse: Lippincott, Williams & Wilkins.

Timby, B. K., & Smith, N. C. (2003). *Introductory medical-
  surgical nursing* (8th ed.). Philadelphia: J. B. Lippincott
  Williams & Wilkins.

4 Urinary Calculi (Renal Calculi)

Patient name: _____   Admission: _____

NRS
DATE INITIAL

I. The client/caregiver can define urinary calculi.

A. Calculi or a kidney stone is a solid mass consisting of a collection of tiny crystals.
B. They can be in the kidney or ureter.
C. Various types of stones include calcium oxide, magnesium-ammonium, uric acid, cystine, and mixed.

II. The client/caregiver can list factors that increase risk of urinary calculi.

A. Familial tendency
B. Dehydration
C. Diet rich in calcium, oxalates, or uric acid
D. Sedentary lifestyles or prolonged immobility
E. Repeated urinary infections
F. Osteoporosis
G. Metabolic disorders (gout)

III. The client/caregiver can recognize signs and symptoms of urinary calculi.

A. Fever and chills
B. Nausea and vomiting
C. Blood in the urine
D. Flank pain or back pain
   • On one or both sides
   • Progressive
   • Severe
   • Spasm-like
   • May radiate or move to pelvic, groin, or genitals
E. Restlessness
F. Cloudy urine with sediment
G. Decreased urine output

IV. The client/caregiver can list measures to prevent or control urinary calculi.

A. Nutritional recommendations are to restrict the following foods to small amounts if stones are composed of calcium oxalate.
   • Apples   • Asparagus
   • Beer   • Beets
   • Berries   • Black pepper

NRS
DATE INITIAL

   • Broccoli   • Cheese
   • Chocolate   • Cocoa
   • Coffee   • Cola
   • Collards   • Figs
   • Grapes   • Ice cream
   • Milk   • Oranges
   • Parsley   • Peanut butter
   • Pineapples   • Rhubarb
   • Spinach   • Swiss chard
   • Tea   • Turnips
   • Vitamin C   • Yogurt

B. If kidney stones are composed of uric acid, then a low-purine diet is recommended. The following list shows foods to use in small amounts.
   • Organ meats   • Anchovies
   • Consommé   • Gravies
   • Lentils   • Whole-grain cereals
   • Beans   • Peas
   • Asparagus   • Cauliflower
   • Mushrooms   • Spinach
   • Butter   • Cola
   • Yeast

C. Increase fluids (water is best) to at least 2.5 quarts per day.
D. Increase activity to decrease urinary stasis:
   1. Use active or passive range of motion exercises.
   2. Change positions frequently.
E. Strain all urine to secure a stone if it passes.
F. Take pain medications as ordered.
G. Take the full course of antibiotics.
H. Consult physician before taking any over-the-counter medications.
I. Avoid alcohol.
J. Urine cultures should be taken periodically as a follow-up to detect any recurrent infections.
K. Report to physician signs of restlessness, flank pain, decreased urine output, and fever, or go to the emergency room if the pain is severe.
L. Keep follow-up appointments with physician.

(Continued)

| NRS |
| DATE | INITIAL |

V. **The client/caregiver is aware of possible complications.**

  A. Urinary tract infection
  B. Urinary obstruction
  C. Renal failure
  D. Pyelonephritis
  E. Kidney damage and scarring

RESOURCES

American Foundation for Urologic Disease
www.afud.org

National Kidney and Urologic Diseases Information
  Clearinghouse
E-mail: nkudic@info.niddk.nih.gov

REFERENCES

Ackley, B. J., & Ladwig, G. B. (2006). *Nursing diagnosis handbook: A guide to planning care.* St. Louis: Mosby Elsevier.

Cohen, B. J., & Taylor, J. J. (2005). *Memmler's the human body in health and disease* (10th ed.). Philadelphia: Lippincott Williams & Wilkins.

Lutz, C., & Przytulski, K. (2001). *Nutrition and diet therapy.* Philadelphia: F. A. Davis Company.

Perry, A., & Potter, P. (2006). *Clinical nursing skills & technique.* St. Louis: Mosby Inc.

Portable RN: The all-in-one nursing reference. (2002). Springhouse: Lippincott, Williams & Wilkins.

Timby, B. K., & Smith, N. C. (2003). *Introductory medical-surgical nursing* (8th ed.). Philadelphia: J. B. Lippincott Williams & Wilkins.

5 Urinary Tract Infection (Cystitis) (Lower Urinary Tract Infection)

Patient name: _____   Admission: _____

NRS DATE INITIAL		

I. The client/caregiver can define urinary tract infection or cystitis.

A. It is an infection of the bladder or urethra frequently caused by bacteria.
B. It is more common in women than men.
C. It can become a chronic problem.

II. The client/caregiver can list factors that increase risk of cystitis.

A. Females
B. Advancing age
C. Obstruction (enlarged prostate, calculi, etc.)
D. Pregnancy
E. Poor personal hygiene
F. Use of catheters
G. Sexual intercourse

III. The client/caregiver can recognize signs and symptoms, although no symptoms may be present.

A. Burning sensation when urinating
B. Strong, persistent urge to urinate
C. Passing frequent, small amounts of urine
D. Low back pain or feeling of pressure in lower abdomen
E. Cloudy or strong-smelling urine
F. Fever

IV. The client/caregiver can list measures to prevent or manage urinary tract infections.

A. Void frequently to empty bladder completely.
B. Always wipe from front to back.
C. Wear cotton underpants and nonrestrictive clothing.
D. Urinate before and after sexual intercourse.
E. Avoid use of feminine sprays and bubble baths.
F. Keep perineal area very clean.
G. Avoid delaying the urge to urinate.
H. Drink fluid intake of 2 to 3 liters per day if not contraindicated.

NRS DATE INITIAL		

I. Eat a well-balanced diet.
   1. Avoid coffee, alcohol, and soft drinks with caffeine, citrus juices, and spicy foods until infection has cleared.
   2. Physician may recommend the use of vitamin C supplements.
   3. Studies have shown cranberry juice to inhibit growth of *E. coli*. Check with physician before using cranberry juice. Cranberry juice may have a negative interaction with the medication Coumadin.
J. Take antibiotics until completed.
K. Report early signs and symptoms of infection to the physician.
L. Take medications as instructed.
M. Shower instead of bathing to decrease possibility of bacteria entrance.
N. Exercise regularly to prevent urinary stasis.
O. Keep follow-up appointments with physician and laboratory.

V. The client/caregiver is aware of possible complications.

A. Recurrent infections
B. Infections of kidney or ureters

REFERENCES

Ackley, B. J., & Ladwig, G. B. (2006). *Nursing diagnosis handbook: A guide to planning care*. St. Louis: Mosby Elsevier.

Cohen, B. J., & Taylor, J. J. (2005). *Memmler's the human body in health and disease* (10th ed.). Philadelphia: Lippincott Williams & Wilkins.

Lutz, C., & Przytulski, K. (2001). *Nutrition and diet therapy*. Philadelphia: F. A. Davis Company.

Perry, A., & Potter, P. (2006). *Clinical nursing skills & technique*. St. Louis: Mosby Inc.

Portable RN: The all-in-one nursing reference. (2002). Springhouse: Lippincott, Williams & Wilkins.

Timby, B. K., & Smith, N. C. (2003). *Introductory medical-surgical nursing* (8th ed.). Philadelphia: J. B. Lippincott Williams & Wilkins.

6   Bladder Control Problems

Patient name: _____   **Admission:** _____

NRS
DATE INITIAL

I.   **The client/caregiver can define types of bladder control caused by nerve damage.**

   A.   Nerves carry signals from the brain to the bladder and sphincter. Damage can cause bladder control problems.
   B.   Overactive bladder
      •   Urinary frequency—eight or more times a day
      •   Urinary urgency—sudden, strong need to urinate immediately
      •   Urge incontinence—leakage of urine that follows a sudden urge
   C.   Poor control of sphincter muscles—may allow leakage of urine
   D.   Urine retention—bladder does not receive message to empty

II.   **The client/caregiver can list causes of this type of nerve damage.**

   A.   Vaginal childbirth
   B.   Diabetes
   C.   Stroke
   D.   Infections of the brain or spinal cord
   E.   Trauma or injury to the brain or spinal cord
   F.   Multiple sclerosis
   G.   Heavy metal poisoning

III.   **The client/caregiver can list measures to manage urinary control problems.**

   A.   Do bladder training (Chapter 23).
   B.   Do Kegel exercises (Chapter 23).
   C.   Use barrier garments or external collection devices (condom catheter).
   D.   Assess for skin breakdown or irritation.
   E.   Control odors by
      1.   Frequent cleansing of the perineum
      2.   Changing to clean clothes
      3.   Room deodorizer
   F.   Avoid using perfume or scented powders, lotions, or sprays.
   G.   Keep a record of fluid intake. Drink plenty of fluids during morning and early afternoon. Decrease fluid intake during evening.
   H.   Contact the physician if any of the following occurs:
      •   Rash around the perineal area
      •   Pain in lower abdomen
      •   Fever or chills
      •   Cloudy urine

NRS
DATE INITIAL

IV.   **The client/caregiver can list possible complications.**

   A.   Rashes, skin infections, or sores
   B.   Urinary tract infections
   C.   Sleep problems
   D.   Less social and sexual activity
   E.   A loss of self-esteem
   F.   Depression

RESOURCE

National Association for Continence
800-BLADDER (252-3337) or 843-377-0900
E-mail: memberservices@nafc.org
www.nafc.org

REFERENCES

Ackley, B. J., & Ladwig, G. B. (2006). *Nursing diagnosis handbook: A guide to planning care*. St. Louis: Mosby Elsevier.

Cohen, B. J., & Taylor, J. J. (2005). *Memmler's the human body in health and disease* (10th ed.). Philadelphia: Lippincott Williams & Wilkins.

Lutz, C., & Przytulski, K. (2001). *Nutrition and diet therapy*. Philadelphia: F. A. Davis Company.

Perry, A., & Potter, P. (2006). *Clinical nursing skills & technique*. St. Louis: Mosby Inc.

Portable RN: The all-in-one nursing reference. (2002). Springhouse: Lippincott, Williams & Wilkins.

Timby, B. K., & Smith, N. C. (2003). *Introductory medical-surgical nursing* (8th ed.). Philadelphia: J. B. Lippincott Williams & Wilkins.

1 Anemia

Patient name: _____ Admission: _____

DATE | NRS INITIAL

I. The client/caregiver can define iron-deficiency anemia.

A. Anemia is a disorder in which there is an abnormally low amount of hemoglobin or red cells. It can be caused by
- Excessive loss of red blood cells
- Destruction of red blood cells
- Impaired production of red blood cells or hemoglobin

B. Hemoglobin is essential for carrying oxygen to the cells.

II. The client/caregiver can list factors that may increase the risk of anemia.

A. Excessive loss of red blood cells
- Loss that can be acute or chronic
- Gastrointestinal blood loss
- Excessive menstrual flow
- Trauma resulting in hemorrhage

B. Destruction of red blood cells
- Overactive spleen
- Infections
- Sickle cell anemia

C. Impaired production of red blood cells
- Nutritional deficiencies (iron-deficiency anemia, pernicious anemia [deficiency of vitamin B12], folic acid-deficiency anemia)
- Intestine disorders that interfere with absorption of water-soluble vitamins
- Alcoholism
- Suppression of bone marrow (aplastic anemia)
- Rapid growth stage in infants and children
- Pregnancy

III. The client/caregiver can list high-risk populations.

A. Women of child-bearing age who have blood loss through menstruation
B. Pregnant or lactating women who have an increased requirement for iron
C. Infants, children, and adolescents in rapid growth phases
D. People with poor dietary intake of iron

IV. The client/caregiver can recognize signs and symptoms of iron deficiency anemia (mild cases usually have no symptoms).

A. Fatigue, weakness, and sometimes dizziness
B. Frontal headache
C. Palpitations
D. Paleness of skin
E. Inflammation and soreness of mouth and tongue
F. Increased sensitivity to cold
G. Brittle fingernails and hair
H. Shortness of breath
I. Chest pain and/or rapid heart rate
J. Decreased concentration
K. Menstrual irregularities
L. Unusual food cravings (pica)
M. Irritability
N. Decreased appetite (more in children)
O. Blue tinge to sclerae (whites of eyes)

V. The client/caregiver can list measures to prevent or control iron deficiency.

A. Eat a well-balanced diet, which is from all food groups.
B. Eat foods that are rich in iron.
- Red meats and liver are the best source of iron.
- Vegetables, whole grains, raisins, egg yolk, fish, poultry, peas, beans, and blackstrap molasses are other good sources of iron.
- Read labels in search of iron-enriched foods.
C. Take iron supplements as ordered by physician.
D. Milk and antacids may interfere with absorption of iron.
E. Include foods high in vitamin C (helps with absorption of iron), such as
- Citrus fruits and juices, strawberries, cantaloupe
- Green peppers, tomatoes, broccoli, leafy green vegetables
F. Plan frequent rest periods.

(Continued)

NRS
DATE INITIAL

G. Avoid exposure to respiratory infections.
H. Use good hand washing and personal hygiene.
I. Obtain prompt treatment for infections.
J. Have stools checked for occult blood.
K. Keep follow-up appointments with physician and laboratory tests. Continue prescribed medications.
L. Perform good oral hygiene.
M. Follow safety precautions to prevent falls/injuries because of possible dizziness.
   1. Have assistance with ambulation.
   2. Change positions slowly.
N. Provide good skin care because of poor wound healing.

VI. **The client/caregiver is aware of factors important when taking oral iron supplements.**

A. Stool will be dark green or black.
B. Iron is best absorbed when taken on empty stomach. Because of complaints of upset stomach, it may need to be taken with food.
C. Side effects possible from iron supplements that should be reported to the physician include nausea, constipation, and diarrhea.
D. Frequent oral hygiene is important if taking ferrous sulfate because deposits may form on teeth.

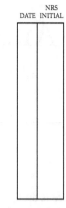

NRS
DATE INITIAL

E. Take liquid iron through a straw, and rinse mouth to avoid staining teeth.
F. Iron supplements should be continued for at least 6 months after hemoglobin levels are normal.

VII. **The client/caregiver is aware of possible complications from untreated anemia.**

A. Heart failure
B. Infection
C. A chronic lack of oxygen

RESOURCES

Nutritionist

Counseling

REFERENCES

Ackley, B. J., & Ladwig, G. B. (2006). *Nursing diagnosis handbook: A guide to planning care.* St. Louis: Mosby Elsevier.

Cohen, B. J., & Taylor, J. J. (2005). *Memmler's the human body in health and disease* (10th ed.). Philadelphia: Lippincott Williams & Wilkins.

Lutz, C., & Przytulski, K. (2001). *Nutrition and diet therapy.* Philadelphia: F. A. Davis Company.

Nutrition made incredibly easy. (2003). Philadelphia: Lippincott Williams & Wilkins.

Taylor, C., Lillis, C., & LeMone, P. (2005). *Fundamentals of nursing.* Philadelphia: Lippincott, Williams & Wilkins.

2 Pernicious Anemia

Patient name: _____ Admission: _____

NRS
DATE INITIAL

I. **The client/caregiver can define pernicious anemia.**

A. It is a decreased absorption of vitamin B12 caused by a deficiency of an intrinsic factor.
B. This causes cell destruction and low hemoglobin levels.
C. Vitamin B12 is necessary for gastric, intestinal, and nervous system functioning.

II. **The client/caregiver can list factors that may increase risk of pernicious anemia.**

A. Age (it typically affects people over 50 years old)
B. Race (it typically affects those of Scandinavian origin with blue eyes)
C. Autoimmune diseases
D. Diet insufficient in folic acid
E. Familial history
F. Malabsorption syndromes
G. Strict vegetarian diet without B12 supplements
H. Pregnancy due to increased need in third trimester
I. Surgical removal of the stomach
J. Celiac disease
K. Metabolic disorders
L. Alcoholism

III. **The client/caregiver can recognize signs and symptoms of pernicious anemia.**

A. Smooth, sore, red tongue and bleeding gums
B. Impaired sense of smell
C. Loss of appetite
D. Abdominal pain
E. Decreased sensation in hands and feet
F. Fatigue and weakness
G. Shortness of breath
H. Constipation or diarrhea
I. A lack of coordination and difficulty walking
J. Nausea and vomiting
K. Poor memory

NRS
DATE INITIAL

IV. **The client/caregiver can list measures to control pernicious anemia.**

A. Take medications as prescribed. Injections of B12 are the treatment of choice. Oral supplements of vitamin B12 can be added. Vitamin B12 can be administered intranasally.
B. Eat a well-balanced diet that is high in vitamin B12 (i.e., eggs, fish, meat, and milk).
C. Avoid injury due to decreased sensations in hands and feet.
D. Perform good oral and personal hygiene.
E. Exercise regularly with regular rest periods.
F. Keep follow-up appointments with physician and laboratory.
G. Report signs and symptoms of infection or any reoccurrence to physician.

V. **The client/caregiver is aware of possible complications of untreated disease.**

A. Heart failure
B. Increased risk for gastric polyps and gastric cancer
C. Persistent neurological defects if treatment is delayed

RESOURCE
Nutritionist or dietitian

REFERENCES
Ackley, B. J., & Ladwig, G. B. (2006). *Nursing diagnosis handbook: A guide to planning care.* St. Louis: Mosby Elsevier.
Cohen, B. J., & Taylor, J. J. (2005). *Memmler's the human body in health and disease* (10th ed.). Philadelphia: Lippincott Williams & Wilkins.
Lutz, C., & Przytulski, K. (2001). *Nutrition and diet therapy.* Philadelphia: F. A. Davis Company.
Nutrition made incredibly easy. (2003). Philadelphia: Lippincott Williams & Wilkins.
Taylor, C., Lillis, C., & LeMone, P. (2005). *Fundamentals of nursing.* Philadelphia: Lippincott, Williams & Wilkins.

3 Folic Acid Deficiency

Patient name: _____ Admission: _____

NRS
DATE INITIAL

I. **The client/caregiver can define folic acid deficiency.**

   A. It is a decrease in red blood cells caused by folate deficiency.
   B. It can result from
      • Poor dietary intake of folic acid
      • Malabsorption diseases such as celiac disease
      • Some medications
      • Increased need for folic acid during pregnancy
   C. Additional risk factors include
      • Poor diet (frequently seen in older or poor populations)
      • Alcoholism

II. **The client/caregiver can list signs and symptoms of this disease.**

   A. Fatigue
   B. Headache
   C. Sore mouth and tongue
   D. Pallor (paleness)

III. **The client/caregiver can list measures used to treat folic acid deficiency.**

   A. Replacement therapy may used on a short-term basis or may be lifelong.
   B. Dietary treatment uses increased intake of green, leafy vegetables and citrus fruits.

NRS
DATE INITIAL

IV. **The client/caregiver can discuss complications of untreated folate deficiency.**

   A. In a pregnant woman, this deficiency has been associated with neural tube or spinal defects such as spina bifida in the infant.

RESOURCES

March of Dimes
www.marchofdimes.com

National Institutes of Health (folic acid facts)
www.nlm.nih.gov.medlineplus/folicacid

REFERENCES

Ackley, B. J., & Ladwig, G. B. (2006). *Nursing diagnosis handbook: A guide to planning care.* St. Louis: Mosby Elsevier.

Cohen, B. J., & Taylor, J. J. (2005). *Memmler's the human body in health and disease* (10th ed.). Philadelphia: Lippincott Williams & Wilkins.

Folic Acid IQ (March of Dimes Birth Defects Foundation). *www.marchofdimes.com/pnhec/1808_1945.asp.*

Folic Acid Quiz (National Center on Birth Defects and Developmental Disabilities). *www.cdc.gov/ncbddd/folicacid/quiz.htm.*

Lutz, C., & Przytulski, K. (2001). *Nutrition and diet therapy.* Philadelphia: F. A. Davis Company.

Nutrition made incredibly easy. (2003). Philadelphia: Lippincott Williams & Wilkins.

Taylor, C., Lillis, C., & LeMone, P. (2005). *Fundamentals of nursing.* Philadelphia: Lippincott, Williams & Wilkins.

4 Sickle Cell Anemia

Patient name: _____ **Admission:** _____

NRS
DATE INITIAL

I. **The client/caregiver can define sickle cell anemia.**

   A. The red blood cells, normally disc shaped, become crescent shaped.

   B. They do not function correctly and can cause small blood clots. This can result in sickle cell pain crisis.

   C. It is an inherited disease. Genetic counseling is recommended for all carriers of sickle cell disease.

   D. It is much more common in African Americans. One in 12 African Americans have a sickle cell trait.

II. **The client/caregiver can list symptoms of sickle cell anemia.**

   A. They are
- Yellow eyes/skin and/or jaundice
- Paleness
- Fatigue
- Breathlessness
- Rapid heart rate
- Delayed growth and puberty
- Greater susceptibility to infections
- Ulcers on lower legs (adolescents and adults)
- Bone pain
- Fever
- Attacks of abdominal pain

   B. They may also have
- Bloody urine
- Frequent urination
- Excessive thirst
- Chest pain
- Poor eyesight/blindness

III. **The client/caregiver can define and list symptoms of sickle cell pain crisis.**

   A. Sickle cell disease is present at birth. Symptoms usually do not occur until after 4 months of age.

B. The malformed cells can block blood vessels and damage organs, resulting in "crisis." This can be life threatening.

C. The three types of "crisis" are as follows:
1. Hemolytic crisis (damaged red blood cells break down)
2. Splenic sequestration crisis (spleen enlarges and traps blood cells)
3. Aplastic crisis (infection causes bone marrow to stop producing red blood cells

D. These painful crises can last from hours to days. Some episodes can require hospitalization for hydration and pain control.

E. Pain is in bones of back, chest, and long bones (such as femur or thigh).

IV. **The client/caregiver can define complications of untreated sickle cell disease.**

   A. Complication of untreated or poorly managed sickle cell disease can result in
- Multisystem disease and failure (kidney, liver, lung, and spleen)
- Recurrent crises resulting in severe anemia and gallstones
- Narcotic abuse
- Joint destruction
- Blindness/visual impairment
- Central nervous system (neurologic symptoms and stroke)
- Infection, including pneumonia, cholecystitis (gallbladder), osteomyelitis (bone), and urinary tract infections

V. **The client/caregiver can list treatment measures for sickle cell anemia/crisis.**

   A. Treatment and medical supervision should be ongoing.

   B. Folic acid supplements are used.

   C. During sickle crisis, pain control and adequate fluid intake are required.

(Continued)

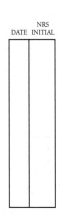

D. Antibiotics and vaccines are used to prevent bacteria infections.

E. Psychosocial counseling is important.

F. Specific actions to prevent crises are to avoid the following:
- Strenuous physical activity, especially if the spleen is enlarged
- Emotional stress
- Environments with low oxygen content (high altitudes, etc.)
- Known sources of infection

RESOURCES

American Sickle Cell Anemia Association

www.ascaa.org

Support groups

Mental health counseling

Genetic counseling

REFERENCES

Ackley, B. J., & Ladwig, G. B. (2006). *Nursing diagnosis handbook: A guide to planning care*. St. Louis: Mosby Elsevier.

Cohen, B. J., & Taylor, J. J. (2005). *Memmler's the human body in health and disease* (10th ed.). Philadelphia: Lippincott Williams & Wilkins.

Lutz, C., & Przytulski, K. (2001). *Nutrition and diet therapy*. Philadelphia: F. A. Davis Company.

Nutrition made incredibly easy. (2003). Philadelphia: Lippincott Williams & Wilkins.

Taylor, C., Lillis, C., & LeMone, P. (2005). *Fundamentals of nursing*. Philadelphia: Lippincott, Williams & Wilkins.

5

Polycythemia Vera

Patient name: _____   **Admission:** _____

NRS
DATE INITIAL

I. The client/caregiver can define polycythemia vera.

A. It is an abnormal increase in blood cells (white blood cells, red blood cells, and platelets).
B. It happens when the bone marrow overproduces all three blood cells. The blood will thicken and can form clots.
C. It occurs more often in men than women. Most patients with this disorder are over 40 years old.
D. The cause is unknown.

II. The client/caregiver can list symptoms of polycythemia vera.

A. Symptoms are due to increased blood viscosity (thickness) and clotting.
- Headache
- Dizziness
- Itchiness, especially after a warm bath
- Fullness in left upper abdomen
- Shortness of breath
- Breathing difficulty when lying down
- Symptoms of phlebitis (inflammation from blood clot)
- Vision abnormalities
- Skin discoloration (red or bluish)
- Fatigue

III. The client/caregiver can list possible complications of polycythemia vera.

A. Leukemia
B. Heart failure
C. Gastric bleeding or peptic ulcer disease
D. Gout
E. Blood clots which increase risk of strokes and heart attacks

NRS
DATE INITIAL

IV. The client/caregiver can list measures to manage this disease.

A. This disease can be treated but not cured.
B. Measures to prevent complications are as follows:
1. Do moderate exercise such as walking.
2. Do leg and ankle stretching exercises.
3. Use cooler water and gentle soap for bathing.
4. Dry skin carefully and use moisturizing lotion.
5. Avoid exposure of your hands and feet to extremes in temperature.
6. Avoid hot tubs, tanning salons, and so forth.
7. Drink plenty of liquids.
8. Check your feet regularly, and report any open areas to physician.

RESOURCES

Support groups

National Library of Medicine MedlinePlus
www.medlineplus.gov

National Institutes of Health
www.nlm.nih.gov/

REFERENCE

Ackley, B. J., & Ladwig, G. B. (2006). *Nursing diagnosis handbook: A guide to planning care.* St. Louis: Mosby Elsevier.

Cohen, B. J., & Taylor, J. J. (2005). *Memmler's the human body in health and disease* (10th ed.). Philadelphia: Lippincott Williams & Wilkins.

Taylor, C., Lillis, C., & LeMone, P. (2005). *Fundamentals of nursing.* Philadelphia: Lippincott, Williams & Wilkins.

Timby, B. K., & Smith, N. C. (2003). *Introductory medical-surgical nursing* (8th ed.). Philadelphia: J. B. Lippincott Williams & Wilkins.

6 Thrombocytopenia

Patient name: _____ Admission: _____

NRS
DATE INITIAL

I. **The client/caregiver can explain disease process of thrombocytopenia.**

   A. It is a disorder in which there are not enough platelets.

   B. Platelets are necessary to help blood clot.

   C. It can result in abnormal bleeding.

II. **The client/caregiver can list symptoms and possible complications of thrombocytopenia.**

   A. Symptoms are
- Bruising easily
- Nosebleeds or bleeding in the mouth
- Rash that resembles pinpoint red spots

   B. Possible complications are
- Hemorrhage
- Bleeding in the brain (intracranial hemorrhage)
- Bleeding in the gastrointestinal system (blood in stool or vomit)

III. **The client/caregiver can explain self-care measures.**

   A. Report to physician or to emergency care if any unexplained bleeding or excessive bruising should occur.

NRS
DATE INITIAL

   B. If you have been told that your platelet count is low, you should
1. Avoid drugs such as aspirin
2. Avoid alcohol
3. Seek physician approval before participating in contact sports

RESOURCES

National Institutes of Health
www.nlm.nih.gov/

National Library of Medicine MedlinePlus
www.medlineplus.gov

REFERENCES

Ackley, B. J., & Ladwig, G. B. (2006). *Nursing diagnosis handbook: A guide to planning care.* St. Louis: Mosby Elsevier.

Cohen, B. J., & Taylor, J. J. (2005). *Memmler's the human body in health and disease* (10th ed.). Philadelphia: Lippincott Williams & Wilkins.

Taylor, C., Lillis, C., & LeMone, P. (2005). *Fundamentals of nursing.* Philadelphia: Lippincott, Williams & Wilkins.

Timby, B. K., & Smith, N. C. (2003). *Introductory medical-surgical nursing* (8th ed.). Philadelphia: J. B. Lippincott Williams & Wilkins.

Disseminated Intravascular Coagulation

7

Patient name: _____   Admission: _____

NRS
DATE INITIAL

I. **The client/caregiver can define disseminated intravascular coagulation and list risk factors.**

A. It is a disorder of the clotting factors. Small blood clots can form throughout the body and deplete the clotting mechanism. This leaves the body unprotected at sites of real tissue injury and unable to clot.

B. Risk factors include the following:
- Blood infections
- Severe tissue injury (burns, etc.)
- Cancer
- Reactions to blood transfusions
- Obstetrical complications
- Severe liver disease

II. **The client/caregiver can describe symptoms and possible complications.**

A. Symptoms are as follows:
- Bleeding, possibly from multiple site in the body
- Clot formation evidenced by bluish coloration of the fingers
- Sudden and unexplained bruising

NRS
DATE INITIAL

B. Possible complications are as follows:
- Severe bleeding
- Stroke
- A lack of blood flow to arms, legs, or major organs can cause tissue damage

C. Seek emergency assistance if symptoms or complications occur.

RESOURCES

National Library of Medicine, MedlinePlus
www.medlineplus.gov

National Institutes of Health
www.nlm.nih.gov/

REFERENCES

Ackley, B. J., & Ladwig, G. B. (2006). *Nursing diagnosis handbook: A guide to planning care.* St. Louis: Mosby Elsevier.

Cohen, B. J., & Taylor, J. J. (2005). *Memmler's the human body in health and disease* (10th ed.). Philadelphia: Lippincott Williams & Wilkins.

Taylor, C., Lillis, C., & LeMone, P. (2005). *Fundamentals of nursing.* Philadelphia: Lippincott, Williams & Wilkins.

Timby, B. K., & Smith, N. C. (2003). *Introductory medical-surgical nursing* (8th ed.). Philadelphia: J. B. Lippincott Williams & Wilkins.

Methicillin-Resistant *Staphylococcus aureus* (MRSA)

1

Patient name: _____ Admission: _____

NRS
DATE INITIAL

I. **The client/caregiver can define MSRA.**

A. MRSA is an infection caused by *Staphylococcus aureus* bacteria or "staph."
B. It was one of the first infections to prove resistant to the broad-spectrum antibiotics.
C. Staph infections are seen mostly in hospitals or health care facilities. They are hospital-acquired infections.
D. The infection can also be acquired in a community setting.
E. Staph can enter the body via a cut or wound. Unfortunately, the client with an impaired immune system or the older client can have a more serious infection.
F. Vancomycin is currently effective against MRSA.

II. **The client/caregiver can list signs and symptoms of MRSA infection.**

A. Staph infections usually start as red bumps that resemble pimples, boils, or spider bites.
B. They can evolve into deep, painful abscesses that require surgical intervention.
C. They can also cause infections in bones, joints, surgical wounds, bloodstream, heart valves, and lungs.

III. **The client/caregiver can list causes of MRSA infections.**

A. Excessive and unnecessary use of antibiotics
B. Antibiotic in food (beef, cattle, pigs, and chickens) and water supplies
C. Bacteria (germs) that can quickly change and evolve to resist antibiotics

IV. **The client/caregiver can list risk factors for MRSA infections.**

A. Risk factors for hospital-acquired infections
• Recent or current stay in hospital
• Living in a long-term care facility

NRS
DATE INITIAL

• Invasive procedures such as dialysis
• Recent use of antibiotics
B. Risks for community-acquired infections
• Young age
• Participating in contact sports
• Sharing sports equipment or personal items such as towels or razors
• Impaired immune system
• Living in crowded or unsanitary conditions
• Close contact with health care workers

V. **The client/caregiver can list measures to prevent or manage a hospital-acquired MRSA infection.**

A. Wash your hands frequently.
B. Ask health care workers to wash their hands before touching you.
C. Ask to use disposable washcloths/disinfectant rather than soap and water.
D. Insist that sterile conditions are used when any procedure is performed.
E. Insist that the health care workers and visitors follow any isolation precautions as set up by the hospital.

VI. **The client/caregiver can list measures to prevent or manage community-acquired MRSA infections.**

A. Avoid sharing personal items such as
• Towels and sheets
• Razors and toothbrushes
• Clothing and athletic equipment
B. Keep all cuts or abrasions clean and covered.
C. Avoid contact with others' wounds or items touching the wound such as towels or bandages.
D. Sanitize linens. Wash gym and athletic clothes after each use.
E. Wash your hands frequently. Carry hand sanitizer containing at least 62% alcohol for times when you cannot wash.

(Continued)

NRS
DATE	INITIAL

F. Ask your physician whether you should be tested for MRSA if there is need to treat a skin infection.

RESOURCES

Centers for Disease Control and Prevention
www.cdc.gov/

State or county health department

REFERENCES

Hitchcock, J. E., Schubert, P. E., & Thomas, S. A. (2003). *Community health nursing: Caring in action.* Clifton Park, NY: Thomson Delmar Learning.

Perry, A., & Potter, P. (2006). *Clinical nursing skills & technique.* St. Louis: Mosby Inc.

Taylor, C., Lillis, C., & LeMone, P. (2005). *Fundamentals of nursing.* Philadelphia: Lippincott, Williams & Wilkins.

Timby, B. K., & Smith, N. C. (2003). *Introductory medical-surgical nursing* (8th ed.). Philadelphia: J. B. Lippincott Williams & Wilkins.

2 West Nile Virus

Patient name: _____ **Admission:** _____

NRS
DATE INITIAL

I. The client/caregiver can explain West Nile Virus (WNV), its symptoms, and its method of transmission.

A. It is an infectious disease spread by infected mosquitoes.

B. People infected with WNV usually have mild or no symptoms.

C. Symptoms that may appear are as follows:
- Fever
- Headache
- Body aches
- Skin rash
- Swollen lymph glands

D. Complications of WNV occur if the infection spreads to the brain and causes inflammation resulting in encephalitis or meningitis.

E. WNV primarily circulates between infected birds and mosquitoes that bite them. The infected mosquitoes can then bite and infect other animals and humans.

II. The client/caregiver can list ways to prevent WNV.

A. Prevent mosquito bites by
1. Using insect repellent
2. Wearing loose-fitting clothing that covers the legs and arms
3. Cleaning clogged rain gutters to avoid standing water where mosquitoes can lay eggs
4. Emptying water once or twice a week from flowerpots, pet food and water dishes, birdbaths, swimming pool covers, and any other items that can collect water
5. Staying indoors between dusk and dawn (when mosquitoes are most active)

NRS
DATE INITIAL

III. The client/caregiver can list new warnings regarding the spread of WNV.

A. In 2002, the Centers for Disease Control and Prevention, the U.S. Food and Drug Administration, and other government agencies confirmed the spread of WNV by infected blood and/or organ transplantation.

B. Blood blanks will ask potential blood donors whether they have had a fever and headache during the previous week. The donor will not be allowed to give blood donations at that time.

RESOURCES

Links to State and Local Government West Nile Virus
www.cdc.gov/ncidod/dvbid/westnile/city_states.htm

Centers for Disease Control and Prevention
www.cdc.gov/

REFERENCES

Hitchcock, J. E., Schubert, P. E., & Thomas, S. A. (2003). *Community health nursing: Caring in action.* Clifton Park, NY: Thomson Delmar Learning.

Hunt, R. (2005). *Introduction to community based nursing.* Philadelphia: Lippincott Williams & Wilkins.

Perry, A., & Potter, P. (2006). *Clinical nursing skills & technique.* St. Louis: Mosby Inc.

Taylor, C., Lillis, C., & LeMone, P. (2005). *Fundamentals of nursing.* Philadelphia: Lippincott, Williams & Wilkins.

Timby, B. K., & Smith, N. C. (2003). *Introductory medical-surgical nursing* (8th ed.). Philadelphia: J. B. Lippincott Williams & Wilkins.

West Nile Virus: Reducing the risk. (2003). *FDA Consumer Magazine,* January–February, Issue Pub No. FDA 03-1326C.

3   Lyme Disease

Patient name: _____   **Admission:** _____

NRS
DATE INITIAL

I. The client/caregiver can explain Lyme disease.

A. It is a disease caused by bacterium and is transmitted to humans by the bite of an infected black-legged tick.

B. Symptoms are as follows:
- Fever
- Headache
- Fatigue
- Skin rash called erythema migrans (bull's eye appearance)
- Muscle pains
- Stiff neck
- Joint inflammation (particularly in knees and large joints)
- Overall itching
- Change in behavior

C. Complications of Lyme disease are infections that can spread to joints, heart, and nervous system, such as:
- Arthritis
- Meningitis and encephalitis
- Bell's palsy
- Heart complications

II. The client/caregiver can list risk factors for Lyme disease.

A. Walking in tall grasses
B. Other outdoor activities that risk exposure to ticks
C. Having a pet that goes outdoors and may carry ticks

III. The client/caregiver can list measures to prevent or manage Lyme disease.

A. Contact physician for testing.
B. Take medications as ordered by physician.
C. Have regular checkups with physician.
D. Avoid fatigue.
E. If walking in wooded or grassy areas, tuck long pants into socks to protect legs.

NRS
DATE INITIAL

F. Wear shoes and long-sleeved shirts.
G. Wear white or light colored clothing, making it easier to identify ticks.
H. Use insect repellant on skin and spray your clothes.
I. Check for ticks on yourself (even your scalp) and pets.
J. Remove tick immediately with tweezers using steady traction. Swab area with antiseptic after removing tick.
K. Signs and symptoms to report to physician are as follows:
- Headache
- Muscle weakness
- Altered mental functioning
- Excessive drowsiness
- Flu-like symptoms

RESOURCES

Lyme Disease Association
www.lymediseaseassociation.org/

Local or state department of health

Centers for Disease Control and Prevention
www.cdc.gov/

REFERENCES

Canobbio, M. M. (2006). *Mosby's handbook of patient teaching.* St. Louis: Mosby Inc.

Hitchcock, J. E., Schubert, P. E., & Thomas, S. A. (2003). *Community health nursing: Caring in action.* Clifton Park, NY: Thomson Delmar Learning.

Perry, A., & Potter, P. (2006). *Clinical nursing skills & technique.* St. Louis: Mosby Inc.

Taylor, C., Lillis, C., & LeMone, P. (2005). *Fundamentals of nursing.* Philadelphia: Lippincott, Williams & Wilkins.

Timby, B. K., & Smith, N. C. (2003). *Introductory medical-surgical nursing* (8th ed.). Philadelphia: J. B. Lippincott Williams & Wilkins.

Toxic Shock Syndrome

4

Patient name: _____   Admission: _____

I.   **The client/caregiver can define toxic shock syndrome and causes.**

   A. It is a rare but life-threatening staph bacterial infection.
   B. It is most often seen with the use of superabsorbent tampons and contraceptive sponges.
   C. It can also affect men, children, and postmenopausal women who have skin wounds and surgery.

II. **The client/caregiver can list signs and symptoms of toxic shock syndrome.**

   A. Sudden high fever
   B. Vomiting or diarrhea
   C. A rash that resembles a sunburn and appears mostly on palms of hands and soles of feet
   D. Confusion
   E. Muscle aches
   F. Redness of your eyes, mouth, and throat
   G. Seizure activity
   H. Headaches

III. **The client/caregiver can list possible complications.**

   A. Hypotension
   B. Kidney damage/failure

IV. **The client/caregiver can list measures to prevent or manage this disease.**

   A. Contact physician for previously listed symptoms.
   B. If using tampons
     • Change frequently
     • Use lowest absorbency tampon
     • Alternate use of tampon and sanitary napkins when possible
     • Physician may recommend avoiding tampons after you have experienced toxic shock syndrome or a prior staph infection.

RESOURCES

The National Women's Health Information Center

U.S. Department of Health and Human Services, Office on Women's Health
www.4woman.gov/

REFERENCES

Novak, J. C., & Broom, B. L. (1999). *Maternal and child health nursing.* St. Louis: Mosby, Inc.

Taylor, C., Lillis, C., & LeMone, P. (2005). *Fundamentals of nursing.* Philadelphia: Lippincott, Williams & Wilkins.

Timby, B. K., & Smith, N. C. (2003). *Introductory medical-surgical nursing* (8th ed.). Philadelphia: J. B. Lippincott Williams & Wilkins.

5 | Herpes Zoster (Shingles)

Patient name: _____   **Admission:** _____

I.   The client/caregiver can define herpes zoster (shingles).

A. It is caused by the varicella-zoster virus, the same virus that causes the chicken pox.

B. After you have had chicken pox, the virus lies dormant (not active) in your nerves. Years later, the virus may reactivate in the form of shingles.

C. Pain from this disease can be severe.

D. Risk factors are aging, stress, and an impaired immune system.

II.   The client/caregiver can describe the symptoms of herpes zoster.

A. It spreads along the nerve tract and causes pain and/or a burning sensation.

B. Symptoms appear on one side of the body or face.

C. A red rash appears with fluid-filled blisters that begin a few days after the pain.

D. Fever appears.

E. Headaches occur.

F. Upset stomach occurs.

III.   The client/caregiver can list measures to prevent the spread of shingles and how to manage the symptoms.

A. Measures to prevent spread
  1. Until blisters dry and have scabs, avoid contact with anyone who has never had chicken pox, has a weak immune system, newborns, and pregnant women.
  2. Varivax was approved in 1995 as immunization for prevention of shingles. Children got immunized between the ages 12 and 18 months. Older children and adults who have never had chicken pox can receive this vaccine.
  3. The Zostavax vaccine was approved in 2006 for use to prevent shingles. It is recommended for adults over 60 years of age who have had chicken pox but not shingles.

B. Measures to manage disease
  1. Physician may order pain medication, antidepressants, or anticonvulsant medication for relief of pain.
  2. Keep the affected area clean.
  3. Apply cool, wet compresses to affected areas.
  4. Soak in a tub of lukewarm water or use calamine lotion to relieve itching and discomfort.
  5. Get plenty of rest.
  6. Maintain a healthy diet.
  7. Consult the physician regarding the use of over-the-counter pain relievers.

IV.   The client/caregiver can describe possible complications.

A. Postherpetic neuralgia, which occurs when the skin remains painful and sensitive to the touch for months or even years

B. Inflammation of the brain (encephalitis)

C. Hearing problems

D. Temporary or permanent blindness

E. Loss of facial movement

F. Secondary skin infections

RESOURCES

National Institute of Neurologic Disorders and Stroke
www.ninds.nih.gov

National Institute of Health for Seniors
www.nihseniorhealth.gov

REFERENCES

Ackley, B. J., & Ladwig, G. B. (2006). *Nursing diagnosis handbook: A guide to planning care.* St. Louis: Mosby Elsevier.

Perry, A., & Potter, P. (2006). *Clinical nursing skills & technique.* St. Louis: Mosby Inc.

Taylor, C., Lillis, C., & LeMone, P. (2005). *Fundamentals of nursing.* Philadelphia: Lippincott, Williams & Wilkins.

Timby, B. K., & Smith, N. C. (2003). *Introductory medical-surgical nursing* (8th ed.). Philadelphia: J. B. Lippincott Williams & Wilkins.

Cellulitis

Patient name: _____ **Admission:** _____

NRS
DATE INITIAL

I. **The client/caregiver will be able to define cellulitis.**

A. It is an inflammation of dermis and subcutaneous tissues.
B. It is usually caused by streptococcal or staphylococcal infection.
C. Common locations for cellulites are the face and lower legs, but it can occur anywhere on the body.
D. Bacteria may enter through a break in the skin, or an area of dry, flaky skin.

II. **The client/caregiver can list risk factors for cellulitis.**

A. Increasing age
B. Impaired immune system
C. Diabetes mellitus
D. Chicken pox or shingles
E. Chronic swelling of arms or legs (lymphedema)
F. Chronic fungal infections of feet and toes

III. **The client/caregiver will be able to list signs and symptoms of cellulitis.**

A. Redness, warmth
B. Localized pain and tenderness
C. Fever, chills, and malaise
D. Swelling
E. Skin resembling that of an orange (peau d'orange)
F. Lesion or open wounds
G. Drainage

IV. **The client/caregiver can list treatments to promote healing.**

A. Immobilize and elevate affected limb
B. High-protein diet
C. Antibiotics (local ointments and/or system antibiotics) as ordered

NRS
DATE INITIAL

D. Pain management
   1. Cool wet packs, which may promote comfort
   2. Pain medications as needed
E. Wound care
   1. Wash hands well before and after changing dressing.
   2. Wash wound with soap and water or ordered solution.
   3. Use aseptic technique.
   4. Wash soiled linens separately.
   5. Cover wound with bandage. Change bandages often.
F. Preventive measures
   1. Moisturize skin regularly—prevent cracking and peeling.
   2. Watch for signs of infection—redness, pain, or drainage.
   3. Trim fingernails and toenails carefully. Consult with podiatrist if necessary.
   4. Protect hands and feet with gloves and proper footwear.
   5. Seek prompt treatment for open areas or signs of infection.

V. **The client/caregiver will be able to list possible complications of cellulitis.**

A. Gangrene
B. Sepsis
C. Metastatic abscess
D. Flesh-eating strep (necrotizing fascitis)

REFERENCES

Canobbio, M. M. (2006). *Mosby's handbook of patient teaching.* St. Louis: Mosby Inc.

Cohen, B. J., & Taylor, J. J. (2005). *Memmler's the human body in health and disease* (10th ed.). Philadelphia: Lippincott Williams & Wilkins.

2 | Psoriasis

Patient name: _____   **Admission:** _____

NRS
DATE INITIAL

I.   The client/caregiver can define psoriasis.

A. It is a skin disease characterized by rapid growth of epidermal cells.

B. Cells are replaced in four days instead of the normal 28 days.

C. It is chronic with periods of remission and exacerbation.

D. Psoriasis is not contagious.

II. The client/caregiver can recognize signs and symptoms of psoriasis.

A. Red patches of skin covered with silvery scales

B. Dry, cracked skin that may bleed

C. Itching, burning, or soreness

D. Thickened, pitted, or ridged nails

E. Swollen and stiff joints

F. Psoriasis patches that can range in size

III. The client/caregiver can list some triggers of psoriasis.

A. Factors that may trigger psoriasis
   • Infections, such as strep throat
   • Injury to the skin, such as cuts, bug bites, or severe sunburn
   • Stress
   • Cold weather
   • Smoking
   • Heavy alcohol consumption
   • Certain medications

IV. The client/caregiver can list factors that may increase risk of psoriasis.

A. Familial history of psoriasis

B. Depressed immune systems

C. Trauma, burns, lacerations, or chemical injuries

D. Anxiety and stress

E. Certain systemic drugs such as steroids

F. Low-humidity environment

V.   The client/caregiver can list measures to prevent or control psoriasis.

A. Bathing
   1. Soak in warm tub baths to remove scales and promote cleanliness.

NRS
DATE INITIAL

   2. Add bath oil, oiled oatmeal, and Epsom salts to water and soak for 15 minutes.
   3. Avoid hot water and harsh soaps.
   4. Use lukewarm water and mild soaps with added oils or fats.
   5. Blot the skin dry. Apply ointment-based moisturizer while skin is moist.

B. Avoid or manage factors that may exacerbate condition.
   1. Obtain early treatment for any type of infection.
   2. Use safety precautions to avoid irritation or trauma.
   3. Use stress-management techniques.
   4. Avoid excessive sunlight. Small amounts of sunlight can improve lesions.

C. Obtain adequate rest, nutrition, and exercise.

D. Humidify the air in the winter.

E. Apply treatments as ordered using precautions as directed (topical corticosteroids, anthralin preparations, salicylic acid, crude coal tar, occlusive wraps, photochemotherapy, etc.).

F. Provide scalp care as ordered (tar shampoo, topical steroids, etc.).

G. Avoid drinking alcohol.

VI. The client/caregiver is aware of possible complications.

A. Severe itching, which can lead to secondary infections

B. Exfoliative psoriatic state (covers entire body)

C. Arthritis

D. Depression and low self-esteem

E. Stress and anxiety

RESOURCES

National Psoriasis Foundation
www.psoriasis.org/home/

Support groups

REFERENCE

Cohen, B. J., & Taylor, J. J. (2005). *Memmler's the human body in health and disease* (10th ed.). Philadelphia: Lippincott Williams & Wilkins.

3 Dermatitis

Patient name: _____ **Admission:** _____

NRS
DATE INITIAL

I. **The client/caregiver can define dermatitis.**

A. Contact dermatitis is an inflammation of the skin caused by contact with an irritating or allergy-causing substance.

B. The reaction to a substance is the result of repeated exposure.

C. Common allergens causing contact dermatitis include the following:
   - Plants such as poison ivy
   - Nickel or other metals
   - Some medications
   - Rubber
   - Cosmetics
   - Fabrics and clothing
   - Adhesives
   - Fragrance and perfumes
   - Detergents

D. Atopic dermatitis or eczema occurs with allergies and can run in families. It usually begins in infancy and continues thru childhood and adolescence. It is less of a problem in adulthood, unless exposed to allergens or irritants.

II. **The client/caregiver can define symptoms of dermatitis.**

A. Symptoms are as follows:
   - Itching of the skin in exposed areas
   - Skin redness, warmth, or inflammation at exposed areas
   - Localized swelling of the skin
   - Skin lesion or rash that may appear as pimple-like vesicles or blisters
   - Lesions that may ooze, drain, or form crusts
   - Lesions that may become scaly, raw, or thickened area of skin

III. **The client/caregiver can list possible complications.**

A. Secondary infections

B. Cellulitis

NRS
DATE INITIAL

IV. **The client/caregiver can list measures to prevent or manage symptoms.**

A. Identify allergen/irritant and avoid contact.

B. Avoid scratching whenever possible. Trim nails. Cover affected areas. Wear gloves at night.

C. Dress in clothing to avoid excessive sweating. Wear soft, smooth-textured clothing.

D. Avoid dry skin by doing the following:
   1. Choose mild soaps and deodorants. Wash clothing in mild detergent.
   2. Use soap only on face, underarms, genital areas, hands, and feet.
   3. Avoid hot water by using only warm water.
   4. Gently pat skin dry after bathing.
   5. Moisturize your skin. Ask physician for suggestions of lubricating cream.

RESOURCES

American Academy of Dermatology
www.aad.org/default.htm

National Institute of Allergy and Infectious Diseases
www.niaid.nih.gov

REFERENCES

Cohen, B. J., & Taylor, J. J. (2005). *Memmler's the human body in health and disease* (10th ed.). Philadelphia: Lippincott Williams & Wilkins.

Mayo clinic guide to self-care (5th ed.). (1999). Rochester, MN: Mayo Clinic.

Muscari, M. E. (2005). *Pediatric nursing*. Philadelphia: Lippincott Williams & Wilkins.

Timby, B. K., & Smith, N. C. (2003). *Introductory medical-surgical nursing* (8th ed.). Philadelphia: J. B. Lippincott Williams & Wilkins.

4 Burns

Patient name: _____

Admission: _____

NRS
DATE INITIAL

I. The client/caregiver can list signs and symptoms of burns.

A. First degree (superficial)—pain, redness, and blanching with pressure
B. Second degree (partial thickness)—pain, blisters, redness, firm texture, and blanching with pressure
C. Third and fourth degree (full thickness)—dryness, pale, red or brown color, no pain, firm, and leathery skin texture

II. The client/caregiver can list actions to take with minor burns.

A. Cool the burn. Hold under cold running water. If this is not possible, immerse the area in cold water or use cold compresses. Do not put ice on the burn (can produce further injury by causing frostbite).
B. Loosely cover area with sterile gauze bandage.
C. Watch for signs of infection.
D. Do not break blisters.
E. After healing, use sunscreen on area for at least a year.
F. Use proper handwashing before and after care.

III. The client/caregiver can list actions needed if third-degree burn.

A. Call for emergency assistance.
B. Do not remove burnt clothing.
C. Do not immerse severe burns in cold water. This could produce shock.
D. Check for signs of circulation and respiration. Begin CPR if needed.
E. Cover area with a cool, moist, sterile bandage; a clean, moist cloth; or moist towels.

IV. The client/caregiver can list treatment measures to promote healing.

A. Eat a high-protein, high-calorie diet.
B. Take vitamin C and vitamin B complex supplements.
C. Increase fluids to 2000 to 3000 ml per day unless contraindicated.

NRS
DATE INITIAL

D. Avoid contact with persons with infections (especially upper-respiratory infections).
E. Use proper handwashing and wound care to prevent contamination or infection.
F. Exercise as tolerated with planned rest periods.
G. Keep follow-up appointment with physician, laboratory, and physical therapy.

V. The client/caregiver can list measures to prevent muscle shortening or contractures.

A. Perform range of motion exercises.
B. Position in good body alignment.

VI. The client/caregiver can list measures to decrease pain.

A. Take pain medication before painful procedures and as directed by physician.
B. Use relaxation techniques.
C. Wear loose-fitting cotton garments.

VII. The client/caregiver can list symptoms related to burns that need immediate attention.

A. Seek medical attention for symptoms such as
  • Fever
  • Pus-like or foul-smelling drainage
  • Excessive swelling
  • Blisters filled with greenish or brownish fluid
  • Burns that do not heal in 10 days to 2 weeks

VIII. The client/caregiver can list possible complications.

A. Dehydration
B. Acute respiratory distress
C. Septic shock (infection)
D. Circulatory collapse
E. Anemia
F. Disuse atrophy and contractures
G. Scarring
H. Stress diabetes
I. Depression

(Continued)

RESOURCES

The Phoenix Society for Burn Survivors
www.phoenix-society.org/

Child safety: Prevent burns, 2007
www.mayoclinic.com/health/child-safety/CC00044

American College of Emergency Physicians on "Avoiding Household Burns"
www.acep.org/webportal/PatientsConsumers/HealthSubjectsBy Topic/Burns/default.htm

Support groups

Counseling services

Clergy

REFERENCES

Ackley, B. J., & Ladwig, G. B. (2006). *Nursing diagnosis handbook: A guide to planning care.* St. Louis: Mosby Inc.

Avoiding household burns. (2007). Irving, TX: American College of Emergency Physicians.

Canobbio, M. M. (2006). *Mosby's handbook of patient teaching.* St. Louis: Mosby Inc.

Cohen, B. J., & Taylor, J. J. (2005). *Memmler's the human body in health and disease* (10th ed.). Philadelphia: Lippincott Williams & Wilkins.

Lutz, C., & Przytulski, K. (2001). *Nutrition and diet therapy.* Philadelphia: F. A. Davis Company.

Nutrition made incredibly easy. (2003). Philadelphia: Lippincott Williams & Wilkins.

Taylor, C., Lillis, C., & LeMone, P. (2005). *Fundamentals of nursing.* Philadelphia: Lippincott, Williams & Wilkins.

5

Decubitus Ulcer (Pressure Ulcer)

Patient name: _____ Admission: _____

NRS DATE INITIAL		

I. **The client/caregiver can define pressure ulcer.**

A. It is an area of skin where a lack of blood flow has caused tissue destruction.

B. It is caused by pressure, friction, or shearing (a combination of pressure and friction) force on the skin.

II. **The client/caregiver has a basic understanding of the anatomy and physiology of the skin.**

A. The outer skin, the epidermis, is made up of layered cells. It contains the pigment that makes up our skin color.

B. The next layer is the dermis, which contains the oil and sweat glands, hair follicles, blood vessels, and nerves.

C. Below the dermis is the subcutaneous layer, which contains fat cells and connective tissue to act as a shock absorber and insulator for the body.

III. **The client/caregiver can list factors that may increase risk of pressure ulcer.**

A. Impaired circulation and sensation

B. Immobility

C. Incontinence of feces or urine

D. Malnutrition

E. Skin pressure, friction, and shearing

F. Edema

G. Certain medical conditions, such as diabetes, dementia, and peripheral vascular disease

H. Overweight or underweight

IV. **The client/caregiver can recognize signs of a pressure ulcer.**

A. Stage I
1. Redness and warmth
2. No break in skin

B. Stage II
1. Partial thickness
2. Loss of skin involving epidermis and often into dermis

C. Stage III
1. Full-thickness skin break
2. Involves epidermis, dermis, and subcutaneous tissue

D. Stage IV
1. Deep-tissue destruction
2. Fascia, muscle, and bone involved

V. **The client/caregiver can list measures to prevent pressure areas and to promote wound healing.**

A. Eliminate or decrease the force causing the skin breakdown.
1. Use pressure-relief devices (many types of mattresses and chair cushions can be rented or purchased).
2. Keep linens clean, dry, and free of wrinkles and crumbs.
3. Move client with a draw sheet to prevent shearing action.
4. Do not massage-reddened areas.
5. Protect heels, elbows, back of head, iliac crest, sacrum, and coccyx by using foam pads.
6. Avoid use of alcohol (because of drying properties).
7. If incontinent, change and cleanse frequently. Encourage the use of a commode.

B. Provide cleanliness of wound.
1. Cleanse hands and put on gloves.
2. Wash wound carefully and pat dry.
3. Cover wound with dressing as ordered.
4. Debride wound if necessary.
5. Avoid using tape directly on the skin.

C. Promote circulation and nutrition.
1. Eat a high-calorie, high-protein diet and smaller, more frequent meals. Use supplemental nutritional feedings.
2. Take vitamin and mineral supplements including multivitamins, vitamin C, and zinc.

(Continued)

NRS
DATE INITIAL

3. Exercise to increase circulation and bring nutrients to the wound.
4. Avoid alcohol and cold temperatures, which constrict blood vessels.

D. Provide a controlled moist environment.
1. Lubricate dry skin.
2. Use ointments to protect skin from excessive moisture and incontinence.
3. Use skin-care products as recommended (i.e., hydrocolloid dressings and Tegaderm).
4. Deep wounds require packing to absorb drainage.

E. Activity
1. Change position every 2 to 3 hours while in bed or chair.
2. Increase activity as tolerated.
3. Teach safe transfer methods.
4. Teach active and passive range of motion.

F. Stress the importance of frequent checks of pressure points (sacrum, hips, heels, elbows, ears, and thoracic spine).

VI. The client/caregiver can list possible complications.

A. Infection
B. Septicemia

RESOURCES

Durable medical equipment companies for pressure-relief devices

Nurse wound therapist consult

Occupational or physical therapist consult

Dietician consult

Home health aid

REFERENCES

Ackley, B. J., & Ladwig, G. B. (2006). *Nursing diagnosis handbook: A guide to planning care.* St. Louis: Mosby Inc.

Canobbio, M. M. (2006). *Mosby's handbook of patient teaching.* St. Louis: Mosby Inc.

Cohen, B. J., & Taylor, J. J. (2005). *Memmler's the human body in health and disease* (10th ed.). Philadelphia: Lippincott Williams & Wilkins.

Lutz, C., & Przytulski, K. (2001). *Nutrition and diet therapy.* Philadelphia: F. A. Davis Company.

Perry, A., & Potter, P. (2006). *Clinical nursing skills & technique.* St. Louis: Mosby Inc.

Timby, B. K., & Smith, N. C. (2003). *Introductory medical-surgical nursing* (8th ed.). Philadelphia: J. B. Lippincott Williams & Wilkins.

1 Fracture

Patient name: _____

Admission: _____

NRS
DATE INITIAL

I.   The client/caregiver can define fracture.

A. It is a break in the bone.
B. Surrounding soft-tissue injury can also occur.
C. Fractures can be caused by trauma or disease.

II.   The client/caregiver can state type of fracture that occurred.

A. Open (skin pierced over the fracture)
B. Closed (skin intact over the fracture)
C. Complete (break across entire bone)
D. Incomplete (fracture extends only part way through the bone), also called greenstick fracture
E. Impacted (one bone fragment forcibly driven into another bone fragment)
F. Comminuted (bone broken in several places)
G. Displaced (bone fragments are separated at the fracture line)
H. Complicated (a body organ or other body tissues injured at the time of the fracture)

III. The client/caregiver can recognize signs and symptoms.

A. Deformity
B. Pain and tenderness
C. Restricted or limited mobility
D. Swelling
E. Bruising
F. Muscle spasm
G. Pallor
H. Numbness and tingling
I. Shortening of a limb

IV. The caregiver can administer first aid to a fracture victim.

A. Move the victim no more than absolutely necessary to prevent further tissue damage.
B. Assess client's total condition.

NRS
DATE INITIAL

C. Remove constricting clothing or jewelry.
D. Cover open wounds with sterile dressing before splinting.
E. Splint injured site before moving to immobilize the joints above and below the fracture.
F. Apply well-padded splints and bandage splints over clothing.

V.   The client/caregiver understands possible medical/surgical treatment of fractures.

A. Closed reduction (manual realignment of bones)
B. Immobilization of bone
C. Electrical bone stimulation
D. Cast, splint, traction, sling, or external fixator
E. Total joint replacement

VI. The client/caregiver can list measures to promote healing and prevent complications of a fracture.

A. Report to physician any signs of coolness, pallor, redness, blueness, numbness, or signs of infection.
B. Eat a well-balanced diet that is high in carbohydrates and proteins. Eat foods that are high in calcium.
C. Take vitamin (A, B, C, and D) and mineral (calcium and zinc) supplements as recommended.
D. Increase fluids to 8 to 10 glasses per day unless contraindicated.
E. Use medications (analgesics, antibiotics, muscle relaxants, etc.) as ordered.
F. Follow activity and weight-bearing instructions as ordered.
G. Use ambulatory aids (cane, walker, and crutches) as ordered.
H. Follow an exercise program as ordered.
I. Follow referral to physical or occupational therapy.

(Continued)

NRS
DATE INITIAL

J. Use safety precautions in environment to prevent falls or injury.

K. Keep follow-up appointments with physician.

VII. The client/caregiver is aware of possible complications.

A. Infection
B. Peripheral nerve damage
C. Fat embolism
D. Shock
E. Compartment syndrome
F. Venous thrombus

REFERENCES

Ackley, B. J., & Ladwig, G. B. (2006). *Nursing diagnosis handbook: A guide to planning care.* St. Louis: Mosby Inc.

Canobbio, M. M. (2006). *Mosby's handbook of patient teaching.* St. Louis: Mosby Inc.

Cohen, B. J., & Taylor, J. J. (2005). *Memmler's the human body in health and disease* (10th ed.). Philadelphia: Lippincott Williams & Wilkins.

Lutz, C., & Przytulski, K. (2001). *Nutrition and diet therapy.* Philadelphia: F. A. Davis Company.

Taylor, C., Lillis, C., & LeMone, P. (2005). *Fundamentals of nursing.* Philadelphia: Lippincott, Williams & Wilkins.

2 Gout

Patient name: _____ Admission: _____

NRS
DATE INITIAL

NRS
DATE INITIAL

I. The client/caregiver can define gout.

A. It is a metabolic condition in which there is excess uric acid in the blood, causing sodium urate crystals to be deposited in or near the joints.
B. The urate crystals form masses called tophi that cause irritation or inflammation of the joint.
C. Deposits are found in joints and other body tissues such as ear, cartilage, and kidneys. The joint most often affected is first metatarsal joint of the great toe.
D. Gout may be primary or secondary.
  1. Primary gout occurs because of an inherited defect in purine metabolism, resulting in excess uric acid.
  2. Secondary gout occurs because of increased uric acid secondary to lead poisoning, diuretics, renal disease, alcohol, surgery effects, and so forth.
E. Gout may be acute or chronic.

II. The client/caregiver can list factors that may cause exacerbation.

A. Prolonged fasting
B. Stress
C. Alcohol
D. Certain medication such as aspirin or thiazide diuretics

III. The client/caregiver can recognize signs and symptoms.

A. Intense pain
B. Swelling and tenderness
C. Limited motion of joint
D. Increased heart rate and blood pressure
E. Headache
F. Fever and chills
G. Malaise
H. Tophi: crystallized deposits accumulating in articular tissues

IV. The client/caregiver can list measures to prevent or control gout.

A. Dietary measures
  1. Eat a high-fiber, low-fat diet.
  2. Reduce intake of refined sugars.
  3. Drink fluids such as water and herbal teas. Drink 8 to 12 glasses of fluid per day.
  4. Avoid foods high in purine such as glandular meats, shellfish, sardines, kidney, liver, lentils, mushrooms, and peas.
  5. Avoid alcoholic beverages.
B. Check urine pH. If pH is less than six, increase fluids. Avoid high purine foods and eat alkaline foods such as potatoes or milk.
C. Avoid stress.
D. Avoid fasting.
E. Protect nodular tophi areas to prevent skin breakdown.
F. Use bed cradle to keep pressure off the affected part.
G. Apply ice to inflamed joints.
H. Obtain adequate rest (bedrest during acute stage).
I. Achieve and maintain ideal weight.
J. Take medications as ordered. Physician may want to avoid diuretics, aspirin, and nicotinic acid. Report nausea, rash, or constipation to physician.
K. Perform range of motion exercise as instructed.
L. Keep follow-up appointments with physician.
M. Notify physician of symptoms of kidney stones (nausea, vomiting, urinary retention, flank pain, fever, etc.).

V. The client/caregiver is aware of possible complications.

A. Permanent joint disability
B. Kidney stones
C. Hypertension
D. Gouty arthritis
E. Infection of ruptured deposits

(Continued)

RESOURCE

National Institute of Arthritis and Musculoskeletal and Skin
   Diseases
www.niams.nih.gov

REFERENCES

Ackley, B. J., & Ladwig, G. B. (2006). *Nursing diagnosis
   handbook: A guide to planning care.* St. Louis: Mosby
   Inc.

Canobbio, M. M. (2006). *Mosby's handbook of patient teaching.*
   St. Louis: Mosby Inc.

Cohen, B. J., & Taylor, J. J. (2005). *Memmler's the human body
   in health and disease* (10th ed.). Philadelphia: Lippincott
   Williams & Wilkins.

Lutz, C., & Przytulski, K. (2001). *Nutrition and diet therapy.*
   Philadelphia: F. A. Davis Company.

Taylor, C., Lillis, C., & LeMone, P. (2005). *Fundamentals of
   nursing.* Philadelphia: Lippincott, Williams & Wilkins.

3 Osteoarthritis

Patient name: _____

Admission: _____

| NRS |
| DATE INITIAL |

I. The client/caregiver can define osteoarthritis.

A. It is a degenerative, noninflammatory joint disease.
B. The cartilage that protects the ends of bones is worn away.
C. It can affect all mobile joints, especially weight-bearing joints: hip, knee, and spinal column.

II. The client/caregiver can list factors that may increase risk of osteoarthritis.

A. Advanced age
B. Trauma
C. Overuse of joints
D. Genetic tendency
E. Obesity
F. Metabolic or endocrine abnormalities

III. The client/caregiver can recognize signs and symptoms of osteoarthritis.

A. Aching pain that increases with activity and is usually relieved with rest
B. Stiffness on rising
C. Heberden's nodes (nodular bony enlargements within the joint)
D. Fatigue
E. Decreased exercise tolerance
F. Crepitus (creaking or grating upon joint movement)
G. Restriction of joint movement

IV. The client/caregiver can list measures to prevent or manage osteoarthritis.

A. Exercise regularly.
   1. Always get physician's permission.
   2. Exercise daily at a slow steady pace using range of motion.
   3. Never exercise a hot, inflamed joint.

| NRS |
| DATE INITIAL |

   4. Set realistic goals.
   5. Balance work with rest.
   6. Stop exercise if pain occurs.
   7. Avoid prolonged walking, sitting, or standing.
B. Obtain adequate nutrition.
   1. Control weight to prevent increased pressure on the joints.
   2. Eat well-balanced meals.
   3. Avoid quackery diets.
   4. Avoid excess sugar and salt.
C. Use stress-management techniques.
D. Apply heat or cold as ordered by physician.
E. Follow safety measures to prevent falls and injury.
F. Take medications as ordered by physician.
   1. Discuss pain control issues with physician.
G. Use joint protection principals.
H. Use assistive and supportive devices as ordered (i.e., splints, braces, walker, and cane).
I. Use self-help hints and devices.
J. Follow good body mechanics and proper posture.
K. Obtain adequate rest.
L. Dress warmly and wear gloves in cold weather.
M. Report to physician increased pain, edema, or fatigue.
N. Keep follow-up appointments with physician.

V. The client/caregiver is aware of possible complications.

A. Loss of range of motion
B. Muscle wasting
C. Decreases mobility
D. Contractures

(Continued)

RESOURCES

American Chronic Pain Association
www.theacpa.org

Arthritis Foundation
www.arthritis.org

Healthy People 2010
www.health.gov/healthypeople

National Institute on Aging
www.nia.nih.gov/

National Institute of Arthritis and Musculoskeletal and Skin
Diseases
www.niams.nih.gov

REFERENCES

Ackley, B. J., & Ladwig, G. B. (2006). *Nursing diagnosis handbook: A guide to planning care.* St. Louis: Mosby Inc.

Canobbio, M. M. (2006). *Mosby's handbook of patient teaching.* St. Louis: Mosby Inc.

Cohen, B. J., & Taylor, J. J. (2005). *Memmler's the human body in health and disease* (10th ed.). Philadelphia: Lippincott Williams & Wilkins.

Lutz, C., & Przytulski, K. (2001). *Nutrition and diet therapy.* Philadelphia: F. A. Davis Company.

Taylor, C., Lillis, C., & LeMone, P. (2005). *Fundamentals of nursing.* Philadelphia: Lippincott, Williams & Wilkins.

4 Osteoporosis

Patient name: _____ Admission: _____

NRS
DATE INITIAL

I. **The client/caregiver can define osteoporosis.**

A. It is a bone disorder in which the reabsorption of bone exceeds the formation of bone.
B. It results in decreased bone mass and bone density causing bones to be brittle.

II. **The client/caregiver can list factors that increase risk.**

A. Menopause
B. Advancing age
C. Limited mobility or sedentary lifestyle
D. Alcohol and nicotine abuse (decreases calcium absorption and retention)
E. Family history
F. Eating disorders
G. Inadequate dietary intake of calcium
H. High intake of caffeine
I. Various diseases, such as liver or kidney disease and chronic obstructive pulmonary disease
J. Certain medications such as antacids, corticosteroids, and heparin
K. A diet low in calcium and vitamin D and high in phosphorous
L. Following bariatric surgery
M. Men, who can develop osteoporosis but much less often

III. **The client/caregiver can recognize signs and symptoms.**

A. Curvature of the spine
B. Loss of height
C. Backache
D. Frequent fractures—most often fractures of spine, hips, or wrists
E. Decreased density of bone
F. Decreased strength in muscles and joints

IV. **The client/caregiver can list measures to prevent or manage osteoporosis.**

A. Bone density tests for evaluation and diagnosis.
B. Exercise can help build bone strength and slow bone loss.

NRS
DATE INITIAL

Exercise suggestions
1. Do weight-bearing exercises such as walking, jogging, running, and stair climbing.
2. Avoid types of exercise that may increase fractures.
3. Increase exercise gradually, and plan regular rest periods.
4. Exercise in the sunlight to increase vitamin D.

C. Eat a well-balanced diet high in calcium, protein, and vitamin D.
1. Foods high in calcium include milk, yogurt, cheese, salmon, sardines, and dark green vegetables.
2. Sources of vitamin D include fortified milk, liver, butter, and eggs.
3. Sources of protein include eggs, milk, and meat.
4. Read labels for products enriched with calcium and vitamin D.
5. Take calcium and vitamin D supplements as ordered.
6. Limit caffeine.
7. Avoid excessive alcohol.
8. Add soy products to diet.
9. Drink plenty of fluids and increase fiber. Calcium supplements can cause gas and constipation. Start supplements gradually to help with these symptoms.

D. Follow safety precautions to prevent falls and injuries.
1. Use good body mechanics and proper posture.
2. Wear well-fitting nonskid shoes.
3. Use a cane or walker as indicated to prevent falls.
4. Use handrails.
5. Use good lighting and night lights.
6. Avoid clutter and keep walkways clear.

E. Use a firm, supportive mattress.
F. Take medications as ordered.
1. Discuss with your physician the benefits of hormone therapy for

(Continued)

you and your individual health
needs.
2. Discuss pain control issues.
G. Keep follow-up appointments with
physician.
H. Do not smoke.
I. Report to physician signs and symptoms of
deformity, pain, edema, decreased range of
motion, or paralysis.

V. **The client/caregiver is aware of possible
complications.**

A. Fractures
B. Respiratory compromise caused by
kyphosis (curved spine)
C. Bone deformity

RESOURCES

National Osteoporosis Foundation
www.nof.org/

National Institute on Aging
www.nihseniorhealth.gov

National Institute of Arthritis and Musculoskeletal and Skin
Diseases
www.niams.nih.gov

The National Women's Health Information Center
www.4woman.gov/

REFERENCES

Ackley, B. J., & Ladwig, G. B. (2006). *Nursing diagnosis
handbook: A guide to planning care.* St. Louis: Mosby
Inc.
Canobbio, M. M. (2006). *Mosby's handbook of patient teaching.*
St. Louis: Mosby Inc.
Cohen, B. J., & Taylor, J. J. (2005). *Memmler's the human body
in health and disease* (10th ed.). Philadelphia: Lippincott
Williams & Wilkins.
Lutz, C., & Przytulski, K. (2001). *Nutrition and diet therapy.*
Philadelphia: F. A. Davis Company.
Taylor, C., Lillis, C., & LeMone, P. (2005). *Fundamentals
of nursing.* Philadelphia: Lippincott, Williams &
Wilkins.

5 Osteomyelitis

Patient name: _____   Admission: _____

DATE | NRS INITIAL

I. **The client/caregiver can define osteomyelitis.**

A. It is an acute or chronic infection of the bone.
B. It can be difficult to cure because of limited blood supply and may persist for years.

II. **The client/caregiver can list possible causes.**

A. Direct infection caused by surgery, penetrating wound, or compound fracture.
B. Indirect infection caused by an infection elsewhere in the body.

III. **The client/caregiver can list signs and symptoms.**

A. Fever
B. Pain in the area of the infection
C. Warmth
D. Swelling and redness over the area of the infection
E. Tiredness
F. Drainage from an open wound near the area of the infection

IV. **The client/caregiver can list risk factors.**

A. Malnourishment
B. Older
C. Diseases that may cause decreased resistance (i.e., diabetes, kidney disease, liver cirrhosis, and rheumatoid arthritis)
D. Situations that can create more risk for bone infections are as follows:
- Illegally injectable drug use
- Dialysis
- Use of Foley catheters
- Central lines for intravenous therapies

V. **The client/caregiver can state measures for management of disease.**

A. Obtain adequate nutrition.
1. Eat foods high in vitamin D, B vitamin complex, vitamin C, phosphorous, and magnesium.

DATE | NRS INITIAL

2. Take vitamin and mineral supplements as needed.
3. Eat a well-balanced diet high in protein.
4. Drink fluids to 3 liters per day unless contraindicated.
B. Provide relief of pain.
1. Take pain medication as needed.
2. Splint or immobilize affected part as needed.
3. Use a foot cradle to keep weight of blankets off extremity.
4. Use good body alignment.
C. Prevent infection.
1. Avoid exposure to persons with infections.
2. Change dressing with sterile technique as instructed.
3. Use good hand-washing techniques.
D. Take medications as ordered (long-term antibiotic therapy).
E. Elevate extremity to decrease swelling.
F. Follow limited weight-bearing ambulation as ordered. Use assistive devices as instructed.
G. Plan frequent rest periods to promote healing.
H. Keep follow-up appointments with physician as instructed.
I. Report signs of infection's getting worse (i.e., additional tender areas, increase in fever, or increase in drainage).
J. Do not smoke. Smoking decreases blood flow to hands and feet.

VI. **The client/caregiver can list possible complications.**

A. Pathological fracture
B. Bone deformity
C. Sepsis
D. Bone abscess

(Continued)

RESOURCE

National Institute of Arthritis and Musculoskeletal and Skin
Diseases
www.niams.nih.gov

REFERENCES

Ackley, B. J., & Ladwig, G. B. (2006). *Nursing diagnosis handbook: A guide to planning care*. St. Louis: Mosby Inc.

Canobbio, M. M. (2006). *Mosby's handbook of patient teaching*. St. Louis: Mosby Inc.

Cohen, B. J., & Taylor, J. J. (2005). *Memmler's the human body in health and disease* (10th ed.). Philadelphia: Lippincott Williams & Wilkins.

Lutz, C., & Przytulski, K. (2001). *Nutrition and diet therapy*. Philadelphia: F. A. Davis Company.

Taylor, C., Lillis, C., & LeMone, P. (2005). *Fundamentals of nursing*. Philadelphia: Lippincott, Williams & Wilkins.

1 Alzheimer's Disease

Patient name: _____   **Admission:** _____

I. The client/caregiver can define Alzheimer's disease.

A. Alzheimer's disease is the most common cause of dementia.

B. Dementia is the loss of intellectual and social abilities severe enough to interfere with activities of daily living.

C. Healthy brain tissue degenerates and causes a steady decline in memory and mental abilities.

D. It leads to irreversible mental impairment. The person's ability to remember, reason, learn, and even imagine is destroyed.

E. The course of the disease varies, but 8 years is the average length of time from diagnosis to death.

F. Alzheimer's disease takes the mental ability to make decisions as the disease progresses. It is important to talk with client and family regarding advance directives and living wills when they are still able to express their decisions.

II. The client/caregiver can recognize signs and symptoms of Alzheimer's.

A. Increasing and persistent forgetfulness, eventually forgetting the names of family members and everyday objects

B. Difficulties with abstract thinking such as writing checks or even recognizing numbers

C. Difficulty finding the right word, meaning the inability to express thoughts and participate in conversation. The ability to read and write is eventually lost.

D. Loss of sense of time, dates, and surroundings

E. Loss of judgment and ability to plan and make decisions

F. Loss of ability to perform familiar tasks such as cooking, dressing, and so forth

G. Personality changes such as
- Mood swings
- Distrust in others
- Increased stubbornness and frustration
- Withdrawal from social situations

- Depression
- Restlessness
- Anxiety
- Aggressive or inappropriate behavior

III. The client/caregiver can list the stages of functional loss.

A. Stage I: early confusion
- Forgetful and loses or misplaces things
- Expresses awareness of loss (depression may be present)

B. Stage II: late confusion
- Increased difficulty with money, work, driving, housekeeping, and shopping
- Social withdrawal from routine activities and friends
- Increased fatigue and depression
- Denies symptoms of forgetfulness but also displays concern
- May require 24-hour supervision

C. Stage III: ambulatory dementia
- Increased loss of abilities to perform activities of daily living
- Worsening of symptoms as day progresses
- Withdrawal from family and friends
- Appears unaware of losses
- Increasing confusion and possibly agitation, wandering, pacing, and so forth
- Speech and writing difficult to understand

D. Stage IV: late-stage dementia
- Difficult or inability to ambulate
- Trouble eating, chewing, or swallowing
- Little or no recognition of caregivers or family
- Total dependence for physical care
- Loss of speech

IV. The client/caregiver can list risk factors for Alzheimer's disease.

A. Alzheimer's disease usually affects people older than 65 years.

B. The risk is higher if a first-degree relative has the disease.

(Continued)

C. Women are more likely than men to develop Alzheimer's disease (partially because they live longer).

D. Lifestyle choices such as poorly controlled diabetes, obesity, and inactivity can increase the risks.

E. Currently, there is no evidence that any particular substance is toxic or increases the risk for Alzheimer's disease.

F. Other risk factors that are being investigated are as follows:
- Difference in education levels
- History of head injury
- Hormone replacement therapy

V. **The client/caregiver can list possible complications in advanced stages.**

A. People with advanced Alzheimer's disease lose the ability to care for themselves and are prone to additional health problems, such as
- Pneumonia resulting from difficulty swallowing and possible aspiration
- Infections mainly caused by urinary incontinence and infections
- Falls resulting in fractures or head injuries
- Prolonged immobility, which increases the risk of blood clots

VI. **The client/caregiver can list possible triggers or causes for behavior problems such as agitation, aggression, and "sundowning."**

A. Physical discomfort caused by illness, injury, a lack of sleep, or negative reactions to medications

B. Overstimulation from noise or busy environment

C. Unfamiliar surroundings or people

D. Complicated task or unclear instructions

E. Change in routine or caregiver

F. Frustration caused by an impaired ability to communicate

G. Misperceived threats

VII. **The caregiver can list measures beneficial in care of the client with Alzheimer's disease.**

A. Measures to aid in general communication
1. Use good eye contact, and let them know that you are listening.
2. Allow time for person to think and speak. Do not interrupt.
3. Avoid criticizing, correcting, and arguing.
4. If you do not understand speech, ask them to point or gesture.
5. Approach a person from the front, and identify yourself.
6. Address the person by name.
7. Use short, simple words and sentences.
8. Ask one question at a time.
9. Avoid quizzing. Reminisce without demanding information or agreement.
10. Give simple explanations, but avoid trying logic and reason to gain acceptance.

B. Measures to decrease confusion, agitation, or aggression
1. Identify the immediate cause that could have triggered behavior.
2. Respond without anger or taking behavior personally.
3. Limit distractions.
4. Try relaxing activity such as music, massage, exercise, and so forth.
5. Shift focus or try something different.
6. Assess level of danger and act accordingly.
7. Unless the situation is critical, avoid using restraint or force.
8. Create calm environment (modify or move).
9. Avoid noise, glare, distractions, visitors, and so forth.
10. Check for pain, hunger, thirst, full bladder, fatigue, and so forth.
11. Simplify tasks and routines.
12. Provide outlet for energy such as exercise or taking a walk.

C. Measures to manage confusion
1. Stay calm.
2. Show photos or reminders of important relationships or places.
3. Do not make corrections, but suggest the correct answer.

D. Measures to reduce "sundowning" (evening agitation and nighttime sleeplessness)
1. Plan active days and discourage afternoon napping.
2. Monitor diet. Restrict sugar and caffeine intake. Serve dinner early and offer a light meal before bedtime.

(Continued)

NRS
DATE INITIAL

3. Allow a person to sleep wherever comfortable. Keep room partially lit to reduce agitation from a dark or unfamiliar place.
4. Establish a daily routine, but be flexible when needed.
5. Use warm baths, back rubs, aromatherapy, quiet music, and so forth.

E. Measures to promote self-esteem
1. Encourage independence.
2. Allow time needed for bathing, dressing, eating, and so forth.
3. Show acceptance verbally and nonverbally.
4. Encourage socialization.

F. Measures to promote good nutrition
1. Present one course at a time.
2. Offer snacks and fluids frequently.
3. Give high-calorie, high-fiber, nutritious meals.
4. Provide finger foods as needed.
5. Make sure dentures or dental appliances fit properly. Make sure that they are used. Label them to prevent loss.
6. Review medications for possible impact on appetite.
7. Reduce distractions at meal time.
8. Allow plenty of time to eat.
9. Choose dinnerware that is without pattern but brightly colored.
10. Choose foods that contrast with the color of the plate.
11. Be careful when serving hot foods and drinks.

G. Measures to use if client is "wandering" or "exit seeking"
1. The Alzheimer's Association Safe Return program is designed to help identify people who wander and become lost locally or far from home and return them to caregiver.
2. Many skilled care facilities and long-term care facilities have a specialty unit that is secure, and they have staff with special training to deal with clients with dementia.

H. Measures to promote independence in self-care
1. Use home safety teaching guide to evaluate environment for safety factors.
2. Give assistance only as needed.

NRS
DATE INITIAL

3. Give verbal cues as needed.
4. Bathing suggestions
   a. Find a time of day and method of bathing (shower versus tub) that the client prefers. Be flexible, and never force someone.
   b. Keep bathroom warm and towels convenient.
   c. Maintain privacy and dignity.
   d. Explain each step and allow them to participate.
5. Dressing suggestions
   a. Limit choices. Clear closet of rarely worn clothes.
   b. Provide directions or give cues regarding dressing.
   c. Do not rush the process.
   d. Do not argue over selections whenever possible.
   e. Use clothing that has elastic waists or fabric closure (Velcro).
6. Toileting suggestions
   a. Place sign or picture of a toilet on the door to make it easy to find.
   b. Observe for signs of restlessness or tugging at clothes that may signal the need to use the bathroom.
   c. Create a schedule. Take the person to the bathroom before and after meals and every 2 hours in between.
   d. Use easy-to-open clothing.

VIII. **The caregiver can list resources specific to their needs.**

A. Be informed and learn as much about the disease as possible.
B. Take care of your own physical and mental health. Signs of caregiver stress are
   • Depressed mood
   • Frequent crying
   • A decrease in energy
   • Sleeping too little or too much
   • Unintended weight gain or loss
   • Increased irritability and anger
C. Ask friends, family, and others for help when needed.
D. Join a support group of other caregivers.
E. Seek counseling or help from clergy.
F. Connect to referrals for home care agencies, nursing care facilities, respite care, educational seminars, and so forth.

(Continued)

IX. **The caregiver can list types of in-home care services.**

A. Companion services

B. Personal care or home health aide services to assist with bathing, dressing, toileting, and exercising.

C. Homemaker or maid services to help with laundry, shopping, and preparing meals.

D. Skilled care services can help with medications, treatment, and health assessments.

E. Adult day care center is a place where the client can be in a safe environment during the day. Planned activities, meals, and transportation are often provided.

RESOURCES

Administration on Aging
www.aoa.dhhs.gov

Centers for Medicare and Medicaid Services
www.cms.hhs.gov

Alzheimer's Association
24-hour contact center, 800-272-3900

National Institute on Aging
www.nia.nih.gov

Alzheimer's Disease Education and Referral Center
www.nia.nih.gov/Alzheimers/

National Association of Adult Day Care
www.nadsa.org/adsfacts

Alzheimer's Association Safe Return
A nationwide identification, support, and enrollment program that provides assistance when a person with Alzheimer's disease or a related dementia wanders and becomes lost locally or far from home.

Support group

Respite care

REFERENCES

Ackley, B. J., & Ladwig, G. B. (2006). *Nursing diagnosis handbook: A guide to planning care.* St. Louis: Mosby Inc.

Canobbio, M. M. (2006). *Mosby's handbook of patient teaching.* St. Louis: Mosby Inc.

Cohen, B. J., & Taylor, J. J. (2005). *Memmler's the human body in health and disease* (10th ed.). Philadelphia: Lippincott Williams & Wilkins.

Home safety for people with Alzheimer's disease. (2005, February). U.S. Department of Health and Human Services. National Institute of Health. National Institute on Aging. NIH Publication No.02-5179. Washington, DC.

Hunt, R. (2005). *Introduction to community based nursing.* Philadelphia: Lippincott Williams & Wilkins.

Lutz, C., & Przytulski, K. (2001). *Nutrition and diet therapy.* Philadelphia: F. A. Davis Company.

Taylor, C., Lillis, C., & LeMone, P. (2005). *Fundamentals of nursing.* Philadelphia: Lippincott, Williams & Wilkins.

Timby, B. K. (2005). *Fundamental nursing skills and concepts.* Philadelphia: J. B. Lippincott Williams & Wilkins.

2 Dementia/Delirium

Patient name: _____ **Admission:** _____

NRS
DATE INITIAL

I. **The caregiver can define dementia and delirium.**

A. Dementia is any condition that creates a decline in memory and other mental functions that is severe enough to affect the daily life.
B. Dementia shows as a gradual, irreversible loss of intellectual abilities.
C. Delirium has similar symptoms but
    - Has sudden onset
    - Is temporary
    - Is curable after specific cause is treated
D. Various conditions are characterized by dementia, such as
    - Alzheimer's disease
    - Parkinson's disease
    - Cerebrovascular disorders
E. Delirium can be caused by
    - Drugs or alcohol abuse
    - Infection (usually urinary or respiratory infections)
    - Medication changes or new combinations
    - Sleep deprivation
    - Electrolyte imbalances (such as severe dehydration)
    - Cardiac or respiratory problems
    - Urinary of fecal problems
    - Complications of medical illness, recovery, or surgery

II. **The caregiver can list signs and symptoms of dementia.**

A. Loss of memory
B. Loss of intellect
C. Loss of judgment
D. Disorientation
E. Anger, agitation, anxiety, and depression
F. Sundowning syndrome (confusion increases at night)
G. Decreased attention span
H. Limited speech

NRS
DATE INITIAL

III. **The caregiver can list measures to decrease confusion.**

A. Follow a routine.
B. Do not rearrange furniture.
C. Label objects.
D. Clarify misperceptions.
E. Reorient as needed.
F. Use clocks, calendars, etc.
G. Remind client to wear glasses/hearing aids.
H. Write reminder notes.
I. Provide adequate lighting.

IV. **The caregiver can list measures to decrease verbal and physical aggression.**

A. Reduce sensory stimulation.
B. Redirect to another room or activity.
C. Praise good behavior.
D. Encourage timeout.
E. Reduce stimuli (lights, noise, etc.).

V. **The caregiver can state measures to increase independence in activities of daily living.**

A. Keep choices of clothing to a minimum.
B. Give verbal cues as needed.
C. Give finger foods.
D. Give one bowl at a time at mealtime.
E. Give assistance only as needed.
F. Use clothing that has elastic waists or Velcro for closures.

VI. **The caregiver can state measures to promote safety.**

A. Precautions while eating
    1. Use unbreakable dishes.
B. Poison prevention
    1. Keep medications out of reach.
    2. Do not keep poisonous plants in the house.
    3. Keep poison control number within reach.

(Continued)

C. Prevention of burns
  1. Keep water temperature 120°F or less to prevent burns.
  2. Watch closely with hot beverages—may use thermal cup with a lid.
  3. Watch closely if smoking.
D. Prevention of falls
  1. Avoid throw rugs.
  2. Assist with walking as needed.
  3. Place gate in front of stairs.
  4. Use low-heeled, nonskid shoes.
E. Prevention of cuts or injuries
  1. Keep sharp objects out of reach.
F. Prevention of client getting lost
  1. Use alarms on doors.
  2. Use identification bracelet.
  3. Place pictures on doors of each room to identify.
G. Prevention of medication errors
  1. Use pill box for early stages.
  2. Keep medications in locked cupboard.

RESOURCES

National Association of Adult Day Care
www.nadsa.org/adsfacts

National Institute on Aging
www.nia.nih.gov

Alzheimer's Disease and Related Disorders Association
800-621-0379

REFERENCES

Ackley, B. J., & Ladwig, G. B. (2006). *Nursing diagnosis handbook: A guide to planning care.* St. Louis: Mosby Inc.

Canobbio, M. M. (2006). *Mosby's handbook of patient teaching.* St. Louis: Mosby Inc.

Cohen, B. J., & Taylor, J. J. (2005). *Memmler's the human body in health and disease* (10th ed.). Philadelphia: Lippincott Williams & Wilkins.

Timby, B. K. (2005). *Fundamental nursing skills and concepts.* Philadelphia: J. B. Lippincott Williams & Wilkins.

Timby, B. K., & Smith, N. C. (2003). *Introductory medical-surgical nursing* (8th ed.). Philadelphia: J. B. Lippincott Williams & Wilkins.

3 Amyotrophic Lateral Sclerosis (Lou Gehrig Disease)

Patient name: _____

Admission: _____

NRS
DATE INITIAL

I. **The client/caregiver can define amyotrophic lateral sclerosis or Lou Gehrig disease.**

A. It is a motor neuron disease affecting nerves of brain and/or spinal cord with progressive degeneration.
B. Death frequently occurs from respiratory failure in 2 to 5 years.
C. The onset of the disease usually occurs in middle age.

II. **The client/caregiver can list signs and symptoms of disease.**

A. Muscle weakness and atrophy
B. Cramping
C. Incoordination of hand and fingers
D. Slurred speech
E. Loss of reflexes
F. Difficulty swallowing
G. Fatigue
H. Spasticity of muscles

III. **The client/caregiver can list measures to promote independence and maintain muscle strength.**

A. Participate in physical and occupational therapy as ordered.
B. Plan activities with rest periods to avoid overexertion.
C. Use adaptive devices to promote independence in activities of daily living.
D. Use assistive devices to promote mobility (i.e., wheelchair, lift chair, and walker).

IV. **The client/caregiver can list measures to meet nutritional needs due to difficulty swallowing.**

A. Adjust diet consistency as needed.
B. Use a high-calorie, high-protein diet.

NRS
DATE INITIAL

C. Allow ample time for eating.
D. Sit in upright position to eat, and do not lie down after eating.
E. Discuss use of feeding tube when unable to take food by mouth.
F. Keep suction equipment nearby.
G. Weigh weekly.

V. **The client/caregiver can list measures to promote communications.**

A. Speech therapy
B. Communication boards or alternative methods of communication
C. Cognitive abilities are not altered.
D. Encourage client to participate in plan of care and urge expressing feeling to condition.
E. Encourage client to plan for future, such as advance directives, living will, and hospice.

VI. **The client/caregiver can list measures to avoid complications.**

A. Avoid people with upper-respiratory infections to prevent infection.
B. Provide good skin care and positioning to prevent breakdown.
C. Provide good oral care.

VII. **The client/caregiver can state possible complications.**

A. Respiratory infection
B. Respiratory failure
C. Use of mechanical ventilation
D. Injury
E. Aspiration pneumonia

(Continued)

RESOURCES

ALS Association
www.alsa.org

National Institute of Neurological Disorders and Stroke
*www.ninds.nih.gov/disorders/amyotrophiclateralsclerosis/
amyotrophiclateralsclerosis*

Support groups for client and caregiver

Agencies for help in provision of home care

Sources of financial assistance

Counseling

REFERENCES

Ackley, B. J., & Ladwig, G. B. (2006). *Nursing diagnosis handbook: A guide to planning care.* St. Louis: Mosby Inc.

Canobbio, M. M. (2006). *Mosby's handbook of patient teaching.* St. Louis: Mosby Inc.

Cohen, B. J., & Taylor, J. J. (2005). *Memmler's the human body in health and disease* (10th ed.). Philadelphia: Lippincott Williams & Wilkins.

Timby, B. K., & Smith, N. C. (2003). *Introductory medical-surgical nursing* (8th ed.). Philadelphia: J. B. Lippincott Williams & Wilkins.

Cerebrovascular Accident (Stroke)/ Transient Ischemic Attack

4

Patient name: _____ Admission: _____

I. **The client/caregiver can define cerebral vascular accident or stroke.**

A. It is a loss of brain function resulting from a disruption of oxygen supply (blood) to a part of the brain.

B. Causes of cerebrovascular accident are
1. Ischemic strokes are caused by a blood clot that blocks the blood flow to area of the brain causing damage.
   - Thrombosis (atherosclerosis, hypertension, and hematologic disorders are typical causes)
   - Embolus (atrial fibrillation, extracranial clot formation, and valvular heart disease are typical causes)
2. Hemorrhagic strokes are usually caused by the rupture of a blood vessel that can block blood flow to the brain and result in destruction of brain tissue. Hypertension, aneurysm, trauma, vacular malformation, and so forth can be responsible for this type of stroke.

C. Damage from a stroke depends on the location of the blockage and the extent of tissue damage.

D. Stroke is the third leading cause of death in the United States.

II. **The client/caregiver can define transient ischemic attack.**

A. It is caused by a temporary decrease in blood supply (oxygen) to a part of the brain.

B. Signs and symptoms vary depending on the area of the brain affected.

C. Signs and symptoms resolve within 24 hours, causing no permanent damage.

D. They can be considered a warning sign of impending cerebral vascular accident and should be evaluated promptly.

E. At least one third of persons with transient ischemic attacks will have a stroke in the next 3 to 5 years.

III. **The client/caregiver can list factors that increase risk of cerebral vascular accident.**

A. Noncontrollable factors
1. Advancing age
2. Positive family history
3. Race (blacks have a higher incidence than whites)
4. Gender (men have a higher incidence than women)
5. History of prior stroke

B. Controllable factors
1. Hypertension
2. Obesity
3. Diabetes mellitus
4. Physical inactivity
5. Elevated blood cholesterol
6. Smoking
7. Oral contraceptives
8. Alcohol consumption abuse

IV. **The client/caregiver can list signs and symptoms of a stroke. Knowing these symptoms will enable prompt evaluation and treatment. The symptoms can be the same for transient ischemic attacks but last for a shorter period of time and then disappear.**

A. Sudden numbness, weakness, or paralysis of face, arm, or leg (usually only on one side of the body)

B. Sudden blurred, double, or decreased vision

C. Sudden difficulty speaking or understanding speech

D. Sudden dizziness and loss of balance or coordination

E. Confusion or problems with memory

F. Sudden severe and unusual headache with stiff neck, facial pain, vomiting, or altered consciousness

V. **The client/caregiver can list possible effects of a stroke, which depend on size and location of the injury.**

A. Physical effects
- Muscles that involuntarily contract (spasticity), creating stiffness and tightness

(Continued)

NRS
DATE INITIAL

- Forty percent of stroke survivors have balance problems
- Weakness or paralysis of one side of body (hemiplegia)
- Defects in vision: hemianopia, which is seeing only half of the normal vision field
- Bowel and bladder incontinence

B. Communication and swallowing
- Expressive aphasia—inability to speak
- Receptive aphasia—inability to understand spoken or written language, damage to language center of brain
- Dysarthria (slurred speech)
- Agnosia—inability to recognize familiar people or objects
- Dysphagia (swallowing problems)
- Short retention of information
- Difficulty with new learning and impaired short-term memory
- Problems with abstract thinking

C. Behavioral
- Depression
- One-sided neglect
- Changes in thinking, memory, solving problems, and communication challenges, which can be frustrating to person
- Easily distracted
- Impulsive behavior or slow, cautious behavior

VI. **The client/caregiver can list measures to prevent a stroke.**

A. Use diet that is low in saturated fat and cholesterol. Cholesterol-lowering medication may be prescribed by physician.
B. Do not smoke.
C. If a diabetic, use good management techniques.
D. Maintain healthy weight. Lose weight if necessary.
E. Exercise regularly.
F. Reduce stress.
G. Drink only in moderation.
H. Avoid use of illicit drugs.
I. Discuss risk of using oral contraceptives with physician.
J. The American Heart Association recommends that risk factor screening (blood pressure, body mass index, waist

NRS
DATE INITIAL

circumference, and pulse every 2 years) and cholesterol and glucose testing should be done every 5 years after the patient is 20 years old.

VII. **The client/caregiver can list measures important in treatment of stroke.**

A. Encouragement and early treatment, which are important
B. Early rehabilitation program, including physical therapy, occupational therapy, and speech therapy
C. Active and passive range of motion exercises
D. Prevention of skin breakdown
E. Bowel and bladder training
F. Good nutrition
G. Emotional support
H. Safe environment
I. The use of adaptive equipment for eating, toileting, mobility, and communication

VIII. **The client/caregiver can list possible complications.**

A. Seizures
B. Contractures and pressure sores
C. Aspiration
D. Respiratory and cardiac complications
E. Thrombophlebitis

RESOURCES

American Stroke Association
www.strokeassociation.org

National Institute of Neurological Disorders and Stroke
National Stroke Association
www.stroke.org/

American Heart Association
www.americanheart.org

Support group

Administration on Aging
www.aoa.dhhs.gov

(Continued)

Centers for Medicare & Medicaid Services
www.cms.hhs.gov

National Institute on Aging
www.nia.nih.gov

REFERENCES

Ackley, B. J., & Ladwig, G. B. (2006). *Nursing diagnosis handbook: A guide to planning care.* St. Louis: Mosby Inc.

Canobbio, M. M. (2006). *Mosby's handbook of patient teaching.* St. Louis: Mosby Inc.

Cohen, B. J., & Taylor, J. J. (2005). *Memmler's the human body in health and disease* (10th ed.). Philadelphia: Lippincott Williams & Wilkins.

Lutz, C., & Przytulski, K. (2001). *Nutrition and diet therapy.* Philadelphia: F. A. Davis Company.

Timby, B. K., & Smith, N. C. (2003). *Introductory medical-surgical nursing* (8th ed.). Philadelphia: J. B. Lippincott Williams & Wilkins.

5

Head Injury

Patient name: _____   Admission: _____

I. **The client/caregiver can list general facts about head injury.**

A. It causes about 80,000 deaths per year.
B. Half of traumatic brain injuries are caused by collisions involving cars, motorcycles, or bicycles.
C. It is the major cause of death in individuals who are 1 to 35 years old but affects all ages.
D. Infants and small children can receive brain injuries as a result of being shaken violently.
E. The brain swells after injury, causing pressure.
F. The risk of traumatic brain injury is highest in children (0 to 4 years old) and adolescents (15 to 19 years old).
G. All persons with head injuries should be examined by a physician.

II. **The client/caregiver can list various types of head injury.**

A. Scalp injury—lacerations, abrasions, and hematomas
B. Skull fractures—may have drainage from ears and nose, headache, hearing impairment, bruising around the eyes
C. Concussions—may cause amnesia, headache, nausea, vomiting, dizziness, and a loss of consciousness for 5 minutes or less
D. Contusions—may cause mental changes, paresis or paralysis, unequal pupils
E. Subdural hematoma—blood that accumulates between brain and skull

III. **The client/caregiver can list symptoms of a mild brain injury.**

A. Brief period of unconsciousness
B. Headache
C. Confusion
D. Dizziness
E. Blurred vision, ringing in the ears, or a bad taste in the mouth

F. Mood changes
G. Memory or concentration problems

IV. **The client/caregiver can list signs and symptoms of a moderate or severe injury.**

A. Persistent headache
B. Repeated vomiting or nausea
C. Convulsions or seizures
D. Inability to awaken from sleep
E. Dilation of one or both pupils of the eyes
F. Slurred speech
G. Weakness or numbness in the extremities
H. A loss of coordination
I. Increased confusion or agitation

V. **The client/caregiver can list symptoms and signs to watch for in a child with a brain injury.**

A. They may refuse to eat.
B. They may appear listless or cranky.
C. Sleep patterns and performance in school may change.

VI. **The client/caregiver can list symptoms that indicate need for evaluation by a physician.**

A. Increased confusion, lethargy, and behavior changes
B. Incoordination, weakness in extremities
C. Leakage of clear fluid from ear, nose, or throat
D. Visual changes, blurred vision, double vision, and so forth
E. Change in judgment, memory, and concentration
F. Slurred speech
G. Change in size of one pupil
H. Vomiting
I. Restlessness

VII. **The client/caregiver can list measures to prevent brain injuries.**

A. Always use seat belts in motor vehicle. Use appropriate car seats for children.

(Continued)

B. Never drive under the influence of drugs or alcohol.

C. Store firearms (unloaded) in locked cabinet. Store bullets somewhere else.

D. Wear helmets when
  • Riding bike, skateboard, motorcycle, snowmobile, or all-terrain vehicles
  • Batting or running bases or playing contact sports

E. Use home safety teaching guide to safety proof home for adults and children.

F. Inspect playground equipment and supervise children using it.

G. Regular vision tests can reduce risk of falling.

VIII. The client/caregiver can state measures for management of a head injury.

A. Give medications as ordered and report any side effects.

B. Keep follow-up appointments with physician and therapists.

C. Avoid alcohol, driving, unsupervised smoking, and the use of hazardous equipment.

IX. The client/caregiver can state possible complications.

A. Coma

B. Seizures

C. Infections (meningitis most common)

D. Nerve damage to facial muscles or nerves involving eye movements

E. Cognitive losses (short-term memory is most common)

F. Sensory problems (clumsy, double vision, taste, and smell changes)

G. Swallowing problems

H. Trouble with spoken and written language

I. Personality change (impulse control and inappropriate behavior common)

RESOURCES

Brain Injury Association of America
www.biausa.org

Counseling for prolonged stress to the family

Rehabilitation centers

Agencies for financial assistance

REFERENCES

Ackley, B. J., & Ladwig, G. B. (2006). *Nursing diagnosis handbook: A guide to planning care.* St. Louis: Mosby Inc.

Canobbio, M. M. (2006). *Mosby's handbook of patient teaching.* St. Louis: Mosby Inc.

Cohen, B. J., & Taylor, J. J. (2005). *Memmler's the human body in health and disease* (10th ed.). Philadelphia: Lippincott Williams & Wilkins.

Perry, A., & Potter, P. (2006). *Clinical nursing skills & technique.* St. Louis: Mosby Inc.

6   Multiple Sclerosis

Patient name: _____   **Admission:** _____

NRS
DATE INITIAL

I.   **The client/caregiver can define multiple sclerosis.**

A. It is a progressive degenerative disease caused by the destruction of the myelin sheath of the nerve tissue, which interrupts nerve impulses.
B. It is characterized by remissions and exacerbations.
C. It usually affects adults between the ages of 20 and 40 years.

II.   **The client/caregiver can list factors that increase risk of multiple sclerosis.**

A. Cool, temperate climates
B. Allergic reactions to infections
C. Familial tendency
D. Viral infection

III.   **The client/caregiver can recognize signs and symptoms.**

A. Slow, monotonous slurred speech
B. Visual disturbances
C. Weakness of lower extremities
D. Dizziness
E. Numbness or tingling in extremities
F. Bladder or bowel dysfunction
G. Impaired sense of touch and pain
H. Spasticity of muscles
I. Mood swings
J. Fatigue
K. Difficulty swallowing or chewing
L. Poor coordination, staggering gait
M. Spasticity of extremities

IV.   **The client/caregiver can list measures for management of multiple sclerosis.**

A. Avoid factors that can cause exacerbation:
   1. Infections
   2. Excess heat: hot tubs or sauna
   3. Excess cold
   4. Physical and emotional stress
   5. Pregnancy
   6. Trauma
B. Exercise regularly with frequent rest periods.
C. Plan regular rest periods to avoid fatigue.
D. Take medications as prescribed.

NRS
DATE INITIAL

E. Avoid over-the-counter medications unless recommended by physician.
F. Consider air conditioning for home.
G. Eat a well-balanced, high-fiber diet with fluid intake of at least six to eight glasses per day to promote bowel function.
H. Use safety measures to prevent injury (safety measures teaching guide).
I. Use assistive and self-help devices as needed to promote maximum independence.
J. Keep follow-up appointments with physician and therapists.
K. Continue hobbies and social interests as tolerated.
L. Be aware of signs of depression and how to seek help.
M. Use stress-management techniques.
N. Report any early signs and symptoms of urinary tract or respiratory infections.
O. Practice bladder and bowel retraining.
P. Wear Medic Alert bracelet.

V.   **The client/caregiver is aware of possible complications.**

A. Renal insufficiency
B. Respiratory infections
C. Suicidal tendencies from depression
D. Falls
E. Constipation
F. Incontinence
G. Urinary tract infections

RESOURCES

National Multiple Sclerosis Society
www.NationalMSSociety.org

Counseling, including sexual counseling

REFERENCES

Ackley, B. J., & Ladwig, G. B. (2006). *Nursing diagnosis handbook: A guide to planning care.* St. Louis: Mosby Inc.

Canobbio, M. M. (2006). *Mosby's handbook of patient teaching.* St. Louis: Mosby Inc.

Cohen, B. J., & Taylor, J. J. (2005). *Memmler's the human body in health and disease* (10th ed.). Philadelphia: Lippincott Williams & Wilkins.

Timby, B. K., & Smith, N. C. (2003). *Introductory medical-surgical nursing* (8th ed.). Philadelphia: J. B. Lippincott Williams & Wilkins.

7 Parkinson's Disease

Patient name: _____ Admission: _____

I. The client/caregiver can define Parkinson's disease.

A. It is a chronic, progressive central nervous system disorder caused by a defect in the cells of the brain that produce dopamine.
B. Dopamine is a chemical substance that enables nerve cells to send messages to other nerve cells.
C. It affects the voluntary muscles causing difficulty with movement and posture.
D. Emotional stress, infection, overwork, and exposure to cold can make symptoms worse.

II. The client/caregiver can list possible risk factors.

A. Carbon monoxide and manganese poisoning
B. Encephalitis
C. Positive family history
D. Tumors of the midbrain
E. Men more likely to have Parkinson's than women
F. Exposure to pesticides and herbicides

III. The client/caregiver can recognize signs and symptoms, which usually begin slowly on one side.

A. Muscle rigidity and weakness
B. Tremors that decrease on purposeful movements
C. Slowed movements
D. Rigid muscles, which are most often seen in limbs and neck and create a mask-like facial expression
E. Loss of automatic movements like blinking, smiling, and swinging arms when walking
F. Impaired balance
G. Shuffling gait and stooped posture
H. Slow, soft, and possibly mumbling speech
I. Difficulty swallowing
J. Dementia, including memory loss, impaired judgment, and personality changes

IV. The client/caregiver can list measures to manage disease.

A. Activity measures
 1. Exercise daily with regular rest periods. Pace yourself.
 2. Pick time to exercise when medication is working well.
 3. Stretch before and after exercise to prevent stiffness and improve flexibility.
 4. Evaluate home environment for potential dangers.
 5. Wear good pair of walking shoes, not running shoes.
 6. Practice taking long steps, and stand up straight with your head over your hips and feet 8 to 10 inches apart.
 7. Advise to use cane or other assistive device for help with balance.
 8. Keep appointments for therapy. Ask physician or physical therapist about exercises that improve balance (especially tai chi).
B. Measures to help with speech
 1. Do speech therapy as indicated.
 2. Face the person you are talking to.
 3. Deliberately speak louder than you think is necessary.
 4. Practice reading or reciting out loud, focusing on your breathing.
 5. Speak for yourself—do not let others speak for you.
C. Measures to help nutrition
 1. Eat small, frequent meals to prevent exhaustion.
 2. Eat a high-calorie diet to prevent weight loss.
 3. Eat a high-fiber diet to prevent constipation. Eat plenty of fruits, vegetables, and whole grains to boost fiber content.
 4. If using fiber supplement, be sure to start gradually and drink plenty of fluids (up to 2,000 ml per day).
 5. Avoid caffeine.

(Continued)

NRS
DATE INITIAL

D. Measures to help with dressing
   1. Allow plenty of time to dress.
   2. Lay clothes nearby.
   3. Use clothes that can be slipped on easily (sweat pants, dresses, or pants with elastic waistbands).
   4. Wear clothes and shoes with fabric fasteners (Velcro, etc.) or replace buttons with fabric fasteners.
E. Build and maintain support system.
F. Engage in social and diversional activities to promote emotional and physical well-being.
G. Minimize work-related stress. The Americans with Disabilities Act requires your employer to make reasonable accommodations.
H. Keep follow-up appointments with physician.
I. Medication considerations
   1. Take as ordered.
   2. Schedule taking medications to achieve peak effect when mobility needed.
   3. Use of chewing gum or eating hard candy to ease mouth dryness (possible side effect of medication).
J. Wear a medical alert bracelet.

V. **The client/caregiver is aware of possible complications.**

A. Injury from falls
B. Urinary problems
C. Constipation
D. Depression
E. Sleep disorders
F. Sexual dysfunction
G. Medication to treat Parkinson's may cause side effects:
   • Involuntary twitching or jerking movements of arms and legs
   • Hallucinations

NRS
DATE INITIAL

   • Sleepiness
   • Orthostatic hypotension (drop in blood pressure when standing up)

RESOURCES

Parkinson's Disease Foundation
www.pdf.org

American Parkinson Disease Association
www.apdaparkinson.org

National Parkinson Foundation
www.parkinson.org

National Institute of Neurological Disorders and Stroke

Local support groups

Counseling/clergy

Americans with Disabilities Act
800-514-0301
www.usdoj.gov/crt/ada/adahom1.htm

REFERENCES

Ackley, B. J., & Ladwig, G. B. (2006). *Nursing diagnosis handbook: A guide to planning care.* St. Louis: Mosby Inc.

Canobbio, M. M. (2006). *Mosby's handbook of patient teaching.* St. Louis: Mosby Inc.

Cohen, B. J., & Taylor, J. J. (2005). *Memmler's the human body in health and disease* (10th ed.). Philadelphia: Lippincott Williams & Wilkins.

Lutz, C., & Przytulski, K. (2001). *Nutrition and diet therapy.* Philadelphia: F. A. Davis Company.

Timby, B. K., & Smith, N. C. (2003). *Introductory medical-surgical nursing* (8th ed.). Philadelphia: J. B. Lippincott Williams & Wilkins.

8   Epilepsy/Seizure

Patient name: _____   **Admission:** _____

I.   **The client/caregiver can define epilepsy and seizure.**

   A.   Epilepsy is a chronic neurological disorder with repeated occurrence of any form of seizure activity.
   B.   Seizures (convulsions) are episodes of abnormal electrical brain activity that produces involuntary muscle contractions.
   C.   These involuntary muscle contraction can cause
   • Disturbances of consciousness
   • Disturbances in behavior
   • Disturbances in sensation
   • Disturbances in anatomic functions
   D.   About 10% of Americans will experience a seizure sometime in their life.
   E.   About 30% will have had a diagnosis of epilepsy by the age of 80 years.

II.   **The client/caregiver can list factors, causes, and risk factors.**

   A.   Idiopathic (no specific cause identified)
   B.   Brain tumor
   C.   Trauma
   D.   Infections (encephalitis and meningitis)
   E.   Fever
   F.   Drug and alcohol intoxication
   G.   Metabolic and nutritional disorders
   H.   Genetic factors
   I.   Toxins
   J.   Extreme fatigue
   K.   Flashing lights

III.   **The client/caregiver can recognize signs and symptoms of various types of seizures.**

   A.   General
   • Involuntary recurrent muscle movements
   • Jerking, patting, and rubbing
   • Sudden contractions of muscle groups
   • Fluttering of eyelids
   • Lip smacking
   • Movements confined to one area or spreading from one side to the other
   • Head and eyes deviating to the side

   B.   Specific
   • Tonic-clonic (grand mal) lasting 2 to 5 minutes. Tonic phase is when the body stiffens. Clonic phase alternates between muscle spasm and relaxation.
   • Other signs are tongue biting, incontinence, dyspnea, apnea, and cyanosis.
   • After seizure is postictal stage with sleepiness and confusion.
   C.   Petit mal
   • Lasts 5 to 30 minutes
   • Blinking, rolling eyes, and blank stare

IV.   **The client/caregiver can explain course of action during and after a grand mal seizure.**

   A.   Remain calm.
   B.   Never try to restrain the client. Prevent or break fall by easing to ground.
   C.   Never leave client alone.
   D.   Note the time and type of seizure activity.
   E.   Do not place anything in person's mouth.
   F.   Protect head by clearing area and place padding.
   G.   After seizure, turn person on side to avoid aspiration.
   H.   Loosen tight clothing.
   I.   Call physician and report seizure activity.
   J.   Maintain quiet environment.
   K.   Reassure and reorient the person.

V.   **The client/caregiver can explain course of action during and after a petit mal seizure.**

   A.   Remain with the person. Do not attempt to awaken or startle them.
   B.   Person will resume normal activity when seizure is over.

VI.   **The client/caregiver can list additional measures to prevent or manage seizures.**

   A.   Take medications as ordered, and avoid over-the-counter medications without approval by physician.
   B.   Keep follow-up appointments with physician.

(Continued)

NRS
DATE INITIAL

C. Identify and avoid possible precipitating factors such as stress, alcohol, fatigue, and so forth.

D. Identify and avoid stimuli that can trigger seizure activity such as flashing lights or loud music.

E. Advise the person to lower water heater temperature to avoid burns if seizure occurs during shower/bath.

F. Check state regulations regarding driving an automobile.

G. Avoid using heavy equipment or dangerous equipment until cleared by physician.

H. Seek vocational counseling or job retraining if needed.

I. For females of childbearing age, discuss risks and options of pregnancy with healthcare provider.

J. Eat a well-balanced diet, avoiding caffeine and alcohol. Space meals and snacks throughout the day to avoid hypo-glycemia.

K. Avoid activities that create excessive visual stimulation such as video games and the use of computer for long periods of time.

L. Wear a Medic Alert bracelet.

NRS
DATE INITIAL

VII. The client/caregiver is aware of possible complications.

A. Status epilepticus (rapid succession of seizures)

B. Physical injury (fracture, tongue or lip laceration)

C. Respiratory impairment

RESOURCES

Epilepsy Foundation of America
www.epilepsyfoundation.org/

Centers for Disease Control and Prevention
www.cdc.gov/epilepsy/resources.htm

National Institute of Neurologic Disorders and Stroke
www.ninds.nih.gov

REFERENCES

Ackley, B. J., & Ladwig, G. B. (2006). *Nursing diagnosis handbook: A guide to planning care.* St. Louis: Mosby Inc.

Canobbio, M. M. (2006). *Mosby's handbook of patient teaching.* St. Louis: Mosby Inc.

Cohen, B. J., & Taylor, J. J. (2005). *Memmler's the human body in health and disease* (10th ed.). Philadelphia: Lippincott Williams & Wilkins.

9   Spinal Cord Injury

Patient name: _____   Admission: _____

NRS DATE INITIAL

I. The client/caregiver can define spinal cord injury.

A. It is an injury to the spinal cord causing loss of function.
1. Paraplegia—paralyzed from the waist down—C7 to T12/L1.
2. Quadriplegia—paralyzed from the neck down—injury above cervical 7.
B. It frequently results from accidents.
C. Causes and risk factors for spinal cord injury are as follows:
- Motor vehicle accidents
- Diving or sports accidents
- Industrial accidents
- Falls
- Assaults (including gun shot wounds)
- Degenerative changes or diseases of the spinal cord

II. The client/caregiver can list measures to prevent skin breakdown.

A. Assess skin daily using a mirror if needed to inspect carefully.
B. Avoid sharp objects, crumbs or wrinkles in the bed or chair.
C. Use preventive devices such as an egg-crate mattress, and gel pads.
D. Keep skin clean and dry.
E. Frequent repositioning. Change position every 15 to 30 minutes when in chair and every 2 hours when in bed.
F. Protect skin from burns.
1. Check bath water temperature carefully.
2. Avoid the use of hot-water bottles.

III. The client/caregiver can list measures to maintain maximum independence.

A. Assistive devices to help with personal care
B. Use of ramps and wheelchairs
C. Use of vehicles with hand controls
D. Adaption of home environment to make wheelchair accessible
E. Lifeline device

NRS DATE INITIAL

IV. The client/caregiver can list measures to promote regular bowel movements.

A. Stool softeners and suppositories
B. Regular evacuation at the same time each day
C. Adequate intake of fluids, fruit, and fiber
D. Massage abdomen from right side to left side for stimulation
E. Signs of rectal fullness, including goose bumps, rising of hair on arms and legs, perspiration, and sense of fullness
F. Upright position or bend forward for defecation

V. The client/caregiver can list measures to maintain muscle integrity and prevent contractures.

A. Range of motion
B. Exercises as instructed
C. Splints/braces
D. High-top sneakers to prevent foot drop

VI. The client/caregiver can list measures for adequate urinary elimination.

A. Do Crede maneuver (application of pressure on the bladder).
B. Have adequate fluid intake.
C. Report signs and symptoms of infections early:
1. UTI—cloudy urine
2. Fever and chills
D. Avoid catheter use if possible.
E. Practice bladder retraining.
F. Drink cranberry juice.

VII. The client/caregiver can list nutritional measures to manage spinal cord injuries.

A. Use high-calorie, high-protein, high-fiber diet.
B. Avoid foods that are gas producing.
C. Drink plenty of fluids, up to 2 liters per day.

(Continued)

NRS
DATE INITIAL

D. Use cranberry juice and/or vitamin C to decrease urine pH.

E. Avoid alcohol and caffeine-containing foods and drinks.

F. Limit milk and dairy products to reduce risk of renal calculi.

G. Use adaptive or assistive utensils to promote independence in eating.

VIII. The client/caregiver can recognize possible complications.

A. Contractures

B. Pressure ulcers

C. Urinary calculi and urinary tract infections

D. Pneumonia

E. Autonomic dysreflexion (may occur if lesion is above T6 level)—severe headache, profuse sweating, nasal congestion, and slow heart rate

F. Sexual dysfunction

G. Paralytic ileus

H. Respiratory failure

I. Sepsis

J. Muscle spasms

RESOURCES

National Spinal Cord Injury Association
www.spinalcord.org

Christopher and Dana Reeve Foundation and Resource Center
www.christopherreeve.org

National Rehabilitation Information Center
www.naric.com

National Institute on Disability and Rehabilitation Research
www.ed.gov/about/offices/list/osers/nidrr

Clearinghouse on Disability Information
www.ed.gov/about/offices/list/osers

Counseling (psychologist, psychiatrist, and clergy)

REFERENCES

Ackley, B. J., & Ladwig, G. B. (2006). *Nursing diagnosis handbook: A guide to planning care.* St. Louis: Mosby Inc.

Canobbio, M. M. (2006). *Mosby's handbook of patient teaching.* St. Louis: Mosby Inc.

Cohen, B. J., & Taylor, J. J. (2005). *Memmler's the human body in health and disease* (10th ed.). Philadelphia: Lippincott Williams & Wilkins.

Timby, B. K., & Smith, N. C. (2003). *Introductory medical-surgical nursing* (8th ed.). Philadelphia: J. B. Lippincott Williams & Wilkins.

1 Asthma

Patient name: _____ **Admission:** _____

I. The client/caregiver has a basic understanding of anatomy and physiology of the lung and respiratory systems.

A. The lungs are two sac-like organs located in the chest cavity.
B. The main windpipe (trachea) breaks into right and left bronchi and then connects to each lung.
C. The bronchi are further divided into smaller branches called bronchioles.

II. The client/caregiver can define asthma.

A. It is a chronic respiratory disorder with irritation and constriction of bronchi and bronchioles.
B. Bronchospasms occur with wheezing, shortness of breath, and increased mucus production.
C. Episodes may last a few minutes to hours and may be relieved with medication or spontaneously.
D. Asthma can range from mild to severe. Some have a chronic set of symptoms: coughing and wheezing with intermittent more severe asthma "attacks."

III. The client/caregiver can list factors that may precipitate an attack of asthma.

A. Allergens, such as pollens, animal dander, or mold
B. Cockroaches and dust mites
C. Air pollution and irritants
D. Smoke
E. Strong odors or scented products or chemicals
F. Respiratory infections and/or sinusitis
G. Physical exercise
H. Strong emotions and stress
I. Cold air
J. Certain medications
K. Preservatives and chemicals added to perishable foods
L. Gastroesophageal reflux disease (GERD)

IV. The client/caregiver can recognize warning signs and symptoms.

A. Wheezing
B. Coughing
C. Shortness of breath
D. Chest tightness or pain
E. Disturbed sleep caused by shortness of breath, coughing, or wheezing
F. Increased need to use bronchodilators
G. Changes in lung function as measured by a peak flow meter
H. Children often present with
   • Audible wheezing or whistling sound when exhaling
   • Frequent coughing spasms

V. The client/caregiver can list measures to manage asthma.

A. Identify and avoid precipitating factors and warning signs.
B. Take long-term medications that are ordered to control chronic symptoms and prevent attacks.
C. Quick relief medications are ordered for rapid, short-term relief of symptoms.
D. Other medications are ordered to decrease sensitivity to allergens and prevent reaction to the allergens.
E. Be careful to keep extra medication on hand. Keep emergency medication available with you in case of asthma attack.
F. Avoid aspirin and over-the-counter drugs that contain aspirin.
G. Prevent upper-respiratory infections:
   1. Avoid exposure to persons with respiratory infections.
   2. Avoid crowds and poorly ventilated areas.
   3. Obtain immunization against influenza and pneumonia.
   4. Report early signs of infection (i.e., increased cough, shortness of breath, fever, and chills).

(Continued)

NRS
DATE INITIAL

H. Eat a well-balanced diet.
I. Drink 2 to 3 quarts of fluid each day to liquefy secretions.
J. Use stress-management techniques.
K. Exercise daily, avoiding overexertion. Avoid exercise in cold temperatures.
L. Obtain allergy shots as recommended.
M. Environmental measures are
1. Use air conditioner.
2. Close windows during pollen season.
3. Use dust-proof covers for bedding. Avoid carpets. Use washable curtains.
4. Use dehumidifier if needed to maintain optimal humidity. Change water daily.
5. Keep air conditioner and furnace serviced and clean.
6. Reduce pet dander by avoiding pets with fur or feathers.
7. Clean home regularly. Wear a mask if doing the cleaning yourself.
8. Limit use of contact lenses when pollen count is high.
9. Control heartburn and GERD to prevent complications.
10. Monitor pollen counts in newspapers, Internet, or radio/television reports.
11. Avoid smoking or being around smoke.
N. Keep follow-up appointments with physician and laboratory.
O. Wear Medic Alert bracelet.
P. For children, communicate the child's condition and treatment plan with school personnel, coaches, and so forth.

NRS
DATE INITIAL

VI. The client/caregiver can list possible complications.

A. Status asthmaticus (prolonged symptoms of asthma)
B. Pneumonia
C. Respiratory arrest
D. Emphysema
E. Bronchitis
F. Right-sided heart failure

RESOURCES

Support groups

American Lung Association
www.lungusa.org

American Academy of Allergy, Asthma, and Immunology
www.aaaai.org

The following two organizations are part of National Institutes of Health:

National Heart, Lung, and Blood Institute
www.nhlbi.nih/gov

National Institute of Allergy and Infectious Diseases
www.niaid.nih.gov

REFERENCES

Ackley, B. J., & Ladwig, G. B. (2006). *Nursing diagnosis handbook: A guide to planning care.* St. Louis: Mosby Inc.

Cohen, B. J., & Taylor, J. J. (2005). *Memmler's the human body in health and disease* (10th ed.). Philadelphia: Lippincott Williams & Wilkins.

Nursing 2006 drug handbook. (2006). Philadelphia: Lippincott Williams and Wilkins.

Perry, A., & Potter, P. (2006). *Clinical nursing skills & technique.* St. Louis: Mosby Inc.

Timby, B. K., & Smith, N. C. (2003). *Introductory medical-surgical nursing* (8th ed.). Philadelphia: J. B. Lippincott Williams & Wilkins.

Chronic Obstructive Pulmonary Disease: Bronchitis/Emphysema

2

Patient name: _____   Admission: _____

I. **The client/caregiver has a basic understanding of anatomy and physiology of the lung and respiratory system.**

  A. The lungs are two sac-like organs located in the chest cavity.

  B. The main windpipe (trachea) breaks into right and left bronchi and then connects to each lung.

  C. The bronchi are further divided into smaller branches called bronchioles.

II. **The client/caregiver can define chronic obstructive pulmonary disease (COPD) and emphysema.**

  A. COPD is the term used to describe several lung disorders, including chronic bronchitis and emphysema.

  B. Both conditions are a result of obstruction to airflow that interferes with normal breathing.

  C. Bronchitis is the inflammation of the bronchi caused by viral, bacterial or mycoplasmal infections. The inflammation and irritation stimulate the production of mucus.

  D. Emphysema is caused by recurrent inflammations that result in destruction of lung tissue. Destruction and loss of elasticity of alveoli result in decreased air exchange. Bronchioles may collapse on expiration causing trapped air, which makes expiration more difficult.

  E. Bronchitis can be acute or chronic. It is considered chronic if a recurrent cough persists at least 3 months of the year for at least 2 successive years.

  F. Emphysema is a chronic disease and damage cannot be reversed.

III. **The client/caregiver can list factors that increase risk of COPD.**

  A. Positive family history

  B. Recurrent respiratory infections

  C. Continual exposure to harmful irritants
- Occupational hazards
- Air pollution
- Cigarette smoking

  D. Allergies

  E. Most people with COPD are at least 40 years old or around middle age.

  F. Impaired immune system

IV. **The client/caregiver can recognize signs and symptoms of COPD.**

  A. The severity of the symptoms depend on how much of the lung has been destroyed. Destruction will continue faster if smoking is continued.

  B. Symptoms
- Cough
- Sputum (mucus) production
- Shortness of breath, especially with exercise
- Wheezing
- Chest tightness
- Barrel chest (emphysema)
- Loss of appetite and weight loss

V. **The client/caregiver can list measures to prevent or manage COPD.**

  A. Stop smoking

  B. Avoid fatigue (energy conservation teaching guide)

  C. Eat healthy foods such as lots of fruits and vegetables. Eat protein foods such as meat, fish, eggs, milk, and soy. Eat smaller, more frequent meals.

  D. Take medications as ordered and make sure you refill them so you do not run out.

  E. Avoid irritants and keep home clean.
1. Avoid newly painted areas or after spraying for insects.
2. Avoid wood or kerosene heaters.
3. Keep windows closed and stay home when pollen count is high or air pollution is high.

(Continued)

NRS
DATE INITIAL

F. Avoid smoking because it destroys ciliary action and increases secretions.
G. Treat all respiratory infections promptly.
H. Receive flu shots and pneumonia immunization.
I. Consult with pulmonary rehabilitation program, which provides
   1. Exercise training
   2. Disease-management training
   3. Counseling
   4. Help with adjusting activities of daily living to disease
   5. Specific instruction with dietician, occupational therapist, respiratory therapist
J. Oxygen therapy as needed or continuously. Oxygen may help
   1. Do activities with less shortness of breath
   2. Protect heart and other organs from damage
   3. Sleep more during the night
   4. Improve alertness during the day
K. Avoid excessive heat, which increases oxygen requirements and avoid excessive cold, which increases possibility of bronchospasm.
L. Use humidifier during winter months.
M. Perform measures to thin or remove secretions to maintain patent airways.
   1. Drink 1.5 to 2 quarts if fluids daily to thin secretions.
   2. Use a humidifier to moisten air.
N. Wear a Medic Alert bracelet.
O. Get emergency help if you have the following symptoms:
   • Heart is beating very fast and irregularly.
   • Lips or fingernails are gray or blue.
   • You are not mentally alert.
   • You are having difficulty talking or walking.

NRS
DATE INITIAL

VI. The client/caregiver is aware of possible complications.

A. Greater risk if respiratory infections and complications
B. Peptic ulcer disease
C. Right-sided heart failure
D. Need of oxygen therapy for hypoxia (lack of oxygen)
E. Need of lung surgery or transplant
F. Acute respiratory failure

RESOURCES

U.S. Office of the Surgeon General
www.surgeongeneral.gov/tobacco/

National Heart, Lung, Blood Institute (National Institutes of Health)
www.nhlbi.nih.gov/

National Lung Education Program
www.nlhep.org/resources

Clearing the Air. (2003). An online guide to quitting.
www.smokefree.gov/quit-smoking/

REFERENCES

Ackley, B. J., & Ladwig, G. B. (2006). *Nursing diagnosis handbook: A guide to planning care.* St. Louis: Mosby Inc.

Cohen, B. J., & Taylor, J. J. (2005). *Memmler's the human body in health and disease* (10th ed.). Philadelphia: Lippincott Williams & Wilkins.

Nursing 2006 drug handbook. (2006). Philadelphia: Lippincott Williams and Wilkins.

Perry, A., & Potter, P. (2006). *Clinical nursing skills & technique.* St. Louis: Mosby Inc.

Timby, B. K., & Smith, N. C. (2003). *Introductory medical-surgical nursing* (8th ed.). Philadelphia: J. B. Lippincott Williams & Wilkins.

Pneumothorax

3

Patient name: _____   Admission: _____

NRS
DATE INITIAL

I.   **The client/caregiver can define pneumothorax.**

A.   Two thin layers of tissue (pleura) separate your lungs and chest wall.
B.   If air leaks through lung tissue into this space, the lung tissue will start to collapse.
C.   Collapse of lung tissue results in pneumothorax. This condition requires immediate medical attention.
D.   Reasons for air to collect in the pleura space are
   • Injuries to the chest wall (stab/gunshot wound)
   • Broken rib that punctures the lung
   • Procedure or surgery that involves the chest or lung
   • Spontaneous pneumothorax

II.   **The client/caregiver can list signs and symptoms of pneumothorax.**

A.   Sudden, sharp chest pain on affected side
B.   Shortness of breath
C.   Chest tightness
D.   Rapid respiratory rate and/or abnormal breathing movement
E.   Bluish color of skin due to lack of oxygen

NRS
DATE INITIAL

III.   **The client/caregiver can list complications.**

A.   Need for chest tube insertion or surgery
B.   Recurrent pneumothorax

IV.   **The client/caregiver can list self-care measures.**

A.   The recurrence rate of pneumothorax can be as high as 40%.
B.   Discontinue smoking, and avoid high altitudes, scuba diving to prevent the recurrence of pneumothorax.

REFERENCES

Ackley, B. J., & Ladwig, G. B. (2006). *Nursing diagnosis handbook: A guide to planning care.* St. Louis: Mosby Inc.

Cohen, B. J., & Taylor, J. J. (2005). *Memmler's the human body in health and disease* (10th ed.). Philadelphia: Lippincott Williams & Wilkins.

Perry, A., & Potter, P. (2006). *Clinical nursing skills & technique.* St. Louis: Mosby Inc.

Timby, B. K., & Smith, N. C. (2003). *Introductory medical-surgical nursing* (8th ed.). Philadelphia: J. B. Lippincott Williams & Wilkins.

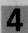

Pulmonary Edema

Patient name: _____   **Admission:** _____

NRS
DATE INITIAL

I. **The client/caregiver can define pulmonary edema.**

A. It is the abnormal accumulation of fluid that results when the heart cannot pump enough blood from the lungs to the rest of the body.
B. Fluid from the small blood vessels of the lungs rapidly oozes from the vessels into the lungs.
C. It typically occurs at night after lying down for several hours.
D. Acute pulmonary edema is a medical emergency.

II. **The client/caregiver can list some of the possible causes of pulmonary edema.**

A. Heart failure (most common)
B. Complications of heart attack
C. Mitral or aortic valve disease
D. Kidney failure
E. Intravenous overload
F. Intravenous drug overdose
G. Drowning
H. Acute respiratory distress syndrome
I. Severe allergic reactions (anaphylaxis)
J. Exposure to toxins
K. High-altitude pulmonary edema

III. **The client/caregiver can recognize the signs and symptoms of pulmonary edema.**

A. Severe and sudden onset symptoms
 • Extreme shortness of breath or difficulty breathing
 • A feeling of suffocating or drowning
 • Wheezing or gasping for breath
 • Anxiety and restlessness
 • A cough that produces frothy sputum (possibly tinged with blood)
 • Excessive sweating
 • Pale skin
 • Chest pain (if caused by coronary artery disease)

NRS
DATE INITIAL

B. Symptoms that develop more gradually include
 • Difficulty when you are lying flat
 • Awakening at night with breathless feeling
 • Increased shortness of breath when physically active
 • Significant weight gain (if result of congestive heart failure)

IV. **The client/caregiver can list measures to prevent a recurrence of pulmonary edema.**

A. Follow activity as ordered with planned rest periods.
B. Eat a heart healthy diet.
 1. Restrict sodium.
 2. Eat plenty of fresh fruits and vegetables.
 3. Restrict cholesterol and fat in diet to prevent hypertension and elevated cholesterol levels.
 4. Limit alcohol and caffeine.
C. Weigh daily (mornings preferred) for early detection of fluid retention. Report a gain of 2 to 3 pounds over one 24-hour period.
D. Exercise regularly as directed by physician.
E. Consult physician before activities that will be at high altitudes (climb or travel).
F. Notify the doctor if the following symptoms occur:
 • Trouble breathing or feeling of suffocating
 • A bubbly, wheezing, or gasping sound when you breathe
 • Pink, frothy sputum when you cough
 • Profuse sweating
 • Lightheadedness
 • A blue or gray tone to your skin

V. **The client/caregiver will know what to do if pulmonary edema occurs.**

A. Call 911 and seek emergency assistance. Do not attempt to drive.

(Continued)

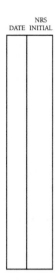

NRS
DATE INITIAL

B. Sit with head and shoulders up and feet down to favor pooling of the blood to lower dependent portions of the body.

C. Do not panic. Have list of your emergency contacts, list of medical conditions, and current medications ready and by the phone.

VI. **The client/caregiver is aware of possible complications.**

A. Respiratory failure
B. Cardiac arrest

REFERENCES

Ackley, B. J., & Ladwig, G. B. (2006). *Nursing diagnosis handbook: A guide to planning care.* St. Louis: Mosby Inc.

Cohen, B. J., & Taylor, J. J. (2005). *Memmler's the human body in health and disease* (10th ed.). Philadelphia: Lippincott Williams & Wilkins.

Lutz, C., & Przytulski, K. (2001). *Nutrition and diet therapy.* Philadelphia: F. A. Davis Company.

Nursing 2006 drug handbook. (2006). Philadelphia: Lippincott Williams and Wilkins.

Perry, A., & Potter, P. (2006). *Clinical nursing skills & technique.* St. Louis: Mosby Inc.

Timby, B. K., & Smith, N. C. (2003). *Introductory medical-surgical nursing* (8th ed.). Philadelphia: J. B. Lippincott Williams & Wilkins.

5 Pulmonary Embolism

Patient name: _____ **Admission:** _____

NRS
DATE INITIAL

I. **The client/caregiver can define pulmonary embolism.**

A. It is an obstruction in the blood vessel of a lung.
B. The obstruction prevents blood flow to a portion of the lung.
C. Without adequate blood supply, the lung cannot function properly, and lung tissue may be destroyed.

II. **The client/caregiver can list factors that may cause pulmonary embolism.**

A. Recent surgery (such as major joint replacement surgery)
B. Immobility or prolonged bedrest
C. Increased levels of clotting factor
D. Smoking
E. Obesity
F. Pregnancy and childbirth
G. Birth control pills
H. Family history
I. Pacemakers
J. Fractures and injury
K. Some medical conditions (certain cancers, heart disease, and inflammatory bowel disease)

III. **The client/caregiver can recognize signs and symptoms.**

A. Symptoms are
- Sudden shortness of breath (active or at rest)
- Chest pain similar to pain with a heart attack that will not ease with rest
- Excessive sweating
- Rapid heartbeat
- Lightheadedness or fainting
- Wheezing
- Clammy or bluish color to skin
- Leg swelling
- Weak pulse

IV. **The client/caregiver can list measures to prevent pulmonary embolism.**

A. Promote good circulation.
1. Exercise regularly especially leg exercises with rest periods.

NRS
DATE INITIAL

2. When traveling, move lower legs and feet while sitting. Change position as able.
3. Wear antiembolism stockings.
4. Avoid crossing legs or sitting for long periods of time.
5. Avoid constrictive clothing.

B. Avoid nicotine.
C. Increase fluid intake to at least six to eight glasses per day.
D. Take medication as prescribed.
E. Follow general safety precautions to prevent injury.
F. Avoid laxatives because they affect vitamin K absorption.
G. Keep follow-up appointments with physician.

V. **The client/caregiver is aware of possible complications.**

A. Pulmonary infarction (death of lung tissue)
B. Pulmonary hypertension
C. Heart failure
D. Collapse of lung
E. Shock
F. Cardiopulmonary arrest (heart stops)

RESOURCES

American Lung Association
www.lungusa.org

National Heart, Lung, and Blood Institute
www.nhlbi.nih.gov

American Heart Association
www.americanheart.org

REFERENCES

Ackley, B. J., & Ladwig, G. B. (2006). *Nursing diagnosis handbook: A guide to planning care.* St. Louis: Mosby Inc.
Cohen, B. J., & Taylor, J. J. (2005). *Memmler's the human body in health and disease* (10th ed.). Philadelphia: Lippincott Williams & Wilkins.
Perry, A., & Potter, P. (2006). *Clinical nursing skills & technique.* St. Louis: Mosby Inc.
Timby, B. K., & Smith, N. C. (2003). *Introductory medical-surgical nursing* (8th ed.). Philadelphia: J. B. Lippincott Williams & Wilkins.

6 Tuberculosis

Patient name: _____ **Admission:** _____

NRS
DATE INITIAL

I. The client/caregiver can define tuberculosis.

 A. It is a chronic, bacterial infectious disease.
 B. It usually infects the respiratory system but can invade other parts of the body.
 C. It is transmitted by airborne droplets. Coughing, sneezing, and spitting can transmit droplets produced from a person with active disease.

II. The client/caregiver can list factors that increase risk of tuberculosis.

 A. People with HIV/AIDS are very vulnerable.
 B. Increased numbers of foreign-born people from countries with high tuberculosis rates
 C. Increased poverty
 D. Crowded facilities with poor hygiene
  • Prisons
  • Homeless shelters
 E. Poor nutrition
 F. Drug addiction
 G. Alcoholism
 H. Failure to take all prescribed antibiotics for tuberculosis
 I. Increased numbers of residents in long-term care facilities are at increased risk because
  • Older
  • General health impaired
  • Weak immune systems
 J. Racial and ethnic minorities

III. The client/caregiver can recognize signs and symptoms although client is frequently without symptoms.

 A. Fatigue
 B. Loss of appetite and weight loss
 C. Low-grade fever
 D. Night sweats
 E. Shortness of breath
 F. Cough, which may be productive
 G. Chest pain

NRS
DATE INITIAL

IV. The client/caregiver can list measures for prevention and management of disease.

 A. Prevent the spread of disease.
  1. Cover nose and mouth when coughing or sneezing.
  2. Dispose of tissues by flushing in toilet or discarding in paper bag that is burned or disposed of in trash.
  3. Wash hands thoroughly.
  4. Keep environment clean and well ventilated.
 B. Keep immune system healthy.
  1. Obtain adequate rest to avoid fatigue.
  2. Eat a nutritious, high-carbohydrate diet with small, frequent feedings.
  3. Exercise regularly.
 C. Get tested regularly as ordered by physician.
 D. Increase fluids to liquefy secretions and maintain hydration to 2000 to 3000 ml per day unless contraindicated.
 E. Take complete course of medications as prescribed and report any side effects.
 F. Keep follow-up appointments with physician.
 G. Avoid crowds and persons with upper respiratory infections.
 H. Ensure adequate ventilation. Open windows whenever possible.
 I. Report to physician any signs of bloody sputum, chest pain, difficulty breathing, fever, increased cough, or night sweats.

V. The client/caregiver is aware of possible complications.

 A. Permanent lung damage
 B. Spread to other parts of body
  • Bone
  • Brain and nervous system
  • Spread throughout entire body (military tuberculosis)
 C. Development of drug-resistant strain of tuberculosis

(Continued)

RESOURCES

Centers for Disease Control and Prevention
www.cdc.gov/

National Center for HIV/AIDS, Viral Hepatitis, STD, and TB Prevention
www.cdc.gov/nchhstp/

Division of Tuberculosis Elimination
www.cdc.gov/nchstp/tb/faqs/qa.htm
www.cdc.gov/nchstp/tb/pubs/tbfactsheets/250010.htm

American Lung Association
www.lungusa.org

Local health department

REFERENCES

Ackley, B. J., & Ladwig, G. B. (2006). *Nursing diagnosis handbook: A guide to planning care.* St. Louis: Mosby Inc.

Cohen, B. J., & Taylor, J. J. (2005). *Memmler's the human body in health and disease* (10th ed.). Philadelphia: Lippincott Williams & Wilkins.

Hitchcock, J. E., Schubert, P. E., & Thomas, S. A. (2003). *Community health nursing: Caring in action.* Clifton Park, NY: Thomson Delmar Learning.

Hunt, R. 2005. *Introduction to community based nursing.* Philadelphia: Lippincott Williams & Wilkins.

Perry, A., & Potter, P. (2006). *Clinical nursing skills & technique.* St. Louis: Mosby Inc.

Timby, B. K., & Smith, N. C. (2003). *Introductory medical-surgical nursing* (8th ed.). Philadelphia: J. B. Lippincott Williams & Wilkins.

7 Pneumonia

Patient name: _____ **Admission:** _____

NRS
DATE INITIAL

NRS
DATE INITIAL

I. **The client/caregiver can define pneumonia.**

   A. It is an inflammation of the lung usually caused by infection with
   - Bacteria
   - Viruses
   - Mycoplasma
   - Chlamydia
   - Fungi
   - Pneumocystis carinii

   B. The disease progresses from filling of the airways and air sacs to hardening of the lung tissue as exudate collects.

II. **The client/caregiver can list factors that increase risk.**

   A. Smoking and air pollution
   B. Upper-respiratory infection
   C. Prolonged immobility
   D. Malnutrition
   E. Chronic diseases (diabetes, heart disease, cancer, renal disease, etc.)
   F. Exposure to intense cold, damp weather
   G. Inhalation of noxious substances
   H. Immunosuppressive drugs
   I. Age (very young or very old)
   J. Alcohol abuse

III. **The client/caregiver can list where and how they can be exposed to organisms that cause pneumonia.**

   A. Community acquired
   B. Hospital acquired
   C. Aspiration pneumonia (foreign matter inhaled into lung)
   D. Opportunistic organisms (when immune system is impaired)

IV. **The client/caregiver can recognize signs and symptoms.**

   A. Chest pain
   B. Fever and chills
   C. Cough (may be productive)
   D. Green-, yellow-, or rust-colored sputum

   E. Muscle pain and weakness
   F. Loss of appetite
   G. Rapid pulse and respirations
   H. Shortness of breath

V. **The client/caregiver can list measures to prevent or manage pneumonia.**

   A. Receive flu and pneumonia vaccinations.
   B. Drink 2 to 3 quarts of fluid daily to thin secretions, and replace fluid loss unless contraindicated.
   C. Avoid the spread of infection.
      1. Wash hands, and use hand sanitizers if not possible to wash.
      2. Cover mouth with tissue when coughing.
      3. Dispose of used tissues properly.
   D. Avoid smoking because it destroys ciliary action and increases secretions.
   E. Avoid excessive alcohol, which lowers resistance to infection.
   F. Allow for plenty of rest during illness.
   G. Encourage deep breathing and coughing every 2 hours.
   H. Prevent aspiration for clients at risk.
   I. Cleanse respiratory equipment on regular basis.
   J. Encourage frequent oral hygiene.
   K. Change position frequently if client is immobilized.
   L. Take all medications prescribed. Avoid sedatives and other medications that cause respiratory depression.
   M. Keep follow-up appointment with physician.

VI. **The client/caregiver is aware of possible complications.**

   A. Pleural effusion
   B. Collapsed lung
   C. Lung abscess
   D. Septic shock
   E. Congestive heart failure

(Continued)

RESOURCE
Smoking cessation support groups

REFERENCES

Ackley, B. J., & Ladwig, G. B. (2006). *Nursing diagnosis handbook: A guide to planning care.* St. Louis: Mosby Inc.

Cohen, B. J., & Taylor, J. J. (2005). *Memmler's the human body in health and disease* (10th ed.). Philadelphia: Lippincott Williams & Wilkins.

Nursing 2006 drug handbook. (2006). Philadelphia: Lippincott Williams and Wilkins.

Perry, A., & Potter, P. (2006). *Clinical nursing skills & technique.* St. Louis: Mosby Inc.

Timby, B. K., & Smith, N. C. (2003). *Introductory medical-surgical nursing* (8th ed.). Philadelphia: J. B. Lippincott Williams & Wilkins.

1 Bacterial Vaginosis

Patient name: _____   Admission: _____

<table>
<tr><td>NRS
DATE INITIAL</td></tr>
</table>

I. The client/caregiver can define bacterial vaginosis.

A. It is a condition in women where the normal balance of bacteria in the vagina is disrupted and certain bacteria produce an overgrowth.

B. It is the most common vaginal infection in women of childbearing age.

C. Symptoms can be
- Abnormal vaginal discharge with an unpleasant odor
- Odor that can have strong fish-like odor, especially after intercourse
- Discharge that is usually thin, white, or gray
- Complaints of burning during urination
- Burning around outside of vagina

II. The client/caregiver can define behaviors that increase risk for this disease.

A. Having a new sex partner or multiple sex partners

B. Douching

C. The use of an intrauterine device for contraception

III. The client/caregiver can list possible complications.

A. Increased susceptibility to HIV infection if exposed

B. Increases chance of HIV-infected woman passing HIV to sex partner

C. Increases the risk of the development of pelvic inflammatory disease, which can cause infertility or increase risk of ectopic pregnancy.

D. If pregnant, an increased risk for complications of pregnancy, such as premature delivery or low birth weight of newborn.

E. Increased susceptibility to other sexually transmitted diseases

IV. The client/caregiver can list treatment and prevention measures.

A. Treatment with antibiotic therapy is recommended.

B. Prevention measures
1. Be abstinent.
2. Limit number of sex partners.
3. Do not douche.
4. Use all medicine prescribed for treatment.

RESOURCES
Community Health Clinic

Centers for Disease Control and Prevention
www.cdc.gov/std/

Healthy People 2010
www.health.gov/healthypeople

REFERENCES
Ackley, B. J., & Ladwig, G. B. (2006). *Nursing diagnosis handbook: A guide to planning care.* St. Louis: Mosby Inc.

Centers for Disease Control and Prevention. (2002). Sexually transmitted diseases treatment guidelines. MMWR 2002;51 (no. RR-6).

Cohen, B. J., & Taylor, J. J. (2005). *Memmler's the human body in health and disease* (10th ed.). Philadelphia: Lippincott Williams & Wilkins.

Hillier, S., & Holmes, K. (1999). Bacterial vaginosis. In: K. Holmes, P. Sparling, P. Mardh, et al. (Eds.). Sexually transmitted diseases (3rd ed., pp. 563–586). New York: McGraw-Hill.

Hitchcock, J. E., Schubert, P. E., & Thomas, S. A. (2003). *Community health nursing: Caring in action.* Clifton Park, NY: Thomson Delmar Learning.

Hunt, R. (2005). *Introduction to community based nursing.* Philadelphia: Lippincott Williams & Wilkins.

Perry, A., & Potter, P. (2006). *Clinical nursing skills & technique.* St. Louis: Mosby Inc.

Timby, B. K., & Smith, N. C. (2003). *Introductory medical-surgical nursing* (8th ed.). Philadelphia: J. B. Lippincott Williams & Wilkins.

2 Chlamydia

Patient name: _____   Admission: _____

NRS
DATE INITIAL

I. **The client/caregiver can define chlamydia.**

   A. It is a sexually transmitted disease caused by the bacterium *Chlamydia trachomatis*.
   B. It can infect both men and women.
   C. It can damage female reproductive organs, including cause infertility. Men rarely have complications.
   D. The bacteria infect the cervix and urethra and can spread to fallopian tubes.
   E. Chlamydia can infect the rectum. Even mouth and throat infection can occur if having oral sex with infected partner.
   F. Testing for chlamydia is done by obtaining cultures of cervix or penis.

II. **The client/caregiver can list symptoms of chlamydia.**

   A. This is a "silent" disease because the majority of infected people have no symptoms.
   B. If symptoms appear, they will show within 1 to 3 weeks after exposure.
   C. Symptoms for women
       • Abnormal vaginal discharge
       • Burning sensation when urinating
       • Lower abdominal pain
       • Low back pain
       • Nausea
       • Fever
       • Pain during intercourse
       • Bleeding between menstrual periods
   D. Symptoms for men
       • Discharge from penis
       • Burning sensation when urinating
       • Burning or itching around opening of the penis
   E. Even mouth and throat infection can occur if having oral sex with infected partner.
   F. If rectal infection, rectal pain, discharge, or bleeding may occur.

III. **The client/caregiver can list treatment options.**

   A. Antibiotic therapy is administered.
   B. Sex partners of infected person should be evaluated, tested, and treated.

NRS
DATE INITIAL

   C. Infected persons should abstain from sexual intercourse until they and their sex partners have completed treatment.
   D. Retesting can be considered 3 to 4 months after treatment.

IV. **The client/caregiver can describe preventive measures.**

   A. Abstain from sexual contact.
   B. Be in a long-term mutually monogamous relationship.
   C. Have correct and consistent use of latex male condoms.
   D. Have annual screening for sexually active women 25 years of age or younger.
   E. Have annual screening for women with new sex partner or multiple sex partners.
   F. All pregnant women should be screened.

RESOURCES

Community Health Clinic

Healthy People 2010
www.health.gov/healthypeople

Centers for Disease Control and Prevention
www.cdc.gov/std/

REFERENCES

Ackley, B. J., & Ladwig, G. B. (2006). *Nursing diagnosis handbook: A guide to planning care*. St. Louis: Mosby Inc.

Centers for Disease Control and Prevention. (2002). Sexually transmitted diseases treatment guidelines. MMWR 2002;51 (no. RR-6).

Centers for Disease Control and Prevention. (2005, September). Sexually transmitted disease surveillance. Atlanta, GA: U.S. Department of Health and Human Services.

Cohen, B. J., & Taylor, J. J. (2005). *Memmler's the human body in health and disease* (10th ed.). Philadelphia: Lippincott Williams & Wilkins.

Hunt, R. (2005). *Introduction to community based nursing*. Philadelphia: Lippincott Williams & Wilkins.

Perry, A., & Potter, P. (2006). *Clinical nursing skills & technique*. St. Louis: Mosby Inc.

Timby, B. K., & Smith, N. C. (2003). *Introductory medical-surgical nursing* (8th ed.). Philadelphia: J. B. Lippincott Williams & Wilkins.

3   Gonorrhea

Patient name: _____ **Admission:** _____

NRS DATE INITIAL	

I. The client/caregiver can define gonorrhea.

A. Gonorrhea is a sexually transmitted disease caused by the bacteria *Neisseria gonorrhoeae*.
B. It can grow and multiply in the reproductive tract of women, and in the urethra of both men and women. It can also grow in the mouth, throat, eyes, and anus.
C. It is spread through contact with penis, vagina, mouth, or anus. Ejaculation does not need to occur for infection to occur.
D. It can also be spread from mother to baby during delivery.
E. The highest reported rates of infection are among sexually active teens, young adults, and blacks.

II. The client/caregiver can list symptoms of gonorrhea.

A. Men can develop symptoms from 2 to 5 days after infection until as long as 30 days. Many men do not develop symptoms.
B. If men develop symptoms, they may be
  - Burning sensation when urinating
  - White, yellow, or green discharge from penis
  - Painful or swollen testicles
C. Most infected women have no symptoms. If they have symptoms, they are mild and consist of
  - Painful or burning sensation when urinating
  - Increased vaginal discharge
  - Vaginal bleeding between periods
D. Symptoms of rectal infection include
  - Rectal discharge
  - Anal itching, soreness, or bleeding
  - Painful bowel movements
E. Infections in the throat may cause a sore throat.

III. The client/caregiver can explain how gonorrhea is diagnosed.

A. A gram stain of a sample from the urethra or cervix under a microscope in a doctors' office or clinic can show bacterium. This is more effective for the male.
B. Samples for testing from parts of the body suspected of infection can be obtained and sent to laboratory.
C. If gonorrhea is present in the cervix or urethra, a urine sample can be sent to the laboratory for testing.
D. Client should be tested for other sexually transmitted diseases.

IV. The client/caregiver can explain the treatment of gonorrhea.

A. Clients positive for gonorrhea should be tested for other sexually transmitted diseases.
B. Antibiotic therapy should be administered, and all medication should be taken as ordered.
C. Drug therapy can stop the infection, but not correct any damage done.

V. The client/caregiver can list possible complications.

A. In women, complications can be
  - Pelvic inflammatory disease
  - Internal pelvic abscesses
  - Chronic pelvic pain
  - Cause infertility
  - Increase risk of ectopic pregnancy
B. In men, complications can be
  - Epididymitis, which can lead to infertility
C. In both men and women
  - Spread to blood or joints
  - Can more easily contract HIV
D. Infants/newborns
  - Blindness
  - Joint infections
  - Life-threatening blood infections

(Continued)

NRS
DATE INITIAL

VI. The client/caregiver can list measures to prevent gonorrhea.

  A. Abstain from sexual intercourse.

  B. Be in a long-term mutually monogamous relationship.

  C. Have sexual partners examined, tested, and treated.

  D. Have consistent and correct use of condoms.

  E. If under treatment, avoid sex until treatment is complete.

  F. Notify physician if symptoms persist or recur.

RESOURCES

Healthy People 2010
www.health.gov/healthypeople

Centers for Disease Control and Prevention
www.cdc.gov/std/

REFERENCES

Ackley, B. J., & Ladwig, G. B. (2006). *Nursing diagnosis handbook: A guide to planning care.* St. Louis: Mosby Inc.

Centers for Disease Control and Prevention. (2002). Sexually transmitted diseases treatment guidelines. MMWR 2002;51 (no. RR-6).

Centers for Disease Control and Prevention. (2005, September). Sexually transmitted disease surveillance. Atlanta, GA: U.S. Department of Health and Human Services.

Cohen, B. J., & Taylor, J. J. (2005). *Memmler's the human body in health and disease* (10th ed.). Philadelphia: Lippincott Williams & Wilkins.

Hunt, R. (2005). *Introduction to community based nursing.* Philadelphia: Lippincott Williams & Wilkins.

Perry, A., & Potter, P. (2006). *Clinical nursing skills & technique.* St. Louis: Mosby Inc.

Timby, B. K., & Smith, N. C. (2003). *Introductory medical-surgical nursing* (8th ed.). Philadelphia: J. B. Lippincott Williams & Wilkins.

4 Herpes Simplex Virus 2

Patient name: _____ **Admission:** _____

I. The client/caregiver can define herpes genitalis.

A. Is a sexually transmitted disease caused by herpes simplex viruses.
B. It is recognized as a chronic, lifelong infection.
C. Herpes simplex viruses have two types: HSV-1 and HSV-2.
D. Most genital herpes is caused by HSV-2.
E. HSV-1 can cause genital herpes, but it more commonly causes infections of the mouth and lips. HSV-1 infections of genitals can be caused by oral–genital or genital–genital contact with a person infected with HSV-1.
F. The infection can stay in the body indefinitely.

II. The client/caregiver can recognize signs and symptoms of genital herpes.

A. Symptoms can range from none to various types.
B. Early symptoms include the following:
  • Burning sensation in the genitals
  • Low-back pain
  • Flu-like symptoms
  • Symptoms that appear with 2 to 20 days after exposure
C. Secondary symptoms
  • Small, red bumps appear.
  • They develop into painful vesicle or blisters.
  • Then they crust over, scab, and heal.
  • The virus remains in body and episodes of active disease can recur.

III. The client/caregiver can list measures to treat and manage genital herpes.

A. There is no treatment to cure herpes, but the use of antiviral medications can shorten and prevent outbreaks.

B. Persons with herpes should abstain from sexual activity when lesions or other symptoms are present.
C. Sex partners of infected persons should be advised that they may become infected. Sex partners can seek testing to determine whether they are infected.
D. Even if a person does not have any symptoms, they can still infect sex partners.
E. During an outbreak
  1. Keep affected areas clean and avoid touching lesions.
  2. Wash hands after contact with lesions to prevent spread.

IV. The client/caregiver can list complications of genital herpes.

A. They can cause recurrent painful genital sores.
B. They can cause psychological distress.
C. Genital HSV can cause potentially fatal infections in babies.
D. There can be a spread of virus to lips, fingers, or breasts.

RESOURCES

Support groups

Counseling

National Herpes Resource Center
www.ashastd.org/hrc/
E-mail: herpesnet@ashastd.org

Healthy People 2010
www.health.gov/healthypeople

Centers for Disease Control and Prevention
www.cdc.gov/std/

(Continued)

REFERENCES

Ackley, B. J., & Ladwig, G. B. (2006). *Nursing diagnosis handbook: A guide to planning care.* St. Louis: Mosby Inc.

Centers for Disease Control and Prevention. (2002). *Sexually transmitted diseases treatment guidelines.* MMWR 2002;51 (no. RR-6).

Centers for Disease Control and Prevention. (2005, September). *Sexually transmitted disease surveillance.* Atlanta, GA: U.S. Department of Health and Human Services.

Cohen, B. J., & Taylor, J. J. (2005). *Memmler's the human body in health and disease* (10th ed.). Philadelphia: Lippincott Williams & Wilkins.

Hunt, R. (2005). *Introduction to community based nursing.* Philadelphia: Lippincott Williams & Wilkins.

Perry, A., & Potter, P. (2006). *Clinical nursing skills & technique.* St. Louis: Mosby Inc.

Timby, B. K., & Smith, N. C. (2003). *Introductory medical-surgical nursing* (8th ed.). Philadelphia: J. B. Lippincott Williams & Wilkins.

5 | Trichomoniasis

Patient name: _____   **Admission:** _____

<table>
<tr><td>DATE</td><td>NRS INITIAL</td></tr>
</table>

I. The client/caregiver can define trichomoniasis.

A. It is caused by the parasite *Trichomonas vaginalis*.
B. Transmission of the organism occurs via sex with an infected person.
C. It is the most common curable STD in young, sexually active women.
D. Diagnosis is made by microscopic exam of culture of penis or vagina.

II. The client/caregiver can list symptoms for this disease.

A. If symptoms occur, they appear within 4 to 20 days of exposure.
B. Most men do not have symptoms. If they do have symptoms, they may have
   • "Tingling" or irritation inside the penis
   • Mild discharge
   • Slight burning after urination or ejaculation
C. Symptoms for women may be
   • Frothy, yellow-green vaginal discharge with strong odor
   • Discomfort during intercourse or urination
   • Itching or irritation to the female genital area

III. The client/caregiver will list treatment and preventive measures for this disease.

A. Metronidazole (Flagyl) is used as an effective medication treatment.
B. Test for other sexually transmitted diseases (especially gonorrhea).

<table>
<tr><td>DATE</td><td>NRS INITIAL</td></tr>
</table>

C. Persons being treated should avoid sex until they and their sex partner(s) complete treatment.
D. People can still be susceptible to reinfection.

RESOURCES

Community Health Clinic

Centers for Disease Control and Prevention
www.cdc.gov/std/

Healthy People 2010
www.health.gov/healthypeople

REFERENCES

Ackley, B. J., & Ladwig, G. B. (2006). *Nursing diagnosis handbook: A guide to planning care.* St. Louis: Mosby Inc.

Centers for Disease Control and Prevention. (2002). *Sexually transmitted diseases treatment guidelines.* MMWR 2002;51 (no. RR-6).

Centers for Disease Control and Prevention. (2005, September). *Sexually transmitted disease surveillance.* Atlanta, GA: U.S. Department of Health and Human Services.

Cohen, B. J., & Taylor, J. J. (2005). *Memmler's the human body in health and disease* (10th ed.). Philadelphia: Lippincott Williams & Wilkins.

Hunt, R. (2005). *Introduction to community based nursing.* Philadelphia: Lippincott Williams & Wilkins.

Perry, A., & Potter, P. (2006). *Clinical nursing skills & technique.* St. Louis: Mosby Inc.

Timby, B. K., & Smith, N. C. (2003). *Introductory medical-surgical nursing* (8th ed.). Philadelphia: J. B. Lippincott Williams & Wilkins.

6   Syphilis

Patient name: _____   **Admission:** _____

NRS
DATE INITIAL

I. **The client/caregiver can define the disease syphilis.**

A. It is a sexually transmitted disease caused by the bacterium *Treponema pallidum*.

B. It is passed from person to person through direct contact with a syphilis sore.

C. These sores occur on the external genitals, vagina, and anus, or in the rectum. They can also occur on the lips and in the mouth.

D. Transmission occurs during sex. Infected pregnant women can pass it to the unborn child.

E. Syphilis is described in three stages.

II. **The client/caregiver can explain stages of syphilis and symptoms for each stage.**

A. First stage of syphilis
   - The first symptom is usually a sore (or chancre).
   - The chancre is firm, round, small, and painless.
   - The first symptom occurs from 10 to 90 days after infection.
   - The chancre can last 3 to 6 weeks and can heal without treatment.
   - Without treatment, disease will progress to stage 2.

B. Second stage of syphilis
   - Rash can occur on one or more areas of the body.
   - Rash does not usually cause itching.
   - Rash may appear as the chancre is healing or several weeks afterward.
   - Most common appearance of rash is a rough, red, or reddish brown spots on palms of hands and bottom of feet.
   - Other symptoms may be fever, swollen lymph glands, sore throat, patchy hair loss, headaches, weight loss, muscle aches, and fatigue.

- These symptoms can pass without treatment, but the disease will progress to the third stage.

C. Late stage of syphilis
   - This is also called latent (hidden) stage.
   - It will start when second-stage symptoms disappear.
   - Infection remains in the body, if not treated.
   - There is damage to brain, nerves, eyes, heart, blood vessels, liver, bones, and joints.
   - Complications if untreated can result in mental deterioration, dementia, loss of vision, loss of balance, and paralysis.

III. **The client/caregiver can list method of testing and treatment.**

A. Testing for syphilis can be done by culture of chancre or by an inexpensive blood test (VDRL or RPR).

B. Treatment by penicillin injection at any stage can cure the disease, but cannot repair damage done to organs before treatment.

C. HIV testing is recommended.

D. Partner should be notified and screening done.

RESOURCES

Community Health Clinic

Centers for Disease Control and Prevention
www.cdc.gov/std/

Healthy People 2010
www.health.gov/healthypeople

(Continued)

REFERENCES

Ackley, B. J., & Ladwig, G. B. (2006). *Nursing diagnosis handbook: A guide to planning care.* St. Louis: Mosby Inc.

Centers for Disease Control and Prevention. (2002). *Sexually transmitted diseases treatment guidelines.* MMWR 2002;51 (no. RR-6).

Centers for Disease Control and Prevention. (2005, September). *Sexually transmitted disease surveillance.* Atlanta, GA: U.S. Department of Health and Human Services.

Cohen, B. J., & Taylor, J. J. (2005). *Memmler's the human body in health and disease* (10th ed.). Philadelphia: Lippincott Williams & Wilkins.

Hunt, R. (2005). *Introduction to community based nursing.* Philadelphia: Lippincott Williams & Wilkins.

Perry, A., & Potter, P. (2006). *Clinical nursing skills & technique.* St. Louis: Mosby Inc.

Timby, B. K., & Smith, N. C. (2003). *Introductory medical-surgical nursing* (8th ed.). Philadelphia: J. B. Lippincott Williams & Wilkins.

Genital Human Papillomavirus (HPV) Infection

7

Patient name: _____ Admission: _____

NRS
DATE INITIAL

I. The client/caregiver will define genital HPV infection.

A. It is caused by human papillomavirus (HPV).
B. HPV can refer to a group of viruses that include more than 100 different strains or types.
C. It infects the genital area of men and women including the skin of the penis, vulva (area outside vagina), anus, and lining of the vagina, cervix, or rectum.
D. Some people have precancerous changes in the cervix, vulva, anus, or penis.

II. The client/caregiver can list symptoms of HPV infections.

A. Most people infected with HPV will not have any symptoms, and the infection will clear on its own.
B. Some of the viruses are called "high-risk" types and may cause abnormal Pap tests. They may also lead to cancer of the cervix, vulva, vagina, anus, or penis.
C. Other viruses are called "low-risk" types. They may cause mild Pap test abnormalities or genital warts.
D. Genital warts are
   1. Soft, moist, pink, or flesh-colored swellings, usually in the genital area
   2. Raised or flat, single or multiple, small or large, and sometimes cauliflower shaped
   3. Growths on the vulva, in or around the vagina or anus, on the cervix, on the penis, scrotum, groin, or thigh

III. The client/caregiver can show how to diagnose HPV infections.

A. Genital warts are diagnosed by visual inspection.
B. Most women are diagnosed on the basis of abnormal Pap tests.
C. No HPV tests are available for men.

NRS
DATE INITIAL

IV. The client/caregiver can list treatment and prevention measures for HPV infections.

A. Warts are removed. This does not cure the infection, and new outbreaks may occur.
B. The Centers for Disease Control recommends patient-applied medications to help treat the symptoms of lesions.
C. Routine Pap tests and careful medical follow-up to monitor cervical infections are important.
D. Recommend HIV testing and routine Pap tests are important.
E. Partner should be notified.

RESOURCES

Community Health Clinic

Healthy People 2010
www.health.gov/healthypeople

Centers for Disease Control and Prevention
www.cdc.gov/std/

REFERENCES

Ackley, B. J., & Ladwig, G. B. (2006). *Nursing diagnosis handbook: A guide to planning care.* St. Louis: Mosby Inc.

Cohen, B. J., & Taylor, J. J. (2005). *Memmler's the human body in health and disease* (10th ed.). Philadelphia: Lippincott Williams & Wilkins.

Hunt, R. (2005). *Introduction to community based nursing.* Philadelphia: Lippincott Williams & Wilkins.

Perry, A., & Potter, P. (2006). *Clinical nursing skills & technique.* St. Louis: Mosby Inc.

Timby, B. K., & Smith, N. C. (2003). *Introductory medical-surgical nursing* (8th ed.). Philadelphia: J. B. Lippincott Williams & Wilkins.

1 Menstruation

Patient name: _____   **Admission:** _____

<table>
<tr><td>DATE</td><td>NRS INITIAL</td></tr>
</table>

I. The client can define normal menstruation.

A. Menstruation is a woman's monthly bleeding. Menstrual blood is partly blood and partly tissue from the inside or lining of the uterus. It flows from the uterus through the cervix and passes outside the body through the vagina.

B. Menstruation is also called menses, menstrual period, or "period."

C. Puberty is the onset of sexual maturation. For females, this is when menstruation (menarche = first menstruation) begins.

D. Menopause is the termination of female fertility (and menstruation).

E. Menstrual cycle
   • Menses or bleeding usually starts around age 12.
   • It starts on the first day of bleeding.
   • Most periods of bleeding last 3 to 5 days.
   • The average cycle is 28 days but can range from 23 to 35 days.

II. The client can list possible problems with menstruation and menses.

A. Amenorrhea—lack of menstrual period. Causes of amenorrhea can be
   • Pregnancy or breastfeeding, which are normal situations
   • Extreme weight loss caused by illness or eating disorders
   • Excessive exercising
   • Stress
   • Hormonal problems

B. Dysmenorrhea—painful periods or severe cramps. Causes can be
   • Uterine fibroids
   • Endometriosis
   • Sometimes no cause that can be identified

C. Abnormal bleeding such as
   • Very heavy bleeding
   • Unusually long periods (menorrhagia)

   • Dysfunctional uterine bleeding periods too close together or bleeding between periods

D. Premenstrual syndrome—experience symptoms such as mood swings, tender breasts, swollen abdomen, food cravings, fatigue, irritability, and depression in days before monthly period

E. Premenstrual dysphoric disorder—a more severe form of premenstrual syndrome

III. The client can list reasons to consult health care provider.

A. If menstruation has not started by the age of 16 years

B. If period suddenly stopped

C. If bleeding for more days than usual

D. If bleeding is excessive

E. Sudden sickness after using tampons (toxic shock syndrome teaching guide)

F. If bleeding between periods (more than just drops)

G. If having severe pain during period

IV. The client can list measure to prevent or manage menstrual problems.

A. Take medication as ordered by physician.

B. Dietary suggestions include the following:
   1. Eat smaller, more frequent meals to reduce bloating and feelings of fullness.
   2. Limit salt and sodium.
   3. Choose foods high in complex carbohydrates (fruits, vegetables, and whole grains).
   4. Choose foods rich in calcium. If dairy products are not well

(Continued)

tolerated, consider calcium supplements.
5. Use multivitamin as suggested by physician.
6. Avoid caffeine and alcohol.
C. Regular daily exercise will help with fatigue and depression.
D. Reduce stress.
E. Get plenty of sleep.
F. Record symptoms and interventions to evaluate effectiveness.
G. Discuss any herbal supplements or over-the-counter medications with physician before use.

RESOURCES

American College of Obstetricians and Gynecologists Resource Center
800-762-2264 x192 (for publications requests only)
www.acog.org
National Women's Health Information Center
800-994-9662

REFERENCES

Lutz, C., & Przytulski, K. (2001). *Nutrition and diet therapy.* Philadelphia: F. A. Davis Company.
Timby, B. K., & Smith, N. C. (2003). *Introductory medical-surgical nursing* (8th ed.). Philadelphia: J. B. Lippincott Williams & Wilkins.

2   Endometriosis

Patient name: _____   **Admission:** _____

NRS
DATE INITIAL

I. **The client/caregiver can define endometriosis.**

A. Tissue that resembles and acts like the lining of the uterus grows outside the uterus. This misplaced tissue can cause pain, infertility, and heavy bleeding.
B. Other areas that it can grow are
   • On or under the ovaries
   • Behind the uterus
   • On tissue that supports the uterus
   • On the bowels or bladder
C. On average, women have symptoms for 2 to 5 years before diagnosis is made.
D. Postmenopause, symptoms disappear.

II. **The client/caregiver can list signs and symptoms of endometriosis.**

A. Very painful menstrual cramps that grow worse over time.
B. Chronic pain in lower back and pelvis
C. Pain during or after sex
D. Intestinal pain
E. Painful bowel movements or urination during menstrual periods
F. Heavy and/or long menstrual periods
G. Spotting or bleeding between periods
H. Infertility
I. Fatigue
J. Diarrhea, constipation, or bloating, especially during periods

III. **The client/caregiver can list risk factors for getting endometriosis.**

A. Began menstruation at an early age
B. Have heavy periods
C. Have periods that last more than 7 days
D. Have a short monthly cycle (27 days or less)
E. Have close relatives (mother, aunt, and sister) with endometriosis

NRS
DATE INITIAL

IV. **The client/caregiver can list measures to treat and cope with endometriosis.**

A. Pain medication is given as prescribed by physician.
B. Hormone treatment is given as prescribed by physician.
C. Health care provider may suggest surgery, such as laparoscopy, major abdominal surgery, or hysterectomy.
D. To cope with this condition
   1. Exercise regularly.
   2. Avoid alcohol and caffeine.
   3. Be informed.
   4. Join support groups.

RESOURCES

The Federal Government Source for Women's Health Information
www.4woman.gov

National Women's Health Information Center
800-994-9662

Endometriosis Association
414-355-2200
www.endometriosisassn.org/

The American College of Obstetricians and Gynecologists
800-762-2264 x192 (for publication requests only)
www.acog.org/

REFERENCES

Ackley, B. J., & Ladwig, G. B. (2006). *Nursing diagnosis handbook: A guide to planning care.* St. Louis: Mosby Inc.
Canobbio, M. M. (2006). *Mosby's handbook of patient teaching.* St. Louis: Mosby Inc.
Cohen, B. J., & Taylor, J. J. (2005). *Memmler's the human body in health and disease* (10th ed.). Philadelphia: Lippincott Williams & Wilkins.
Timby, B. K., & Smith, N. C. (2003). *Introductory medical-surgical nursing* (8th ed.). Philadelphia: J. B. Lippincott Williams & Wilkins.

3 Pelvic Inflammatory Disease

Patient name: _____ Admission: _____

NRS
DATE INITIAL

I. **The client/caregiver can define pelvic inflammatory disease (PID).**

A. It is an infection and inflammation of the upper genital tract in women.
B. It affects the
   - Uterus
   - Fallopian tubes
   - Ovaries
C. Damage to these organs result from scarring caused by the infection and inflammation.
D. It is the most common preventable cause of infertility in the United States.
E. The Centers for Disease Control reports that more than 1 million women seek treatment for PID each year. A similar or greater number of women may have pelvic inflammatory disease and not be aware of it.
F. The most common cause is from bacteria that cause chlamydia and gonorrhea.

II. **The client/caregiver can list risk factors for pelvic inflammatory disease.**

A. Same women who are at risk for sexually transmitted infections
B. Women with history of previous pelvic inflammatory disease
C. Sexually active women under the age of 25
D. Douching
E. Occasionally, an intrauterine device
F. Black and Hispanic women

III. **The client/caregiver can list signs and symptoms of pelvic inflammatory disease.**

A. You may not have symptoms.
B. The most common symptom is pain in lower abdomen. Others are
   - Fever
   - Vaginal discharge that may have an odor
   - Painful intercourse

NRS
DATE INITIAL

   - Painful urination
   - Irregular menstrual bleeding
C. Sometimes pelvic inflammatory disease causes symptoms of extreme pain, and a fever will appear suddenly.

IV. **The client/caregiver can list possible complications from pelvic inflammatory disease.**

A. Atopic or tubal pregnancy (rupture of tube causes internal bleeding and is life threatening)
B. Infertility (about one of eight women with pelvic inflammatory disease become infertile)
C. Chronic pelvic pain

V. **The client/caregiver can list treatment and preventive measures for pelvic inflammatory disease.**

A. Know symptoms and report to health care provider promptly if symptoms appear.
B. Take medication as prescribed. Be sure to finish taking all of medications.
C. Surgery may be recommended if medical treatment not effective.
D. Client's sex partner(s) should be treated even if symptoms are not apparent.
E. Avoid sex with partner who has not been treated.
F. Abstain from sex or be in a long-term monogamous relationship.
G. A consistent use of condoms can reduce risk.
H. The Centers for Disease Control recommend
   1. Yearly chlamydia testing of all sexually active women age 25 or younger or older women with new or multiple partners
   2. Retesting after treatment to ensure chlamydia treatment effective

(Continued)

RESOURCES

Centers for Disease Control and Prevention, Division of
 Sexually Transmitted Diseases Prevention
800-CDC-INFO (800-232-4636)
www.cdc.gov/std

Centers for Disease Control and Prevention
National Prevention Information Network
800-458-5231
www.cdcnpin.org

American Social Health Association
www.ashastd.org

The American College of Obstetricians and Gynecologists
www.acog.org/

REFERENCES

Ackley, B. J., & Ladwig, G. B. (2006). *Nursing diagnosis
 handbook: A guide to planning care.* St. Louis: Mosby Inc.
Pelvic inflammatory disease. American Social Health
 Association.
Health matters: Pelvic inflammatory disease. (2005, December).
 National Institutes of Health: U.S. Department of Health
 and Human Services.

4 Menopause

Patient name: _____   **Admission:** _____

NRS
DATE INITIAL

I.   **The client can define menopause.**

A. A female who has not had a period for 12 consecutive months has reached menopause.

B. Symptoms of menopause can start in the 30- to 40-year age group and last into the 50- to 60-year age group.

C. Menopause begins when ovaries start making less estrogen and progesterone.

D. The transition of menopause is divided into two stages:
   • Perimenopause
   • Postmenopause

E. Menopause can also be the result of medical or surgical interventions. They are
   • Hysterectomy
   • Chemotherapy and radiation therapy

II. **The client can list signs and symptoms of menopause.**

A. Irregular periods

B. Decreased fertility, in which ovulation can fluctuate

C. Vaginal and urinary changes

D. Hot flashes

E. Sleep disturbances and night sweats

F. Changes in appearance—usually weight gain

G. Emotional and cognitive changes

III. **The client can list methods of treatment and measures to manage menopause.**

A. Hormone therapy. Estrogen therapy continues to be used to treat hot flashes and vaginal discomfort. Talk with physician regarding benefits versus risk factor for your individual case (personal and family medical history) regarding the use of hormone therapy.

B. Other medications that might be used to treat symptoms of menopause are
   1. Low-dose antidepressants
   2. Neurontin to reduce hot flashes

NRS
DATE INITIAL

   3. Clonidine and other similar medications used to treat high blood pressure and hot flashes

   4. Medications to reduce bone loss and osteoporosis

   5. Vaginal estrogen creams, ring, or tablet to relieve vaginal dryness

   6. Discussion of any side effects with physician to evaluate benefit of medication.

C. Other measures to promote wellness are

   1. To avoid hot flashes dress in layers, and try to pinpoint any triggers for them. Some triggers are hot beverages, spicy foods, alcohol, and hot weather.

   2. For vaginal discomfort or dryness with intercourse, try some of the over-the-counter water-based vaginal lubricants or moisturizers.

   3. Encourage good sleep habits. Avoid caffeinated beverages and exercise before bedtime. Learn more about relaxation exercises and techniques.

   4. Strengthen pelvic floor using Kegel exercises. This can also help avoid urinary incontinence.

   5. Eat a balanced diet. Choose fruits, vegetables, and whole grains and limit saturated fats, oils, and sugars. Talk with your physician about the use of calcium supplements. Strive to lose weight if overweight.

   6. Do not smoke.

   7. Do moderate exercise at least 30 minutes on most days.

   8. Schedule regular checkups for mammograms, Pap tests, and any other indicated testing.

   9. Discuss any herbal products or supplements with physician before using them.

D. The client can list possible complications often associated with menopause.

   1. The risk of cardiovascular disease increases as estrogen levels decrease.

(Continued)

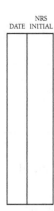

NRS
DATE INITIAL

2. Osteoporosis can occur. Maintain adequate calcium intake. The use of Vitamin D may enhance the absorption of calcium. Weight-bearing exercises also help keep healthy bones.
3. Urinary incontinence may appear as a result of vagina and urethral tissue losing elasticity.
4. Weight gain may be a problem. Try to balance exercise level with caloric intake to prevent weight gain.

RESOURCES

The National Women's Health Information Center
www.4woman.gov/

National Osteoporosis Foundation
www.nof.org/

The American College of Obstetricians and Gynecologists
www.acog.org/

REFERENCES

Ackley, B. J., & Ladwig, G. B. (2006). *Nursing diagnosis handbook: A guide to planning care.* St. Louis: Mosby Inc.

Canobbio, M. M. (2006). *Mosby's handbook of patient teaching.* St. Louis: Mosby Inc.

Cohen, B. J., & Taylor, J. J. (2005). *Memmler's the human body in health and disease* (10th ed.). Philadelphia: Lippincott Williams & Wilkins.

Lutz, C., & Przytulski, K. (2001). *Nutrition and diet therapy.* Philadelphia: F. A. Davis Company.

Timby, B. K., & Smith, N. C. (2003). *Introductory medical-surgical nursing* (8th ed.). Philadelphia: J. B. Lippincott Williams & Wilkins.

5 # Birth Control Methods

Patient name: _____ **Admission:** _____

I. **The client/caregiver can discuss the use of birth control and issues to be considered when choosing a method of birth control.**

A. To have control over if and when to become a parent, birth control, or whether contraception needs to be used.

B. There is no "best" method of birth control. Each method has its pros and cons. Some methods are more effective than others.

C. There is no method of birth control that is 100% effective. Any method of birth control is more effective if used correctly all of the time. Abstinence is the only way never to get pregnant.

D. Things to consider when choosing a birth control method are
   • Your overall health
   • How often you have sex
   • The number of sexual partners you have
   • Whether you want to have children
   • How effective is each method for preventing pregnancy
   • Any possible side effects
   • How comfortable are you or your partner in using the method

E. Most birth control methods do not protect you from HIV or sexually transmitted diseases.

F. Birth control methods may work in different ways. These include
   1. Blocking sperm from getting to the eggs (condoms, diaphragms, etc.).
   2. Keep the woman's ovaries from releasing eggs that could be fertilized (birth control pills).
   3. Prevent the fertilized egg from attaching to the lining of the uterus.
   4. Sterilization is a permanent method for women and men.

G. Margaret Sanger, a public health nurse, opened the first birth control clinic in the United States in Brooklyn, New York in 1971.

II. **The client/caregiver can list birth control methods and their effectiveness.**

A. Periodic abstinence or fertility awareness methods are means for the fertile days of the female menstrual cycle, there is no sex or the use of a "barrier" method of birth control is employed. This method is 75% to 99% effective if done properly. Ask for more information on how to calculate your cycle safely.

B. Use a male condom. If used properly, they are 84% to 98% effective. Latex or polyurethane condoms are the only method (other than abstinence) that protect against HIV or sexually transmitted diseases.

C. Oral contraceptives or the "pill" are taken daily to block the release of eggs from ovary. They are 95% to 99.9% effective. Contraindications for using oral contraceptives are
   1. It may increase risk of heart disease, hypertension, and blood clots.
   2. The risks increase if you smoke.
   3. The risks also increase if over the age of 35, have a history of blood clots and breast, liver, or endometrial cancer.

D. The mini pill has only one hormone, progestin.
   1. One advantage of this method is that it can be used with mothers who are breastfeeding.
   2. It is 92% to 99.9% effective.
   3. It needs to be taken at the same time each day. If more than 3 hours late, a backup method of birth control is needed.

E. Intrauterine devices are placed inside of the uterus. There are different types of intrauterine devices, but they average 98% to 99% effective. Depending on the type of intrauterine device, it can remain from 1 to 12 years.

F. The female condom is worn by the woman, and it uses the barrier method of

(Continued)

NRS
DATE INITIAL

birth control. It is 70% to 95% effective. They can be purchased at drug stores.

G. Depo-Provera is an injection of progestin every 3 months. It should not used for more than 2 years continually because of possible bone loss. It is considered to be 97% effective.

H. A diaphragm, cervical cap, or shield is also an example of the barrier method of birth control. The diaphragm and cervical cap require a physician to fit them because they come in different sizes. They are used with spermicide and are placed over cervix prior to sexual intercourse. Both are 84% to 94% effective if used correctly. The effectiveness of the cervical cap drops to 68% to 74% if used after the delivery of a child. The cervical shield needs a prescription for purchase, and it is 85% effective.

I. The contraceptive sponge was reapproved by the Food and Drug Administration in 2005. It is another example of the barrier method of birth control. It is 84% to 91% effective for women who have not had a child and drops to 68% to 80% effective for women who have had a child. There is a risk for toxic shock syndrome if left in place longer than 30 hours. It also can be purchased at the drug store without prescription.

J. Ortho Evra Patch is worn on skin on the lower abdomen, buttocks, or upper body. It uses both progestin and estrogen. It is changed once a week for 3 weeks, and then no patch is used the fourth week. It is 98% to 99% effective (less effective for women who weigh more than 198 pounds).

K. The hormonal vaginal contraceptive ring is inserted into vagina and is worn for 3 weeks. It is 98% to 99% effective. It is not recommended for use if breastfeeding. It needs a prescription.

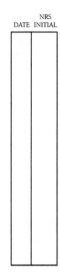

NRS
DATE INITIAL

L. Surgical sterilization for either male or female is used when a permanent method of birth control is desired. They are 99.9% effective.

M. Nonsurgical sterilization (Essure Permanent Birth Control System) is the first nonsurgical method of sterilizing women. An implant is inserted through the vagina and uterus and placed in the fallopian tubes. The implant will irritate and cause scar tissue and block the fallopian tubes. Because it takes up to 3 months to complete, a backup method of birth control is recommended. It has been shown to be 99.8% effective.

RESOURCES

Food and Drug Administration
888-463-6332
www.fda.gov

Planned Parenthood Federation of America
800-230-7526
www.plannedparenthood.org/

American College of Obstetricians and Gynecologists Resource Center
800-762-2264 x192 (for publications requests only)
www.acog.org/

REFERENCES

Ackley, B. J., & Ladwig, G. B. (2006). *Nursing diagnosis handbook: A guide to planning care.* St. Louis: Mosby Inc.

Cohen, B. J., & Taylor, J. J. (2005). *Memmler's the human body in health and disease* (10th ed.). Philadelphia: Lippincott Williams & Wilkins.

Novak, J. C., & Broom, B. L. (1999). *Maternal and child health nursing.* St. Louis: Mosby, Inc.

Taylor, C., Lillis, C., & LeMone, P. (2005). *Fundamentals of nursing.* Philadelphia: Lippincott, Williams & Wilkins.

Cystic Fibrosis

Admission: _____

NRS
DATE INITIAL

I. The client/caregiver can define cystic fibrosis.

A. It is an inherited disease that affects breathing and digestion.
B. Cystic fibrosis affects the movement of sodium (salt) into and out of certain cells.
C. This malfunction results in formation of thick, sticky mucus.
D. It affects multiple systems of the body, such as
    1. Lungs (most common)
    2. Pancreas (also common)
    3. Gastrointestinal tract
    4. Salivary glands
    5. Reproductive tract
E. It is usually diagnosed in early infancy or childhood. Cystic fibrosis rarely occurs in blacks and Asians.

II. The client/caregiver can recognize signs and symptoms.

A. Coughing or wheezing
B. Repeated lung infections
C. Shortness of breath
D. Greasy, foul-smelling, pale stools
E. Excessive appetite but poor weight gain and growth
F. Intestinal blockage in newborns
G. Rectal prolapse
H. Salty sweat, tears, and saliva
I. Infertility
J. Clubbing of the fingers and toes

III. The client/caregiver can list measures to manage cystic fibrosis.

A. Prevent infection.
    1. Avoid persons with respiratory infections.
    2. Take antibiotics as needed.
    3. Obtain immunizations as recommended.

NRS
DATE INITIAL

B. Provide respiratory care.
    1. Be aware of postural drainage and percussion (respiratory care treatments).
    2. Take oxygen as needed.
    3. Use nebulizer treatments.
    4. Take medications as ordered.
    5. Do breathing exercises.
    6. Avoid known irritants such as smoke and air pollution.
C. Provide a well-balanced diet.
    1. Eat food that is high in calories and protein but low in fat.
    2. Increase fluids.
    3. Eat salty foods, and add salt to food at the table as tolerated.
    4. Take pancreatic enzyme supplements. Take supplements with foods especially carbohydrates.
    5. Discuss the use of vitamins A, D, E, and K and zinc with physician.
D. Do daily exercise with rest periods. Use respiratory treatments before exercise. Modify exercise on warm days, and drink plenty of fluids.
E. Keep follow-up appointments.
F. Provide good oral hygiene.

IV. The client/caregiver can list possible complications.

A. Pneumothorax
B. Cor pulmonale
C. Dehydration
D. Salt depletion
E. Rectal prolapse
F. Damage to the eye
G. Osteoporosis

(Continued)

RESOURCES

March of Dimes
www.marchofdimes.com

Cystic Fibrosis Foundation
800-344-4823
www.cff.org/

National Heart, Lung, and Blood Institute Health Information
   Center
301-592-8573
www.nhlbi.nih.gov/health/infoctr/index.htm

Support groups

Dietician

Counseling

REFERENCES

Ackley, B. J., & Ladwig, G. B. (2006). *Nursing diagnosis handbook: A guide to planning care.* St. Louis: Mosby Inc.

Canobbio, M. M. (2006). *Mosby's handbook of patient teaching.* St. Louis: Mosby Inc.

Lutz, C., & Przytulski, K. (2001). *Nutrition and diet therapy.* Philadelphia: F. A. Davis Company.

Muscari, M. E. (2005). *Pediatric nursing.* Philadelphia: Lippincott Williams & Wilkins.

Novak, J. C., & Broom, B. L. (1999). *Maternal and child health nursing.* St. Louis: Mosby, Inc.

2

Hemophilia

Patient name: _____ **Admission:** _____

NRS
DATE INITIAL

I. **The client/caregiver can define hemophilia.**

A. It is a hereditary bleeding disorder caused by a deficiency that is necessary for coagulation of blood.

B. It can be a very mild to a very severe disorder:
1. Clotting factors are between 5% and 25% in mild hemophilia.
2. Clotting factors are between 1% and 5% in moderate hemophilia.
3. Clotting factors are less than 1% in severe hemophilia.

C. Hemophilia can be classified as A or B.
1. Hemophilia A is a deficiency of factor VIII.
2. Hemophilia B is a deficiency of factor IX.

D. It is a recessive disorder transmitted by females and found predominantly in males.

II. **The client/caregiver can recognize signs and/or symptoms of bleeding.**

A. Hemophilia is suspected in newborns if there is excessive bleeding from the umbilical cord or after circumcision.

B. Major signs and symptoms are
• Bleeding
• Bruising

C. The extent of bleeding depends on the type and severity of the hemophilia.

D. In most children with hemophilia, the first signs/symptoms are
• Heavy bruising and bleeding from gums when they cut baby teeth
• Bumps and bruises that appear frequently when they learn to walk
• Joints that have swelling and bruising from bleeding in soft tissue and muscles

E. In older children, the signs/symptoms are
• Bleeding in the joints (hemarthrosis)
• Bleeding and bruising in soft tissue and muscles
• Bleeding in the mouth from cut or bite or loss of a tooth
• Nosebleeds for no reason

NRS
DATE INITIAL

• Blood in the urine (bleeding in kidneys or bladder)
• Blood in the stool (bleeding in intestines or stomach)

F. Children with severe hemophilia have bleeding in the joints as the most common problem.
1. The most common joints to have bleeding are the knees, elbows, and ankles.
2. The signs/symptoms of bleeding in the joints are
• Tightness in the joint without real pain
• Tightness and pain that may occur before visible signs of bleeding
• Joint that becomes swollen and hot to touch; pain that is experienced with any movement
• Swelling and severe pain that can result in a loss of movement
3. If not treated, bleeding can lead to permanent damage and arthritis.

G. Bleeding in the brain is a serious complication and requires emergency treatment. The bleeding can happen after only a small bump or injury to the head.
1. Signs and symptoms of bleeding in the brain are
• Long-lasting and painful headache
• Multiple episodes of vomiting
• Changes in behavior
• Becoming very sleepy
• Sudden weakness or clumsiness of arms or legs, including difficulty walking
• Double vision
• Convulsions or seizures

III. **The client/caregiver can list ongoing medical needs for the person with hemophilia.**

A. Ask for referral to any of the Hemophilia Treatment Centers in the U.S. (Directory of Hemophilia Treatment Centers— *www.cdc.gov/ncbddd/hbd/htc_list.htm*).

(Continued)

NRS
DATE INITIAL

They can help your local care provider to meet your special needs.

B. Continue treatments as prescribed.

C. Have regular checkups and immunizations as recommended.

D. Have regular dental care.

E. Learn the signs and symptoms of bleeding in the joints.

F. Contact your health care provider or go to the emergency room if these symptoms appear:
- Heavy bleeding that cannot be stopped or continues to ooze
- Any of the symptoms of bleeding in the brain

G. Try to keep a record of all treatments with you to appointments or emergency room visits.

IV. **The client/caregiver can list necessary precautions for the young child with hemophilia.**

A. Use kneepads, elbow pads, and protective helmets. Use car seat belts properly.

B. Use the safety belts and straps in highchairs, car seats, shopping carts, and strollers.

C. Remove furniture with sharp corners or pad them carefully.

D. Keep any small and sharp objects out of the reach of child.

E. Use cabinet safety locks, electrical outlet covers, and security gates to keep child away from stairs.

F. Monitor play equipment and outdoor public play areas for possible hazards.

G. Keep cold packs in the freezer to use quickly.

H. Prepare a bag with needed supplies and information if you need to take child to emergency room.

I. Notify anyone who is responsible for your child of his or her condition. That may include the following:
- Babysitters
- Daycare providers
- Teachers
- Coaches

J. Have child wear a medical alert bracelet.

V. **The client/caregiver can list preventive measures for the adolescent with hemophilia.**

A. Teenager should learn signs of bleeding and what are the appropriate actions.

NRS
DATE INITIAL

B. Exercise regularly and safely.

C. Learn not to take unnecessary risks.

D. Take care of teeth and gums.

E. Recognize and eat a healthy diet.

F. Possibly participate in administration of medications needed.

G. Some examples of safer physical activities are as follows:
- Swimming
- Biking (wearing appropriate equipment)
- Walking
- Golf

H. The contact sports such as football, hockey, or wrestling are not usually considered safe.

I. Wear Medical Alert bracelet.

VI. **The client/caregiver can list measures to help with emotional factor of hemophilia.**

A. Educate about disease and treatment in a way that he or she can understand.

B. Reassure that the disease is not the fault of child.

C. Encourage child to participate in their own care (as age of child is appropriate).

D. Offer support group participation for both client and family.

VII. **The client/caregiver can list possible complications.**

A. Joint deformities

B. Life-threatening bleeding

RESOURCES

National Hemophilia Foundation
www.hemophilia.org

National Heart, Lung, and Blood Institute
www.nhlbi.nih/gov

Support groups

REFERENCES

Ackley, B. J., & Ladwig, G. B. (2006). *Nursing diagnosis handbook: A guide to planning care.* St. Louis: Mosby Inc.

Canobbio, M. M. (2006). *Mosby's handbook of patient teaching.* St. Louis: Mosby Inc.

Lutz, C., & Przytulski, K. (2001). *Nutrition and diet therapy.* Philadelphia: F. A. Davis Company.

Muscari, M. E. (2005). *Pediatric nursing.* Philadelphia: Lippincott Williams & Wilkins.

Novak, J. C., & Broom, B. L. (1999). *Maternal and child health nursing.* St. Louis: Mosby, Inc.

3 Hyperbilirubinemia

Patient name: _____ **Admission:** _____

NRS
DATE INITIAL

I. The caregiver can define hyperbilirubinemia.

A. It is the excessive accumulation of bilirubin in blood (12 mg per 100 ml or greater).

B. Bilirubin is caused by the breakdown of hemoglobin in the destruction of red blood cells.

C. If bilirubin is 20 or greater, it is termed kernicterus and can cause permanent brain damage (signs and symptoms of kernicterus include lethargy, feeding difficulties, irritability, and seizures).

D. A symptom of hyperbilirubinemia is jaundice (a yellowish discoloration of the skin).

II. The caregiver can list treatment for hyperbilirubinemia.

A. Phototherapy (most common treatment) is used.

B. In more severe cases, exchange transfusions may be used.

C. Keep newborn hydrated with breast milk or formula.

D. Stop breastfeeding for 1 to 2 days, and give formula, which may reduce jaundice.

III. The caregiver can define and explain purpose of phototherapy.

A. Infant is placed under artificial light in a protected isolette to maintain constant temperature.

B. A fiberoptic blanket (another form of phototherapy) is placed under baby (infant may remain dressed).

C. Lights help break down bilirubin in the skin.

D. Infant is clothed only in a diaper.

E. The infant's eyes are protected from light source by eye patch or headbox.

F. Bilirubin levels need to be taken at least daily.

IV. The caregiver can list measures to protect infant during phototherapy.

A. Increase fluids by 20% to 25%.

B. Turn regularly to expose all parts of body, at least every 2 hours.

C. Make certain that eyelids are closed before applying eye shield.

D. Check eyes for drainage or irritation frequently.

E. Cover male genitalia to prevent damage from heat and light waves.

F. Turn the light off, and unmask eyes at least every 3 to 4 hours (with feedings).

G. Monitor body temperature every 2 hours.

H. Avoid oils and lotions on the skin.

I. Report any signs of increased lethargy, difficulty arousing infant, or changes in stools or urination.

J. Monitor elimination, and weigh twice daily.

K. Keep skin clean and dry.

L. Assess for symptoms of dehydration, such as
   • Poor skin turgor
   • Sunken fontanels
   • Decreased urine output

M. Turn off phototherapy unit before drawing blood for testing.

V. The caregiver can list possible complications of untreated hyperbilirubinemia.

A. Dehydration

B. Brain damage

C. Blindness

D. Loss of hearing

REFERENCES

Ackley, B. J., & Ladwig, G. B. (2006). *Nursing diagnosis handbook: A guide to planning care.* St. Louis: Mosby Inc.

Maternal-neonatal nursing: Lippincott manual of nursing practice pocket guides. (2007). Philadelphia: Lippincott Williams & Wilkins.

Novak, J. C., & Broom, B. L. (1999). *Maternal and child health nursing.* St. Louis: Mosby, Inc.

4 Phenylketonuria (PKU)

Patient name: _____ **Admission:** _____

I. The client/caregiver can define phenyl-ketonuria (PKU).

A. It is a rare condition in which the body does not properly break down an amino acid called phenylalanine.
B. PKU is an inherited disorder.
C. High levels of phenylalanine are harmful to the central nervous system.
D. PKU can lead to mental retardation.

II. The client/caregiver can list signs and symptoms of PKU.

A. Symptoms are as follows:
- Skin rashes
- Tremors
- Jerking movements of arms or legs
- Seizures
- Mental retardation
- Attention deficit hyperactivity disorder
- Light complexion, hair, and eyes
- "Mousy" odor to the urine, breath, and sweat

III. The client/caregiver can list how to test for PKU and standard treatments.

A. Testing for PKU is detected with a simple blood test. Most states require a PKU screening test for all newborns. Ask your health care provider if this is done at the time of your baby's birth.
B. PKU is a treatable disease.
C. Treatment is a diet that is extremely low in phenylalanine. This diet is necessary to prevent or reduce mental retardation.
D. Lofenalac is a special infant formula made for infants with PKU. It can continue to be used throughout life as a source of protein.

IV. The client/caregiver can list measures to manage this disorder.

A. Foods that are high in phenylalanine should be avoided:
  1. High-protein foods, such as milk, ice cream, eggs, nuts, beans, chicken, steak, and fish
  2. Foods, medicine, and beverages containing NutraSweet (aspartame)
B. Lofenalac is a special infant formula made for infants with PKU. It can continue to be used throughout life as a source of protein.
C. Seek genetic testing to determine if you are a carrier of this defective gene.
D. Seek help from dietician because diet can be very restricted. Some suggestions they may make are as follows:
  1. Use diluted nondairy creamer for cereal.
  2. Corn flakes or puffed rice are suggested cereals.
  3. A packed lunch could include rice cakes, grapes, applesauce, lemonade, and jelly beans.
  4. Safe seasonings and herbs to use in cooking are basil, cilantro, lemon juice, sesame oil, maple syrup, or honey.
E. Read labels carefully for PKU listed as an ingredient.
F. Work with child's teachers, daycare providers, and so forth by explaining disorder and proper choices.
G. Be informed. Start children in planning food choices early.
H. Join support groups and learn from others about coping skills and foods.

(Continued)

RESOURCES

March of Dimes
www.marchofdimes.com/

National PKU News
www.pkunews.org/

National Institute of Child Health and Human Development
www.nichd.nih.gov/

Dietician

Support groups

REFERENCES

Ackley, B. J., & Ladwig, G. B. (2006). *Nursing diagnosis handbook: A guide to planning care.* St. Louis: Mosby Inc.

Canobbio, M. M. (2006). *Mosby's handbook of patient teaching.* St. Louis: Mosby Inc.

Lutz, C., & Przytulski, K. (2001). *Nutrition and diet therapy.* Philadelphia: F. A. Davis Company.

Maternal-neonatal nursing: Lippincott manual of nursing practice pocket guides. (2007). Philadelphia: Lippincott Williams & Wilkins.

Muscari, M. E. (2005). *Pediatric nursing.* Philadelphia: Lippincott Williams & Wilkins.

Novak, J. C., & Broom, B. L. (1999). *Maternal and child health nursing.* St. Louis: Mosby, Inc.

5 Spina Bifida

Patient name: _____

Admission: _____

I. **The client/caregiver can define spina bifida.**

 A. It is a neural tube defect involving incomplete development of the brain, spinal cord, and/or the protective coverings.
 B. It is caused by the failure of the fetus's spine to close properly during the first month of pregnancy.
 C. The three types of spina bifida are
  1. Myelomeningocele (most severe)—the spinal cord and its protective covering protrude from an opening in the spine.
  2. Meningocele—the spinal cord develops normally but the meninges protrude from a spinal opening.
  3. Occulta—one or more vertebrae are malformed and covered by a layer of skin.
 D. Spina bifida can cause bowel and bladder complications.
 E. Spina bifida is often associated with hydrocephalus (excessive accumulation of cerebrospinal fluid in the brain).

II. **The client/caregiver can list risk factors for spina bifida.**

 A. Spina bifida is more common among Hispanics and whites of European descent.
 B. Family history of neural tube defects
 C. Folic acid deficiency
 D. Some medications (antiseizure medications) taken during pregnancy can increase risk for neural tube defects.
 E. Diabetes and poor blood sugar control during early pregnancy
 F. Obesity and prepregnancy obesity
 G. Increased body temperature in the early months of pregnancy

III. **The client/caregiver can list methods to screen and diagnose spina bifida.**

 A. Maternal serum alpha-fetoprotein (MSAFP) test. This is a blood test

performed during weeks 16 and 18 of pregnancy.
 B. Based on the results of this test, the physician may suggest amniocentesis or high-resolution ultrasonography.

IV. **The client/caregiver can list current treatment considerations for SB.**

 A. The treatment depends on the severity of the condition.
 B. Often a caesarean birth is planned for the safety of the baby, and it can provide for quick and skilled intervention after birth.
 C. Research is promising regarding prenatal surgery to correct defects before birth.
 D. Treatment can include multiple surgeries and a multidisciplinary team of health care providers.

V. **The client/caregiver can list prevention tips and measures to manage this condition.**

 A. Folic acid supplements taken at least 1 month before conception and during the first trimester of pregnancy will greatly reduce the risk of neural tube defects.
 B. March of Dimes, the Centers for Disease Control and Prevention, and the Institute of Medicine recommend that women of childbearing age take folic acid supplements of 400 micrograms daily.
 C. Be informed. Develop realistic goals.
 D. There is a need for periodic and ongoing medical evaluations and treatment.
 E. Understand medications and treatments.
 F. Prevent infection and injury.
 G. More than 70% of people with spina bifida have a latex allergy. Check Latex allergy information in Chapter 2. The Spina Bifida Association offers a latex update list (2006).
 H. Promote family coping. Seek counseling, education, emotional support, and financial assistance as needed.

(Continued)

RESOURCES

National Institute of Neurological Disorders and Stroke
www.ninds.nih.gov/disorders/spina_bifida/spina_bifida.htm

Spina Bifida Association of America
800-621-3141
www.sbaa.org

March of Dimes Birth Defects Foundation
888-MODIMES (888-663-4637)
www.marchofdimes.com

Support groups

REFERENCES

Ackley, B. J., & Ladwig, G. B. (2006). *Nursing diagnosis handbook: A guide to planning care.* St. Louis: Mosby Inc.

Cohen, B. J., & Taylor, J. J. (2005). *Memmler's the human body in health and disease* (10th ed.). Philadelphia: Lippincott Williams & Wilkins.

Maternal-neonatal nursing: Lippincott manual of nursing practice pocket guides. (2007). Philadelphia: Lippincott Williams & Wilkins.

Muscari, M. E. (2005). *Pediatric nursing.* Philadelphia: Lippincott Williams & Wilkins.

Novak, J. C., & Broom, B. L. (1999). *Maternal and child health nursing.* St. Louis: Mosby, Inc.

6 Scoliosis

Patient name: _____ **Admission:** _____

I. **The client/caregiver can define scoliosis.**

A. Scoliosis is when there is a curve of the spine to one side. Two curves in opposite directions may be present.
B. Most children diagnosed with scoliosis have a mild curve—less than 20 degrees.
C. The onset of scoliosis is rare in adults.
D. It is the most common spinal deformity.

II. **The client/caregiver can list methods used for detection of scoliosis.**

A. Most public schools check for scoliosis in grade school.
B. Ask your physician for a routine exam at regular check-ups.
C. Have x-rays as indicated.

III. **The client/caregiver can list signs and symptoms of spine curvatures.**

A. Signs of scoliosis are
   • Uneven shoulders
   • One shoulder blade that appears more prominent than the other
   • An uneven waist
   • One hip higher than the other
   • Leaning to one side
B. Severe scoliosis can cause back pain and difficulty breathing.

IV. **The client/caregiver can list risk factors for scoliosis.**

A. The cause is unknown.
B. Scoliosis is often noticed before or during adolescence.
C. Growth is the biggest risk factor for worsening of curve.
D. Most forms of scoliosis are more common in girls.
E. The greater the curve when discovered, the more likely it will worsen.

F. Curves in the upper spine are more likely to increase.
G. Scoliosis runs in families.

V. **The client/caregiver can list possible complications of scoliosis.**

A. Lung and heart damage
B. Back problems
C. Impaired body image

VI. **The client/caregiver can list methods of treatment.**

A. Regular systematic observations to measure changes
B. Use of brace
C. Surgery
D. Emotional support and learned coping skills for client
E. Support groups for parents to help them learn ways of helping child

RESOURCES

National Scoliosis Foundation
781-341-6333
www.scoliosis.org/

The Scoliosis Association, Inc.
800-800-0669

REFERENCES

Ackley, B. J., & Ladwig, G. B. (2006). *Nursing diagnosis handbook: A guide to planning care.* St. Louis: Mosby Inc.
Canobbio, M. M. (2006). *Mosby's handbook of patient teaching.* St. Louis: Mosby Inc.
Cohen, B. J., & Taylor, J. J. (2005). *Memmler's the human body in health and disease* (10th ed.). Philadelphia: Lippincott Williams & Wilkins.
Muscari, M. E. (2005). *Pediatric nursing.* Philadelphia: Lippincott Williams & Wilkins.
Taylor, C., Lillis, C., & LeMone, P. (2005). *Fundamentals of nursing.* Philadelphia: Lippincott, Williams & Wilkins.

7

Muscular Dystrophy

Patient name: _____ **Admission:** _____

<table>
<tr><td>NRS
DATE INITIAL</td></tr>
</table>

I. **The client/caregiver can define muscular dystrophy.**

A. It is a group of rare inherited muscle diseases. The muscle fibers are unusually susceptible to damage.

B. Muscles (primarily voluntary) become progressively weaker.

C. In late stages of disease, fat and connective tissue replace muscle fibers.

D. There is no known cure, but medications and therapy can help slow the course of the disease.

E. Duchenne muscular dystrophy is the most severe form. It is the most common form of muscular dystrophy that affects children. Boys are at greater risk.

II. **The client/caregiver can explain symptoms of muscular dystrophy.**

A. Signs and symptoms appear between the ages of 2 and 5.

B. Muscles of the pelvic, upper arms, and upper legs are affected first.

C. Most children by late childhood cannot walk.

D. Life expectancy is only for late teens or early 20s.

E. Signs and symptoms are
- Frequent falls
- Large calf muscles
- Difficulty getting up from a lying or sitting position
- Weakness in lower leg muscles with difficulty running and jumping
- Waddling like gait
- Mild mental retardation sometimes

III. **The client/caregiver can list measures to manage or deal with muscular dystrophy.**

A. Physical and occupational therapy as ordered

B. Range of motion exercises

<table>
<tr><td>NRS
DATE INITIAL</td></tr>
</table>

C. Hydrotherapy (hot baths) for comfort and maintain range of movement

D. Use balanced diet with fruits, vegetables, milk, poultry, and fish. Limit the intake of sugars and saturated fats. Adapt texture of foods as needed if having difficulty chewing or swallowing. Feed smaller, more frequent meals.

E. Take medications as ordered.

F. Assistive devices are available for
1. Prevention of contractures
2. Maintain mobility and independence
3. Possible respiratory equipment to assist respiratory muscles
4. Surgery to relieve contractures and relieve tendons

G. Promote good skin care and positioning if confined to bed or wheelchair.

H. Keep immunizations current.

I. Have regular follow-up visits with physician.

J. Encourage medical alert bracelet.

K. Support groups are available for client and parents/caregivers.

L. Have a medical social consult for financial concerns.

RESOURCES

Muscular Dystrophy Association
800-572-1717
www.mdausa.org/

Support groups

Respite care

Clergy

REFERENCES

Ackley, B. J., & Ladwig, G. B. (2006). *Nursing diagnosis handbook: A guide to planning care.* St. Louis: Mosby Inc.

(Continued)

Canobbio, M. M. (2006). *Mosby's handbook of patient teaching.* St. Louis: Mosby Inc.

Cohen, B. J., & Taylor, J. J. (2005). *Memmler's the human body in health and disease* (10th ed.). Philadelphia: Lippincott Williams & Wilkins.

Lutz, C., & Przytulski, K. (2001). *Nutrition and diet therapy.* Philadelphia: F. A. Davis Company.

Taylor, C., Lillis, C., & LeMone, P. (2005). *Fundamentals of nursing.* Philadelphia: Lippincott, Williams & Wilkins.

8 Fetal Alcohol Syndrome

Patient name: _____ **Admission:** _____

NRS
DATE INITIAL

I. **The client/caregiver can define fetal alcohol syndrome.**

   A. It is when a baby is born with a group of birth defects that is a result of the mother drinking alcohol during pregnancy.

   B. These defects are irreversible and can include physical, mental, and behavioral problems.

II. **The client/caregiver can list signs and symptoms of fetal alcohol syndrome.**

   A. Facial features that include
- Small eyelid openings
- Sunken nasal bridge
- Very thin upper lip
- Short upturned nose
- Smooth skin surface between the nose and upper lip

   B. Small teeth with poor enamel.

   C. Heart defects

   D. Deformity of joints, limbs, and fingers

   E. Slow physical growth before and after birth

   F. Vision problems, including nearsightedness

   G. Small head circumference and brain size

   H. Mental retardation and delayed development

   I. Abnormal behavior, such as
- Short attention span
- Hyperactivity
- Poor impulse control
- Extreme nervousness and anxiety

III. **The client/caregiver can explain causes of fetal alcohol syndrome.**

   A. Any alcohol entering the mother's bloodstream crosses the placenta to the fetus.

   B. The fetus will metabolize alcohol slower and have a higher alcohol concentration.

   C. The risk of alcohol causing defects to the fetus is present at any time during the pregnancy.

NRS
DATE INITIAL

   D. Much of the damage to the fetus can be done during the first trimester, when many of the organs are developing. Stress that damages can occur at any time during pregnancy.

IV. **The client/caregiver can list ways to prevent fetal alcohol syndrome and measures to deal with damage.**

   A. Fetal alcohol syndrome is completely preventable by not drinking alcohol during pregnancy.

   B. If you are sexually active and having unprotected sex, think about giving up alcohol.

   C. Seek professional help to make diagnosis if fetal alcohol syndrome is suspected.

   D. Seek substance abuse counseling and treatment if you have given birth to a child with fetal alcohol syndrome.

   E. Seek help from healthcare professionals and mental health counselors to cope with the health and behavior problems of child.

   F. Possible complications for child with FAS are
- Drug abuse
- Dropping out of school
- Ending up in juvenile justice system

RESOURCES

National Organization on Fetal Alcohol Syndrome
800-66-NOFAS
www.nofas.org

National Institute on Alcohol Abuse and Alcoholism
301-443-3860
www.niaaa.nih.gov

Drinking and Your Pregnancy
http://pubs.niaaa.nih.gov/publications/DrinkingPregnancy_HTML/pregnancy.htm

Substance Abuse and Mental Health Services Administration Treatment Facility Locator
800-662-HELP
www.findtreatment.samhsa.gov

(Continued)

REFERENCES

Ackley, B. J., & Ladwig, G. B. (2006). *Nursing diagnosis handbook: A guide to planning care.* St. Louis: Mosby Inc.

Cohen, B. J., & Taylor, J. J. (2005). *Memmler's the human body in health and disease* (10th ed.). Philadelphia: Lippincott Williams & Wilkins.

Hunt, R. (2005). *Introduction to community based nursing.* Philadelphia: Lippincott Williams & Wilkins.

Maternal-neonatal nursing: Lippincott manual of nursing practice pocket guides. (2007). Philadelphia: Lippincott Williams & Wilkins.

Novak, J. C., & Broom, B. L. (1999). *Maternal and child health nursing.* St. Louis: Mosby, Inc.

Taylor, C., Lillis, C., & LeMone, P. (2005). *Fundamentals of nursing.* Philadelphia: Lippincott, Williams & Wilkins.

9 Lead Poisoning

Patient name: _____   **Admission:** _____

NRS
DATE INITIAL

I. **The client/caregiver can define lead poisoning.**

   A. Lead poisoning is the result of exposure to lead in the environment.

   B. Children are more susceptible to the negative effects of lead.

   C. Lead can accumulate and damage the nervous system. This may result in lower intelligence and problems with school.

   D. Most exposure to lead is from lead pipes and lead-based paint in older homes.

II. **The client/caregiver can list signs and symptoms of lead poisoning.**

   A. Lead poisoning is a gradual build up and symptoms may not appear until levels reach a dangerous level.

   B. Symptoms in children may be
- Irritability
- Loss of appetite
- Weight loss
- Abdominal pain
- Vomiting
- Constipation
- Sluggishness
- Paleness
- Learning difficulties

   C. Symptoms for adults include these plus
- Pain, numbness, or tingling of the extremities
- Muscular weakness
- Headache
- Memory loss
- Mood disorders
- Reduced sperm count

III. **The client/caregiver can list causes or sources of lead poisoning.**

   A. High levels of lead are in soil as a result of gasoline or paint with lead being disposed of improperly.

   B. Prior to 1980, lead pipes, copper pipes, brass plumbing, and solder were used and could allow lead to release into tap water.

NRS
DATE INITIAL

Now theses products are restricted. The Environmental Protection Act recommends not making baby formula with tap water from old plumbing systems.

   C. In 1978, lead-based paints used in homes, children's toys, and furniture were banned. Lead-based paint may still remain on walls and woodwork in older homes.

   D. Dust can contain lead from chipped paint or soil from outside.

   E. Imported canned foods may still have been sealed by lead solder.

   F. Read labels to avoid lead in cosmetics or complementary remedies.

IV. **The client/caregiver can list possible complications from lead poisoning.**

   A. Complications for children include
- Nervous system and kidney damage
- Learning disabilities
- Speech, language, and behavior problems
- Poor muscle coordination
- Decreased muscle and bone growth
- Hearing damage
- Seizures

   B. Complications for adults include
- High blood pressure
- Digestive or nerve disorders
- Cataracts
- Memory and concentration problems
- Muscle and joint problems
- Pregnancy complications (miscarriage, preterm delivery, and still birth)
- Damage to sperm production

V. **The client/caregiver can list measures to prevent lead poisoning.**

   A. Have a professional check your home for lead.

   B. Wash children's hands after they play outside and before eating and going to bed.

   C. Clean floors with wet mop, and wipe furniture, windowsills, and dusty surfaces.

(Continued)

NRS
DATE INITIAL

D. Restrict where your children play.
E. Make sure child's diet is high in iron and calcium (reduces lead absorption).
F. Run cold water for over a minute before using.
G. Fix surfaces with peeling or chipping paint.
H. If doing remodeling or work in an older house
   1. Wear protective equipment and clothing.
   2. Do not eat or drink in area where lead dust is present.
   3. Do not remove lead paint by sanding.
   4. Do not use open-flame torch or heat guns to remove paint.

RESOURCES

Centers for Disease Control and Prevention: Lead Paint Prevention Program
www.cdc.gov/nceh/lead/

Consumer Product Safety Commission: Protect Your Family from Lead in Your Home
www.cpsc.gov/cpscpub/pubs/426.html

U.S. Environmental Protection Agency: Lead in Paint, Dust, and Soil
www.epa.gov/opptintr/lead/index.html

REFERENCES

Ackley, B. J., & Ladwig, G. B. (2006). *Nursing diagnosis handbook: A guide to planning care.* St. Louis: Mosby Inc.

Cohen, B. J., & Taylor, J. J. (2005). *Memmler's the human body in health and disease* (10th ed.). Philadelphia: Lippincott Williams & Wilkins.

Hunt, R. (2005). *Introduction to community based nursing.* Philadelphia: Lippincott Williams & Wilkins.

Maternal-neonatal nursing: Lippincott manual of nursing practice pocket guides. (2007). Philadelphia: Lippincott Williams & Wilkins.

Novak, J. C., & Broom, B. L. (1999). *Maternal and child health nursing.* St. Louis: Mosby, Inc.

Taylor, C., Lillis, C., & LeMone, P. (2005). *Fundamentals of nursing.* Philadelphia: Lippincott, Williams & Wilkins.

10 Sudden Infant Death Syndrome

Admission: _____

NRS
DATE INITIAL

I. **The client/caregiver can define sudden infant death syndrome (SIDS).**

   A. It is the sudden, unexplained death of a seemingly healthy infant younger than 1 year old.

   B. Most SIDS deaths happen to babies between the age of 2 months and 4 months of age.

II. **The client/caregiver can list groups of infants most at risk for SIDS.**

   A. Babies placed on their stomachs or sides to sleep.

   B. African American babies are two times as likely to die of SIDS.

   C. American Indian/Alaska Native babies are three times as likely to die of SIDS.

   D. Babies born to mothers who smoked during pregnancy are a higher risk.

   E. Sharing a bed with adults increases the risk.

   F. Preterm or low birth weight infants are at risk.

   G. Sleeping on soft surface such as waterbed, couch, or pillows increases the risk.

   H. Boy infants have higher risk of SIDS.

III. **The client/caregiver can list measures to prevent or reduce risks of SIDS.**

   A. New guidelines from the American Academy of Pediatrics for preventing SIDS was issued in October 2005.

     1. Place babies on their backs to sleep. Do not place them on their side.

     2. Be consistent to lay baby down to sleep on back.

     3. Place the baby on a safety-approved crib mattress covered with a fitted sheet. Never place him or her on a pillow, quilt, sheepskin, or soft surface.

     4. Do not sleep with your baby. It is okay to bring baby into bed to nurse or comfort, but return baby to crib to sleep.

     5. Keep baby in crib in the same room at first.

     6. Do not use soft items in crib such as
- Pillows
- Blankets
- Quilts
- Sheepskin
- Pillow-like bumpers in sleep area

     7. Use sleep clothing (one piece sleeper) instead of blankets.

     8. Keep soft objects, stuffed toys, or loose bedding out of sleep area.

     9. Make sure that nothing covers the baby's head.

    10. Avoid letting the baby overheat during sleep. Dress him or her in light clothes, and keep the room at comfortable temperature.

    11. Do not let anyone smoke near your baby.

    12. Use tummy time when baby is awake and someone is watching.

    13. Offer a pacifier—do not force. If breastfeeding, wait to offer a pacifier until the age of 1 month.

    14. Avoid products with claims to help prevent SIDS.

    15. Prevent flat spots on baby's head by alternating the direction your baby's head faces.

IV. **The client/caregiver can discuss measures to help cope with the loss of infant.**

   A. Seek emotional support of others.

   B. Support groups can be helpful, but not for everyone. Find a friend or counselor to discuss feelings and emotions.

   C. Keep yourself open to the communication of friends and family. Many people want to help, but they do not know what to say or do.

   D. Keep communication open between parents. Seek help and counseling if needed.

   E. Allow time to grieve. Be kind to yourself, and discuss possible feelings of guilt or helplessness with family or professional grief counselor.

(Continued)

RESOURCES

Back to Sleep
800-505-CRIB
E-mail: NICHDIRC@mail.nih.gov

Support groups

Clergy

REFERENCES

Hunt, R. (2005). *Introduction to community based nursing.* Philadelphia: Lippincott Williams & Wilkins.

Maternal-neonatal nursing: Lippincott manual of nursing practice pocket guides. (2007). Philadelphia: Lippincott Williams & Wilkins.

Muscari, M. E. (2005). *Pediatric nursing.* Philadelphia: Lippincott Williams & Wilkins.

National Institute of Child Health and Human Development. *Safe Sleep for Your Baby: Ten Ways to Reduce the Risk of Sudden Infant Death Syndrome (SIDS).* (2006). Available from: *www.nichd.nih.gov/publications/pubs/safe_sleep_gen.cfm.*

Novak, J. C., & Broom, B. L. (1999). *Maternal and child health nursing.* St. Louis: Mosby, Inc.

Taylor, C., Lillis, C., & LeMone, P. (2005). *Fundamentals of nursing.* Philadelphia: Lippincott, Williams & Wilkins.

11 Otitis Media

Patient name: _____   **Admission:** _____

I. **The client/caregiver can define otitis media.**

   A. The middle ear is an air space containing three small bones (malleus, incus, and stapes).
   B. The Eustachian tube connects the middle ear cavity with the throat. In children, this tube is short and horizontal. Transmission of infection to the middle ear is common.
   C. Otitis media is a bacterial or viral infection in the middle ear.

II. **The client/caregiver can list common signs to watch for when considering otitis media.**

   A. Unusual irritability
   B. Difficulty sleeping
   C. Tugging or pulling at one or both ears
   D. Fever
   E. Fluid draining from the ear
   F. Loss of balance
   G. Signs of hearing difficulty
      • Unresponsiveness to quiet sounds
      • Sitting too close to the television
      • Being inattentive

III. **The client/caregiver can list measures to prevent or manage otitis media.**

   A. Avoid contact with sick playmates.
   B. Avoid environmental tobacco smoke.

   C. Children who nurse from a bottle while lying down appear to develop otitis media more often.
   D. Take medication as ordered and complete all medication cycle.

IV. **The client/caregiver can list possible complications from otitis media.**

   A. Infection can spread to the brain, if untreated.
   B. Hearing loss, possible permanent
   C. Interfere with speech and language development

RESOURCE
American Speech-Language-Hearing Association
www.asha.org

REFERENCES
Cohen, B. J., & Taylor, J. J. (2005). *Memmler's the human body in health and disease* (10th ed.). Philadelphia: Lippincott Williams & Wilkins.

Perry, A., & Potter, P. (2006). *Clinical nursing skills & technique.* St. Louis: Mosby Inc.

Timby, B. K., & Smith, N. C. (2003). *Introductory medical-surgical nursing* (8th ed.). Philadelphia: J. B. Lippincott Williams & Wilkins.

Prenatal Care

■ Patient name: _____   Admission: _____

DATE NRS INITIAL

I. **The client/caregiver can list measures for good nutrition during pregnancy.**

A. Eat well-balanced meals including meats, fruits, vegetables, breads, cereals, and milk.

B. Caloric intake varies according to height and weight but should be at least 1800 calories per day. As a general rule, a healthy pregnant female should consume an additional 300 calories per day during pregnancy.

C. Increase protein with sources, such as milk, meat, eggs, cheese, poultry, and so forth. Be aware that animal sources of protein are complete proteins but can be high in saturated fat and cholesterol.

D. Vegetarian diets can be a problem when trying to meet protein requirements during pregnancy. Understanding how to combine plant proteins (incomplete proteins) to meet the protein requirements of pregnancy may need the assistance of a nutritionist. The physician may also order B12 injections to avoid deficiencies.

E. Evaluate food patterns and choices of other cultures to meet requirements of well-balanced nutrition. Adjust diet as needed to meet standards for pregnancy.

F. Certain vitamins and minerals are even more important during pregnancy. Sources for the following nutrients can be found in the nutrition section.

1. Vitamin A in correct amounts is needed for fetal growth and development.
2. Vitamin E is needed to prevent cell damage and neurological symptoms.
3. Vitamin B6 is needed for the metabolism of protein.
4. Folic acid is necessary to reduce the incidence of neural tube defects such as spina bifida.
5. Iron is needed for the manufacture of hemoglobin in both mother and fetus.

DATE NRS INITIAL

6. Calcium is necessary for the development of the fetal skeleton and teeth. If a pregnant woman is deficient in calcium, the fetus will demand calcium and create an even greater deficiency.
7. Vitamin D is important for the role it plays in calcium metabolism.

G. Only take vitamin supplements as ordered by physician. Do not take megadoses of vitamins or supplements. This can be dangerous to the fetus.

H. Avoid empty calories, such as candy, cakes, soda, and so forth.

II. **The client/caregiver can list measures for exercise and rest.**

A. Avoid becoming overly tired. Get adequate sleep at night and rest periods or naps in the afternoon. Avoid exercise during high heat or humidity.

B. Exercise daily (walking or swimming is beneficial).

C. Limit exercise periods to 30 to 45 minutes.

D. After the fourth month of pregnancy, do not exercise in the supine position (on your back).

E. Perform warm-up and cool-down exercises before and after exercising.

F. Stop exercise immediately if any faintness, shortness of breath, excessively fast heart rate, or chest pain occurs.

G. Kegel exercises (exercises using pelvic floor muscles) can be used.

III. **The client/caregiver can list other general care measures during pregnancy.**

A. Practice good hygiene measures
1. Bathe daily.
2. Tub baths may be taken until membranes rupture.
3. Use safety precautions if using tub baths in late pregnancy to prevent falls.
4. Avoid douching.

(Continued)

B. Learn danger signs for each trimester of pregnancy that should be reported to physician immediately.

C. Avoid over-the-counter medications unless permitted by physician.

D. Keep appointments with physician and obtain laboratory studies as ordered.

E. Travel should allow for rest stops at least every two hours. Proper use and placement of seat belts should be taught. Lap belt should be snug and low across the hip bones. The shoulder belt rides above the pregnant uterus and rests between the breasts.

F. Clothing should not be constrictive.

G. Saunas, hot tubs, and steam rooms should be avoided during pregnancy.

H. Toxoplasmosis is an infection caused by a parasite harmful to the unborn baby. Avoid eating undercooked meat and handling cat litter. Wear gloves when gardening.

IV. **The client/caregiver can list the dangers of smoking, alcohol, and drugs.**

A. Avoid smoking because it restricts blood vessels, causing a decreased oxygen level to the infant. Cigarette smoking during pregnancy can result in low-weight babies.

B. Avoid alcohol and drugs because of possible premature delivery, fetal abnormalities, and low birth weight.

C. Avoid all medications while pregnant unless specifically ordered by physician.

V. **The client/caregiver understands the need for good breast care.**

A. Wear a well-fitting brassiere to relieve discomfort and to prevent sagging after childbirth.

B. Wash breasts with soap and water, rinse, and dry to cleanse secretion of colostrum.

C. If planning to breast feed, nipples should be prepared by rubbing with a rough towel several times a day during the last trimester.

VI. **The client/caregiver is aware of measures to prevent complications.**

A. Backache
   1. Use good body mechanics ("body mechanics" teaching guide).
   2. Use good posture.
   3. Use side-lying position for rest.
   4. Wear low heeled, well-fitting shoes.

B. Constipation
   1. Eat high-fiber food (i.e., fresh fruits and vegetables).
   2. Drink at least 8 to 10 glasses of fluid per day unless contraindicated.
   3. Exercise regularly.

C. Hemorrhoids
   1. Avoid constipation.
   2. Witch hazel compresses to the rectal area, or sitz baths may help.
   3. Use analgesic ointments or suppositories only with physician approval.

D. Leg cramps
   1. Wear loose-fitting clothing to prevent leg cramps.
   2. Practice gentle stretching; do not massage.

E. Nausea and vomiting
   1. Eat bland, dry foods.
   2. Eat small, frequent meals.
   3. Avoid fried, spicy foods.

F. Heartburn
   1. Avoid lying flat after eating.
   2. Use antacids only with physician approval.
   3. Follow the same suggestions as for nausea and vomiting.

G. Urinary frequency
   1. Decrease fluids at bedtime.

H. Varicose veins
   1. Wear support hose.
   2. Avoid long periods of standing or sitting with legs crossed.

I. Swelling of extremities
   1. Elevate feet.
   2. Limit sodium intake.

J. Fatigue
   1. Get a good night's sleep.
   2. Take naps during the day. Elevate legs.

VII. **The client/caregiver is aware of danger signals to be reported immediately.**

A. Vaginal spotting or bleeding at any time

B. Leaking of fluid from vagina

C. Unusual abdominal pain, cramping, pelvic pressure, or persistent backache

D. Persistent nausea or vomiting, especially into the second and third trimester

E. Marked swelling of ankles, face, or hands

F. Persistent headache or changes in vision

G. Chills and fever

H. Muscular irritability or convulsions

(Continued)

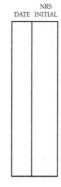

I. Blood in urine, painful or burning urination, or decreased urine output
J. Decreased or absence of fetal movement in third trimester of pregnancy
K. Foul-smelling vaginal discharge
L. Signs of preeclampsia (i.e., rapid weight gain, hypertension, and protein in urine)

VIII. The client/caregiver can list possible complications during pregnancy.

A. Abruptio placentae
B. Cephalopelvic disproportion
C. Cervical insufficiency
D. Gestational diabetes
E. Ectopic pregnancy
F. Gestational hypertension
G. Hyperemesis gravidarum
H. Isoimmunization
I. Multiple gestation
J. Placenta previa
K. Premature labor
L. Prolapsed umbical cord
M. Spontaneous abortion

IX. The client/caregiver can list laboratory tests that may be used during pregnancy.

A. Maternal Serum-Alpha-Fetoprotein (MSAFP). This test is done between week 16 and 18. Screen for neural tube defects or for Down syndrome.
B. Hemoglobin and hematocrit. This is used to screen for iron or folic acid deficiencies.
C. Blood glucose screening. This can screen for diabetes during pregnancy.
D. Antibody titers. This will screen the pregnant client for serious isoimmune condition that is a threat to the life of the fetus.

E. Tests for sexually transmitted diseases. These tests will screen for syphilis, gonorrhea, HIV, and genital herpes.
F. Group B streptococcus. An initial test followed by a test at 35 to 37 weeks gestation will indicate whether there is a need for treatment before delivery. Identification and treatment of this organism can prevent exposing the newborn to overwhelming infection and possibly death.

RESOURCES

National Institutes of Health: National Institute of Child Health and Human Development
www.nichd.nih.gov/health/topics/pregnancy.cfm

U.S. Food & Drug Administration
www.cfsan.fda.gov/~pregnant/ataglanc.html

U.S. Department of Health and Human Services (Office on Women's Health)—The National Women's Health Information Center
http://womenshealth.gov/pregnancy/

REFERENCES

Hitchcock, J. E., Schubert, P. E., & Thomas, S. A. (2003). *Community health nursing: Caring in action.* Clifton Park, NY: Thomson Delmar Learning.

Lutz, C., & Przytulski, K. (2001). *Nutrition and diet therapy.* Philadelphia: F. A. Davis Company.

Maternal-neonatal nursing: Lippincott manual of nursing practice pocket guides. (2007). Philadelphia: Lippincott Williams & Wilkins.

Novak, J. C., & Broom, B. L. (1999). *Maternal and child health nursing.* St. Louis: Mosby, Inc.

2 Postpartum Care

Patient name: _____   **Admission:** _____

I. **The client/caregiver can list measures for general good health habits during postpartum.**

A. Measures to promote good nutrition
1. Eat a well-balanced diet of 2200 to 2300 calories per day with fluids of at least 2000 ml per day.
2. Increase calories to 2700 to 2800 if breast feeding, with fluids at least 3000 ml per day.
3. Eat plenty of fruits, vegetables, and whole grains.

B. Measures to promote exercise to restore muscle tone and promote healing
1. Advance exercises as instructed from very light exercise to more extensive exercise.
2. Avoid fatigue by planning regular rest periods and stopping exercise if tired.
3. Avoid vigorous exercise in early postpartum period because of possible bleeding.

C. Measures to promote healing and comfort of episiotomy
1. Take sitz baths as needed.
2. Use an ice pack or wrap ice in a washcloth to soothe area. Chilled witch hazel pads may also help to promote comfort.
3. Perform good hygiene.
4. Observe episiotomy for signs of infection, such as wound becoming hot, swollen, and production of pus-like discharge.

D. Measures to promote regular bowel regimen and ease hemorrhoid pain
1. Eat a high-fiber diet (i.e., fresh fruits and vegetables).
2. Increase fluid intake.
3. Exercise daily.
4. Use sitz bath, witch hazel compresses, or topical medication prescribed by physician for hemorrhoids.

E. Keep follow-up appointments with physician.

F. Mood swings, irritability, and anxiety are common emotions after giving birth. Even mild depression is normal and stops about 7 to 10 days after delivery. If depression deepens or feelings of hopelessness and sadness are present most of the time, contact your physician.

II. **The client/caregiver can describe normal vaginal discharge.**

A. Vaginal bleeding usually lasts approximately 6 weeks and changes from red to a reddish-brown discharge.
B. Symptoms to report to physician are
  • Discharge has a foul odor
  • Passing clots larger than a golf ball
  • Temperature of 100.3°F or higher
C. Menstruation frequently does not occur during breast feeding period, although pregnancy can still occur.

III. **The client/caregiver can list measures to promote comfort and prevent complication after a caesarean section delivery.**

A. Expect a longer recovery period.
B. Start activity and ambulation as ordered. Allow for plenty of rest.
C. Ask for pain medication if needed.

IV. **The client/caregiver can state instructions regarding sexual activity.**

A. Sexual activity can resume at the comfort of the mother and orders of the physician usually at approximately 4 weeks.
B. Discuss birth control options with your physician. Some form of contraception is needed if pregnancy is not desired.

V. **The client/caregiver is aware of special emotional needs.**

A. Avoid exhaustion, which may increase postpartum blues.

(Continued)

NRS
DATE INITIAL

B. Mood swings, irritability, and anxiety are common emotions after giving birth. Even mild depression is normal and stops about 7 to 10 days after delivery. If depression deepens or feelings of hopelessness and sadness are present most of the time, contact your physician.

C. Obtain counseling if depression is not resolved.

VI. **The client can list postpartum signs to report to physician.**

A. Change in vaginal discharge including an increase in amount, a change to bright-red bleeding, or foul-smelling discharge

B. Pain, redness, and swelling of one leg

C. Sore breasts with areas of pain, redness, or swelling

D. Fever

E. Pain in abdominal area

F. Painful urination

G. Depression

VII. **The client can list measures for successful breastfeeding and care of the breast.**

A. Measures for breast care
1. Wash breasts and rinse and dry well to prevent possible irritation.
2. Try a lanolin-based ointment for dry or cracked nipples.
3. Wear a well-fitting bra.
4. Use cold compresses or ice packs or mild analgesic to decrease discomfort of engorged breasts.

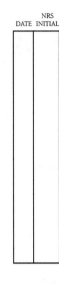

NRS
DATE INITIAL

5. Wear pads inside the bra for leakage. Change the pad often to keep nipples dry.

B. Breastfeeding tips
1. Cradle baby close to breast instead of bending or leaning forward.
2. Beware of caffeine and alcohol. Caffeine can make breastfed babies irritable.
3. Wait 2 hours after intake of alcohol before breastfeeding.
4. Wear loose tops that can be partially unbuttoned (from bottom) for feedings.
5. Only take medications that are approved by physician.
6. Contact lactation consultant.

RESOURCES

Lactation consultant

The National Women's Health Information Center
www.4woman.gov/

REFERENCES

Hitchcock, J. E., Schubert, P. E., & Thomas, S. A. (2003). *Community health nursing: Caring in action.* Clifton Park, NY: Thomson Delmar Learning.

Lutz, C., & Przytulski, K. (2001). *Nutrition and diet therapy.* Philadelphia: F. A. Davis Company.

Maternal-neonatal nursing: Lippincott manual of nursing practice pocket guides. (2007). Philadelphia: Lippincott Williams & Wilkins.

Novak, J. C., & Broom, B. L. (1999). *Maternal and child health nursing.* St. Louis: Mosby, Inc.

3 # Care of Newborn

Patient name: _____ **Admission:** _____

I. **The caregiver can list an infant's basic needs.**

  A. Feeding

  B. Sucking pleasure

  C. Warmth and comfort

  D. Love and security

  E. Sensory stimulation

II. **The client can explain how to properly handle a newborn infant.**

  A. Support your baby's head and neck. Cradle the head when carrying the baby. Support the head when carrying the baby upright or when laying them down.

  B. Be careful not to shake your newborn. Vigorous shaking can cause bleeding in the brain and even death.

  C. Be sure to securely fasten your baby into the carrier, stroller, or car seat.

  D. Newborns are not ready for rough play, such as being jiggled on the knee or thrown in the air.

III. **The caregiver can list general information tips for feeding the infant.**

  A. Feeding should be done "on demand" (when baby is hungry).

  B. Signs that babies are hungry include
    1. Moving head from side to side
    2. Opening mouth and sticking out tongues
    3. Placing hands and fists to mouth
    4. Opening their mouths and puckering their lips as if to suck
    5. Nuzzling against mother's breasts
    6. Showing rooting reflex

  C. Breastfeeding
    1. Mother should be eating a well-balanced diet and drinking at least eight glasses of fluid per day. Avoid smoking and use of caffeine and alcohol.
    2. Breastfeeding promotes bonding.
    3. Nipples should be cleansed carefully once a day, not using soap.
    4. Breast pumps or hand expression of milk can be used.

    5. Infant should be burped after 4 to 5 minutes on each breast.
    6. Infant should take vitamin supplements as recommended, including fluoride.

  D. Bottle feeding
    1. Formula is available in liquid, concentrate, or powder.
    2. Read instructions and prepare different forms of formula per directions.
    3. Never prop a bottle because of possible aspiration and lack of human contact.
    4. Keep the infant in an upright position, and place on his or her right side after feeding.
    5. Bottles and formula should be sterilized the first 5 months.
    6. Infants need to be burped after each ounce of formula and at the end of the feeding.

  E. Burping methods
    1. Hold the baby upright with head on parent's shoulder. Support the baby's head and back while gently patting the back with your other hand.
    2. Sit the baby on your lap. Support the baby's chest and head with one hand and gently rub his or her back with the other hand.

IV. **The client can explain how to change the newborn infant's diaper properly.**

  A. Make sure that you have all supplies within reach so that you will not have to leave your baby unattended on the changing surface.

  B. Plan on needing appropriately 10 diapers a day or 70 diapers per week.

  C. Place the baby on his or her back and remove dirty diaper. Using wipes, gently cleanse the baby's genital area.
    1. When removing a boy's diaper, do so carefully because exposure to air may make him urinate.
    2. When wiping a girl, wipe her bottom from front to back to avoid a urinary tract infection.

(Continued)

NRS
DATE INITIAL

3. If baby has rash or irritation, apply ointment.

4. Always remember to wash your hands after changing a diaper.

V. **The caregiver can demonstrate proper technique for bathing the infant.**

A. For the first year of life, the baby can be bathed two to three times a week. More frequent bathing may be drying to the skin.

B. Make sure that you have all supplies within reach so that you will not have to leave your baby unattended.

C. Make sure that the room where you are bathing is warm and has no drafts.

D. Use warm water (not hot), and test the water temperature with your elbow or wrist.

E. Use unscented baby soap and shampoo.

F. Use a soft baby brush to stimulate baby's scalp and manage potential cradle cap.

G. Use only water when bathing around the face. Soap may be used for the rest of the body.

H. Take care to cleanse the creases under the arm, behind the ears, and around the neck and genital areas.

I. Pat dry, and then diaper and dress baby.

VI. **The caregiver can demonstrate cord care.**

A. Do not bathe infant in the tub until naval area is well healed. Umbilical cord falls off in 1 to 4 weeks.
   • The navel heals completely in 1 to 4 weeks.

B. Clean cord area daily, and apply a drying agent as ordered.

C. Do not try to remove the cord.

D. Notify the physician if any bleeding, discharge, or foul odor is present.

VII. **The caregiver can demonstrate circumcision care.**

A. Wash the area with warm, soapy water.

B. The circumcision heals in 1 to 2 weeks.

C. Report any bleeding, foul odor, or failure to heal.

VIII. **The client can explain sleep basics for the newborn.**

A. Newborns sleep about 16 hours or more a day.

B. Place babies on their backs to sleep.

C. Remove fluffy bedding, quilts, sheepskins, stuffed animals, and pillows from crib.

NRS
DATE INITIAL

IX. **The caregiver can describe normal elimination.**

A. Stools may be greenish brown or yellowish brown.

B. Stools usually move several times per day.

C. Notify nurse or physician if there is blood in the stool or if no bowel movement in several days.

X. **The caregiver can list measures to meet emotional needs of the infant.**

A. The infant needs to be cuddled and held and talked to frequently.

B. Sensory stimulation, such as music, mobiles, and so forth promotes awareness.

C. Infant massage is important.

RESOURCES

Kangaroo Care/Cleveland Clinic
www.clevelandclinic.org

National Institute of Child Health and Human Development
www.nichd.nih.gov/

National Maternal and Child Health Clearinghouse

Health Resources and Services Administration

U.S. Department of Health and Human Resources
888-Ask HRSA (888-275-4772)
www.ask.hrsa.gov/MCH.cfm

La Leche League International
www.lalecheleague.org/

Women, Infants, Children Program
www.fns.usda.gov/wic/

International Association of Infant Massage
www.iaim.ws/home

REFERENCES

Hitchcock, J. E., Schubert, P. E., & Thomas, S. A. (2003). *Community health nursing: Caring in action.* Clifton Park, NY: Thomson Delmar Learning.

Lutz, C., & Przytulski, K. (2001). *Nutrition and diet therapy.* Philadelphia: F. A. Davis Company.

Maternal-neonatal nursing: Lippincott manual of nursing practice pocket guides. (2007). Philadelphia: Lippincott Williams & Wilkins.

Novak, J. C., & Broom, B. L. (1999). *Maternal and child health nursing.* St. Louis: Mosby, Inc.

Conjunctivitis

Patient name: _____

Admission: _____

NRS
DATE INITIAL

I. **The client/caregiver can define conjunctivitis.**

   A. It is an inflammation of the conjunctive, the clear membrane that covers the white part of the eye and inner surface of the eyelids.
   B. Viruses, bacteria, allergies, or substances that irritate the eyes can cause conjunctivitis.
   C. It is commonly called "pink eye."
   D. It is very contagious.

II. **The client/caregiver can recognize signs and symptoms.**

   A. Discomfort or feeling of irritation
   B. Redness
   C. Watery or pus-like drainage
   D. Eyelid swelling
   E. Itching and tearing
   F. Crusting discharge that can mat the eyelashes together

III. **The client/caregiver can list measures to prevent spread of the disease.**

   A. Wash hands (with soap and water) frequently, especially after touching eyes.
   B. Do not share washcloths, towels, eye drops, tissues, make-up, or pillowcases.
   C. Wash items such as towels in hot water and separate from others.

NRS
DATE INITIAL

   D. Discard cotton balls, gauze, or tissues properly.
   E. Avoid smoke or other known items that cause irritation or allergic reactions.
   F. Keep a child home from school and away from other children as directed by the physician.

IV. **The client/caregiver can list measures that relieve symptoms.**

   A. Cleanse eyelids and lashes frequently.
   B. Apply warm or cold compresses.
   C. Use acetaminophen or ibuprofen as directed by physician for discomfort.
   D. Take medication/eye ointments as ordered.
   E. The physician may order antiallergy medication (in pill form) if the child has allergic conjunctivitis.

REFERENCES

Cohen, B. J., & Taylor, J. J. (2005). *Memmler's the human body in health and disease* (10th ed.). Philadelphia: Lippincott Williams & Wilkins.

Perry, A., & Potter, P. (2006). *Clinical nursing skills & technique.* St. Louis: Mosby Inc.

Timby, B. K., & Smith, N. C. (2003). *Introductory medical-surgical nursing* (8th ed.). Philadelphia: J. B. Lippincott Williams & Wilkins.

Glaucoma

2

Patient name: _____ Admission: _____

NRS
DATE INITIAL

I. **The client/caregiver can define glaucoma.**

   A. It is increased fluid pressure within the eyeball.
   B. It is caused by increased production or decreased outflow of aqueous humor.
   C. The optic nerve can be damaged as the result of increased pressure.

II. **The client/caregiver can list signs and symptoms of glaucoma.**

   A. Chronic or open-angle glaucoma (gradual onset)
      1. Reduced peripheral vision
      2. Intermittent and temporary blurred vision
      3. Halos around lights
      4. Dull eye pain or headache, especially in morning
      5. Difficulty adjusting to dark rooms
   B. Acute or closed angle (rapid or sudden onset)
      1. Severe eye pain
      2. Headache
      3. Nausea or vomiting
      4. Loss of sight
      5. Cornea that appears cloudy
      6. Considered medical emergency

III. **The client/caregiver can list factors that increase the risk.**

   A. Blacks over the age of 40 years. Blacks are five times more likely to have glaucoma than whites.
   B. People with family history of glaucoma
   C. Everyone over the age of 60 years, especially Mexican Americans
   D. Trauma to the eye, or eye abnormalities
   E. Prolonged corticosteroid use
   F. Nearsightedness also increases risk of glaucoma.

NRS
DATE INITIAL

IV. **The client/caregiver can list possible treatments.**

   A. Medications
   B. Surgery

V. **The client/caregiver can list measures to prevent or manage glaucoma.**

   A. Obtain early detection with comprehensive dilated eye exam routinely. Comprehensive eye exam includes the following:
      1. Visual acuity testing measures how well you see at various distances.
      2. A dilated eye exam can reveal any damage to retina or optic nerve.
      3. Tonometry uses an instrument to measure pressure inside the eye.
   B. Medication teaching should include the following:
      1. Take medications as ordered.
      2. Teach proper technique to administer medication for eye drops or ocular therapeutic system.
      3. Arrange for assistance in administering medication if client has difficulty in medication administration.
      4. Keep an extra supply of prescribed drugs on hand.
      5. Avoid all drugs that contain atropine.
      6. Check with the physician before using any nonprescription medications. Be cautious about herbal supplements and check with physician before using.
      7. Stress the importance of ongoing need for medication use.
   C. Nutritional considerations are as follows:
      1. Maintain a healthy diet that includes plenty of fruits and vegetables.
      2. Your physician may suggest supplements of vitamins A, C, and E and minerals such as zinc and copper.

(Continued)

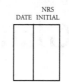

3. Drink fluids in small amounts but frequently over the course of a day.
4. Use caffeine in low to moderate amounts.
D. Exercise regularly. Consult with physician regarding an appropriate exercise program.
E. Learn relaxation techniques. Stress can trigger an attack of acute-angle glaucoma. Avoid emotional upsets, especially crying.
F. Wear proper eye protection when using tools, playing sports, or working with chemicals.
G. Avoid factors that increase pressure in eye:
   • Coughing, sneezing, aggressive nose blowing
   • Strenuous exercise
   • Straining when having bowel movement
   • Bending at the waist
   • Lifting heavy objects
H. Prevent overuse and strain of eyes.
I. Wear identification tag or bracelet.
J. Seek medical attention immediately if pain or visual changes occur.

VI. The client/caregiver can list measures to promote safety, as decreased peripheral vision can be detrimental.

A. Clear pathways.
B. Provide adequate lighting.
C. Turn head to visualize either side.
D. Ask for a referral to a specialist in low vision for help with adaptive equipment or low vision rehabilitation.

RESOURCES
National Eye Institute, National Institutes of Health
www.nei.nih.gov/health/glaucoma/glaucoma_facts.asp

American Academy of Family Physicians

Occupational consult for activities of daily living

REFERENCES
Ackley, B. J., & Ladwig, G. B. (2006). *Nursing diagnosis handbook: A guide to planning care.* St. Louis: Mosby Inc.
Cohen, B. J., & Taylor, J. J. (2005). *Memmler's the human body in health and disease* (10th ed.). Philadelphia: Lippincott Williams & Wilkins.
Hunt, R. (2005). *Introduction to community based nursing.* Philadelphia: Lippincott Williams & Wilkins.
Lutz, C., & Przytulski, K. (2001). *Nutrition and diet therapy.* Philadelphia: F. A. Davis Company.
National Eye Institute. (2007). *Glaucoma resource guide.* Bethesda, MD. Available from: *www.nei.nih.gov/health/glaucoma/glaucoma_facts.asp.*
Timby, B. K., & Smith, N. C. (2003). *Introductory medical-surgical nursing* (8th ed.). Philadelphia: J. B. Lippincott Williams & Wilkins.

3 Cataracts

Patient name: _____ Admission: _____

NRS
DATE INITIAL

I. **The client/caregiver can define cataracts and risks for developing cataracts.**

  A. It is when the lens of the eye becomes cloudy and impairs vision.

  B. Cataracts can occur in one or both eyes.

  C. Cataracts grow slowly, and thus, vision gets worse gradually.

  D. Risk of cataracts increases by
- Aging process
- Diabetes
- Lifestyle behaviors such as smoking or alcohol use
- Prolonged exposure to ultraviolet sunlight

II. **The client/caregiver can list symptoms of a cataract.**

  A. Cloudy or blurry vision

  B. Poor night vision

  C. Glare—sensitivity to bright light or halo may appear around lights

  D. Double vision or multiple images in one eye

  E. Frequent prescription changes in eyeglasses or contact lenses

III. **The client/caregiver can list method of detection for cataracts.**

  A. Comprehensive eye exam that includes
1. Visual acuity testing measures how well you see at various distances.
2. Dilated eye exam can reveal any damage to retina or optic nerve.
3. Tonometry uses an instrument to measure pressure inside the eye.

IV. **The client/caregiver can list methods to manage, treat or prevent cataracts.**

  A. Early symptoms can be improved with
- New eyeglasses/contacts
- Use of brighter indoor lighting

NRS
DATE INITIAL

- Antiglare sunglasses
- Wearing hat with brim to block ultraviolet sunlight
- Use of magnifying lenses

  B. If cataracts interfere with activities such as driving, reading, and watching television, surgery may be indicated.

  C. Surgical treatment would remove cloudy lens and insert replacement artificial lens. Follow postsurgery instructions. and wait for clearance from physician before driving again.

  D. Nutritional suggestions include eating green leafy vegetables, fruits, and other foods with antioxidants.

  E. Routine comprehensive eye exams.

RESOURCE

National Eye Institute
301-496-5248
www.nei.nih.gov

REFERENCES

Ackley, B. J., & Ladwig, G. B. (2006). *Nursing diagnosis handbook: A guide to planning care*. St. Louis: Mosby Inc.

Cohen, B. J., & Taylor, J. J. (2005). *Memmler's the human body in health and disease* (10th ed.). Philadelphia: Lippincott Williams & Wilkins.

Hunt, R. (2005). *Introduction to community based nursing*. Philadelphia: Lippincott Williams & Wilkins.

Lutz, C., & Przytulski, K. (2001). *Nutrition and diet therapy*. Philadelphia: F. A. Davis Company.

Nutrition made incredibly easy. (2003). Philadelphia: Lippincott Williams & Wilkins.

Taylor, C., Lillis, C., & LeMone, P. (2005). *Fundamentals of nursing*. Philadelphia: Lippincott, Williams & Wilkins.

Timby, B. K., & Smith, N. C. (2003). *Introductory medical-surgical nursing* (8th ed.). Philadelphia: J. B. Lippincott Williams & Wilkins.

4 Age-Related Macular Degeneration

Patient name: _____ Admission: _____

NRS
DATE INITIAL

I. **The client/caregiver will define macular degeneration.**

   A. It is the breakdown or damage to the macula (located in retina) of the eye.
   B. It is a disease that gradually destroys sharp, central vision needed for reading and other activities.
   C. It is more common in aging adults.
   D. It usually occurs in both eyes.

II. **The client/caregiver can list symptoms of macular degeneration.**

   A. Blurred or distorted vision is usually the first symptom.
   B. There is a color vision disturbance (become dimmer).
   C. There is difficulty reading or doing close work.
   D. There is a distortion of objects.
   E. There is vision in which the center (or bull's eye) area is absent.
   F. Side vision is not affected.

III. **The client/caregiver can list causes or risk factors for macular degeneration.**

   A. The greatest risk factor is age, especially over the age of 60 years.
   B. Women have a greater risk than men.
   C. Those with a family history of macular degeneration are at higher risk.
   D. Smoking and obesity may increase the risk.

IV. **The client/caregiver can list lifestyle measures to reduce risk of developing disease.**

   A. Eat healthy diet that is high in green leafy vegetables and fish.
   B. Do not smoke.
   C. Maintain a healthy weight.
   D. Maintain a normal blood pressure.
   E. Exercise.

NRS
DATE INITIAL

V. **The client/caregiver can list measures to manage this disease.**

   A. Comprehensive eye exam that includes
      1. Visual acuity testing measures how well you see at various distances.
      2. Dilated eye exam can reveal any damage to retina or optic nerve.
      3. Tonometry uses an instrument to measure pressure inside the eye.
      4. Amsler Grid Testing is specific for macular degeneration.
   B. Photocoagulation (laser surgery) or photodynamic therapy may be an option your physician will suggest if the condition is diagnosed early enough.
   C. Discuss with physician possibility of using specific supplement high in antioxidants. Use zinc to slow the progression of disease.

VI. **The client/caregiver can list complications.**

   A. Blindness

RESOURCES

Macular Degeneration Partnership
www.AMD.org

Occupational therapy consult

Low-vision specialist

National Eye Institute
301-496-5248
www.nei.nih.gov

Association for Macular Diseases
212-605-3719

(Continued)

REFERENCES

Ackley, B. J., & Ladwig, G. B. (2006). *Nursing diagnosis handbook: A guide to planning care.* St. Louis: Mosby Inc.

Lutz, C., & Przytulski, K. *Nutrition and diet therapy.* (2001). Philadelphia: F. A. Davis Company.

National Eye Institute. *Age-Related Eye Disease Study* (2001). Bethesda, MD. Available from: *www.nei.nih.gov/amd/.*

Nutrition made incredibly easy. (2003). Philadelphia: Lippincott Williams & Wilkins.

Taylor, C., Lillis, C., & LeMone, P. (2005). *Fundamentals of nursing.* Philadelphia: Lippincott, Williams & Wilkins.

Timby, B. K., & Smith, N. C. (2003). *Introductory medical-surgical nursing* (8th ed.). Philadelphia: J. B. Lippincott Williams & Wilkins.

5

Blepharitis

Patient name: _____

Admission: _____

NRS
DATE INITIAL

I. **The client/caregiver can define blepharitis.**

  A. It is an inflammation of the lash follicle on the eyelid.

  B. It is caused by an excessive growth of bacteria creating an infection.

II. **The client/caregiver can list other conditions that can be associated with this disease.**

  A. Seborrheic dermatitis

  B. Allergies

  C. Infestation of lice

  D. Styes (inflamed oil gland on edge of eyelid)

  E. Rosacea

III. **The client/caregiver can list symptoms of blepharitis.**

  A. Eyelids will appear
- Crusted
- Reddened
- Swollen

  B. The client will complain of itching and burning or a sensation that sand or dust is in the eye, causing irritation.

IV. **The client/caregiver can list measures to treat or manage this condition.**

  A. Careful and routine cleansing should be done on the eyelid to remove excessive skin oil.

NRS
DATE INITIAL

  B. Physician may recommend use of prescription shampoo or cleansers for hair.

  C. If infection occurs, physician may order antibiotic ointments for use on eyelids.

  D. Treat any condition contributing to the problem.

  E. Maintain a good hand-washing technique.

  F. Avoid rubbing eyes.

  G. Follow the physician's orders regarding use of contact lenses.

  H. Use gauze or soft cloth to cleanse eyelids once and discard or launder after use.

V. **The client/caregiver can list possible complications of blepharitis.**

  A. Styes

  B. Conjunctivitis

  C. Corneal ulcer

  D. Loss of eyelashes

  E. Scarring of eyelids

REFERENCES

Cohen, B. J., & Taylor, J. J. (2005). *Memmler's the human body in health and disease* (10th ed.). Philadelphia: Lippincott Williams & Wilkins.

Perry, A., & Potter, P. (2006). *Clinical nursing skills & technique.* St. Louis: Mosby Inc.

6 Corneal Ulcers or Infection

Patient name: _____ Admission: _____

I. **The client/caregiver can define corneal ulcer**

A. The cornea is the curved, transparent covering on the front of the eye.
B. The cornea can become damaged by injury (trauma), or an infection can cause a sore on the outer layer of cornea.

II. **The client/caregiver can list causes or risk factors for corneal ulcers or infection.**

A. Ulcers can be caused by infections (bacteria, viruses, fungi, or amoebae).
B. Other causes for the creation of sores or abrasions on the cornea can be
- From foreign bodies such as sand or dust
- Severely dry eyes
- Severe allergies
- Overuse of contact lens
- Inflammatory disorders

III. **The client/caregiver can list symptoms of corneal abrasions or infections.**

A. Eye pain
B. Impaired vision
C. Eye redness
D. White patch on the cornea
E. Abnormal sensitivity to light
F. Watery eyes
G. Eye burning, itching, and discharge

IV. **The client/caregiver can list measures to manage or treat corneal injuries.**

A. Physician may use antibiotic, antiviral, or antifungal eye drops to treat any identified infection.
B. Corticosteroid eye drops may be used to reduce inflammation.
C. Wash hands carefully.

D. Use proper technique when handling contact lens.
E. Avoid wearing contact lens during sleep.

V. **The client/caregiver can list measures to prevent injury/infection to eyes.**

A. Wear safety goggles.
- When using hand or power tools
- When using chemicals
- When involved in high impact sports
B. Wear sunglasses designed to screen ultraviolet light.
C. Use good technique when handling contact lens.
D. Avoid wearing contact lens during sleep.
E. Use good hand-washing techniques.

VI. **The client/caregiver can list possible complications.**

A. Corneal scarring
B. Severe vision loss
C. Need for corneal transplant
D. Loss of the eye

RESOURCES

Emergency care facility

Ophthalmologist

National Eye Institute (National Institutes of Health)
www.nei.nih.gov

REFERENCES

Cohen, B. J., & Taylor, J. J. (2005). *Memmler's the human body in health and disease* (10th ed.). Philadelphia: Lippincott Williams & Wilkins.
Perry, A., & Potter, P. (2006). *Clinical nursing skills & technique.* St. Louis: Mosby Inc.
Taylor, C., Lillis, C., & LeMone, P. (2005). *Fundamentals of nursing.* Philadelphia: Lippincott, Williams & Wilkins.

7 Retinal Detachment

Patient name: _____ Admission: _____

NRS
DATE INITIAL

I. The client/caregiver can explain the purpose of retina and possible problems.

A. The retina is the light sensitive layer of tissue that lines the inside of the eye.
B. It sends visual messages to the brain.
C. The optic nerve serves as a go-between for the retina and the brain.
D. If the retina is pulled away or lifted from the lining of the eye, vision loss will occur.
E. Types of retina damage are
   • Retina tear
   • Retina breaks
   • Retina detachment

II. The client/caregiver can describe causes and possible risk factors.

A. Causes of retinal detachment
   1. Fluid accumulates under retina and separates it from underlying layer.
   2. Scarring causes the retina to contract and separate.
   3. Inflammatory disease or trauma allows fluid to leak under the retina and separate.
B. Factors that increase risk for retina detachment
   • Older than the age of 40 years
   • Men more than women
   • Whites more than African Americans
   • Extremely nearsighted
   • Retinal detachment in the other eye
   • Previous cataract surgery
   • Family history of retinal detachment
   • Eye injury or trauma

NRS
DATE INITIAL

III. The client/caregiver can list symptoms and possible complications.

A. Symptoms include
   1. Sudden or gradual increase in the number of "floaters" (specks that float in your field of vision) and/or light flashes in the eye
   2. Appearance of a curtain over field of vision
B. Complication of untreated retina detachment can result in blindness. Consult with physician or eye care professional promptly if symptoms begin.
C. This can become a medical emergency.

RESOURCES
Emergency care facility

National Eye Institute (National Institutes of Health)
www.nei.nih.gov

REFERENCES
Cohen, B. J., & Taylor, J. J. (2005). *Memmler's the human body in health and disease* (10th ed.). Philadelphia: Lippincott Williams & Wilkins.
Perry, A., & Potter, P. (2006). *Clinical nursing skills & technique.* St. Louis: Mosby Inc.
Taylor, C., Lillis, C., & LeMone, P. (2005). *Fundamentals of nursing.* Philadelphia: Lippincott, Williams & Wilkins.

1 Labyrinthitis

Patient name: _____ Admission: _____

NRS
DATE INITIAL

I. **The client/caregiver can define labyrinthitis and list risk factors.**

A. It is an ear disorder that involves irritation and swelling of the labyrinth in the inner ear.
B. When the inner ear does not function properly, the ability to keep your balance is disturbed.
C. Risk factors are as follows:
   - Recent respiratory or ear infection
   - Stress
   - Fatigue
   - History of allergies
   - Smoking
   - Drinking large amounts of alcohol
   - Certain drugs that are dangerous to the inner ear (aspirin, etc.)

II. **The client/caregiver can list symptoms.**

A. Dizziness
B. Vertigo (abnormal sensation of movement), with nausea and vomiting
C. Loss of balance
D. Hearing loss in affected ear
E. Ringing or other noises in ears (tinnitus)
F. Involuntary eye movements (nystagmus)

III. **The client/caregiver can list measures to manage this disease.**

A. Take medication as ordered by physician.
B. Keep still and rest during attacks.

NRS
DATE INITIAL

C. Gradually resume activity.
D. Avoid sudden position changes.
E. Avoid chocolate, coffee, and alcohol.
F. Stop smoking.
G. Reduce sodium and sugar intake.
H. Do not try to read during attacks.
I. Avoid bright lights.
J. Avoid hazardous activities such as driving, operating heavy machinery, and working at heights until 1 week after symptoms have disappeared.

IV. **The client/caregiver can list possible complications.**

A. Injury to self or others during attacks of vertigo
B. Hearing loss

REFERENCES

Cohen, B. J., & Taylor, J. J. (2005). *Memmler's the human body in health and disease* (10th ed.). Philadelphia: Lippincott Williams & Wilkins.

Perry, A., & Potter, P. (2006). *Clinical nursing skills & technique.* St. Louis: Mosby Inc.

Timby, B. K., & Smith, N. C. (2003). *Introductory medical-surgical nursing* (8th ed.). Philadelphia: J. B. Lippincott Williams & Wilkins.

2 Epistaxis

Patient name: _____   **Admission:** _____

I. **The client/caregiver can define epistaxis and common causes.**

  A. Epistaxis is bleeding from the nose.

  B. Common causes of epistaxis are
- Injury or blow to nose
- Inflammation or ulceration from sinusitis
- Growths or polyps in the nose
- Chemical irritants
- Receiving large doses of aspirin or anticoagulants

II. **The client/caregiver can list ways to stop the epistaxis.**

  A. Remain calm with head slightly elevated.

  B. Apply pressure to the nostril of the bleeding side.

  C. Apply cold compresses over the nose.

  D. Notify health care providers of use of any medication such as
- Aspirin
- Nonsteroidal antiinflammatory drugs
- Anticoagulants

  E. Use saline spray or gel to moisten lining of nose.

  F. Remind children not to "pick" nose or use excessive force when blowing nose.

  G. Get emergency help if
1. Bleeding does not stop after 20 minutes
2. Also received injury to the head
3. The nose is misshapen after an injury

RESOURCES
Childcare classes

First aid classes

REFERENCES
Cohen, B. J., & Taylor, J. J. (2005). *Memmler's the human body in health and disease* (10th ed.). Philadelphia: Lippincott Williams & Wilkins.

Perry, A., & Potter, P. (2006). *Clinical nursing skills & technique.* St. Louis: Mosby Inc.

Timby, B. K., & Smith, N. C. (2003). *Introductory medical-surgical nursing* (8th ed.). Philadelphia: J. B. Lippincott Williams & Wilkins.

3 Hearing Loss

Patient name: _____ Admission: _____

NRS
DATE INITIAL

I. **The client/caregiver can list general facts about hearing loss.**

A. It is the most common disability.
B. It affects mostly the older population.
C. According to the Mayo Clinic, one third of Americans older than the age of 60 years has hearing loss, and one half of Americans older than the age of 85 years has some hearing loss.

II. **The client/caregiver can list signs and symptoms of hearing loss.**

A. Muffled quality of speech and other sounds
B. Difficulty understanding words, especially in a crowd
C. Asking others to speak more slowly, clearly, or loudly
D. Needing to turn up the volume of television or radio
E. Withdrawal from conversations
F. Avoidance of some social settings

III. **The client/caregiver can list types of hearing loss.**

A. Conductive is an interference with conduction of sound impulses through external canal, eardrum, or middle ear.
B. Sensorineural is caused by disease or trauma of the inner ear.
C. Mixed hearing loss is a combination of conductive and sensorineural.
D. Central deafness is a rare form affecting the central nervous system causing lack of interpretation of sounds.
E. Sometimes a build-up of wax causing blockage can cause loss of hearing.

NRS
DATE INITIAL

IV. **The client/caregiver can list risk factors for hearing loss.**

A. Aging and the normal wear and tear can cause damage.
B. Loud noises like occupational noise, loud music, shooting firearms can contribute to damage inside your ear.
C. Heredity
D. Some medication such as the antibiotic gentamicin or aspirin
E. Illnesses that result in high fevers may damage the hearing

V. **The client/caregiver can list some treatment options for hearing loss.**

A. Removing wax blockage
B. Using hearing aid
C. Having cochlear implants

VI. **The client/caregiver can list coping skills to promote communication.**

A. Face the person with whom you are speaking.
B. Turn off background noise such as television.
C. Choose quiet settings to talk.
D. Ask others to speak clearly.
E. Avoid covering mouth or chewing gum when speaking.
F. Speak slowly and clearly. Do not shout. Pitch your voice lower (they can be heard better than high tones).
G. Consider using a hearing aid or other hearing devices, such as telephone-amplifying devices.

(Continued)

NRS
DATE   INITIAL

VII. The client/caregiver can list measures to prevent hearing loss.

A. Protect your ears in the workplace.
B. Have your hearing tested.
C. Avoid recreational risks by turning down loud music or wearing ear plugs for protection.

VIII. The client/caregiver can list educational services available to the hearing impaired of any age.

A. Regular speech, language, and auditory training from a specialist
B. Amplification systems
C. Services of an interpreter for those students who use sign language
D. Favorable seating in the class to facilitate lip reading
E. Captioned film, video, and television
F. Assistance of a notetaker for student with a hearing loss
G. Instruction in alternate communication methods, such as sign language
H. Counseling

RESOURCES

National Institutes of Health Senior Health
http://nihseniorhealth.gov/hearingloss/toc.html

National Institute on Deafness and other Communication Disorders
www.nidcd.nih.gov/

Alexander Graham Bell Association for the Deaf and Hard of Hearing
www.agbell.org

Self Help for Hard of Hearing People
www.hearingloss.org

REFERENCES

Ackley, B. J., & Ladwig, G. B. (2006). *Nursing diagnosis handbook: A guide to planning care.* St. Louis: Mosby Elsevier.

Cohen, B. J., & Taylor, J. J. (2005). *Memmler's the human body in health and disease* (10th ed.). Philadelphia: Lippincott Williams & Wilkins.

Hitchcock, J. E., Schubert, P. E., & Thomas, S. A. (2003). *Community health nursing: Caring in action.* Clifton Park, NY: Thomson Delmar Learning.

Hunt, R. (2005). *Introduction to community based nursing.* Philadelphia: Lippincott Williams & Wilkins.

Perry, A., & Potter, P. (2006). *Clinical nursing skills & technique.* St. Louis: Mosby Inc.

Timby, B. K., & Smith, N. C. (2003). *Introductory medical-surgical nursing* (8th ed.). Philadelphia: J. B. Lippincott Williams & Wilkins.

1 Breast Cancer

Patient name: _____ **Admission:** _____

NRS DATE INITIAL	

I. **The client/caregiver can define breast cancer.**

  A. Breast cancer is second only to lung cancer as cause of cancer deaths in American women. One in every nine women may get breast cancer.

  B. It is staged according to size of primary lesion, extent of spread to regional lymph nodes, and metastasis to other parts of body.

  C. Paget's disease is found in 1% to 4% of breast cancer. It involves skin changes in the nipple caused by a tumor growing through the ducts into the nipple.

II. **The client/caregiver can list factors regarding risk of breast cancer.**

  A. Factors that increase risk
   • Females (males also get breast cancer)
   • Aging increases risk (80% of breast cancers occur in women older than 50 years)
   • Personal history of breast cancer
   • Positive family history (mother, sister, or daughter with either breast or ovarian cancer)
   • Genetic predisposition
   • Radiation exposure (the younger the exposure, the greater the risk)
   • Excess weight (especially weight around the waist)
   • Exposure to estrogen (late menopause, after age of 55; early menses, before age of 12; women who have never had children; or first pregnancy after 35)
   • Higher risk of developing breast cancer in white women (but black women are more likely to die of breast cancer)
   • Hormone therapy (especially combination of estrogen plus progestin)
   • Talk with physician about the current reports of birth control pill use as a risk factor.

   • Smoking (even exposure to secondhand smoke)
   • Exposure to pesticides, chemical components of cigarette smoke, and so forth
   • Excessive use of alcohol
   • Breast density

III. **The client/caregiver can list measures for early detection.**

  A. Mammograms. The American Cancer Society (2003) and National Cancer Institute (2004) guidelines suggest an annual mammogram for women 40 years old and older.

  B. Self-breast exams. Know how your breasts normally feel, and report any changes to your doctor. Starting in your 20s, breast self-examination is an option.

  C. A health care professional exam is important every 3 years until the age of 40, and then annual exams should be performed.

IV. **The client/caregiver can list warning signs of breast cancer.**

  A. A lump or thickening (often painless) in the breast or in the underarm area
  B. A change in the size or shape of the breast
  C. Nipple tenderness
  D. A retraction or indentation of nipple or of the skin over breast
  E. Spontaneous clear or bloody discharge from nipple
  F. Redness or pitting of the skin over the breast, areola, or nipple (like the skin of an orange)

V. **The client/caregiver can list treatments for breast cancer.**

  A. Surgery
   • Lumpectomy
   • Partial or segmental mastectomy

(Continued)

NRS
DATE INITIAL

- Simple mastectomy
- Modified radical mastectomy
- Sentinel lymph node biopsy
- Reconstructive surgery
B. Radiation
C. Chemotherapy
D. Hormonal therapy to reduce estrogen

RESOURCES

National Cancer Institute
www.cancer.gov/cancer_information/

National Cancer Society
www.cancer.org/docroot/home/index.asp

Y-ME National Breast Cancer Organization
www.y-me.org/

Susan G. Komen for the Cure
www.komen.org/

Support groups

REFERENCES

Ackley, B. J., & Ladwig, G. B. (2006). *Nursing diagnosis handbook: A guide to planning care.* St. Louis: Mosby Inc.

Canobbio, M. M. (2006). *Mosby's handbook of patient teaching.* St. Louis: Mosby Inc.

Cohen, B. J., & Taylor, J. J. (2005). *Memmler's the human body in health and disease* (10th ed.). Philadelphia: Lippincott Williams & Wilkins.

Mayo Clinic. (2006, December). *Mastectomy vs. lumpectomy.* Available from: *www.mayoclinic.com/health/mastectomy-lumpectomy/BC99999.*

Timby, B. K., & Smith, N. C. (2003). *Introductory medical-surgical nursing* (8th ed.). Philadelphia: J. B. Lippincott Williams & Wilkins.

2

Ovarian Cancer

Patient name: _____   Admission: _____

I. **The client/caregiver can define ovarian cancer.**

   A. Women have two ovaries (each the size of an almond), one on each side of the uterus.
   B. Ovaries produce eggs (ova), estrogen, and progesterone.
   C. Ovarian cancer ranks fifth in cancer deaths among women.
   D. The types of ovarian tumors are
      1. Epithelial tumors develop in the layer of tissue that covers the ovaries. About 80% to 90% of ovarian cancers develop here. It is most common in post-menopausal women.
      2. Germ cell tumors develop in the egg-producing cells and usually occur in younger women.
      3. Stromal tumors develop in the estrogen and progesterone producing tissue.

II. **The client/caregiver can list signs and symptoms of ovarian cancer.**

   A. Symptoms are nonspecific and can appear like those of other common conditions. Symptoms are persistent and gradually worsen.
   B. There is abdominal swelling and sense of bloating or fullness and increased abdominal girth with normal clothing fitting tightly.
   C. There is pain in lower abdomen and pelvic area (sometimes lower back).
   D. There is unexplained weight loss or gain.
   E. There is a lack of energy.
   F. There are gastrointestinal complaints, such as indigestion, gas, nausea, diarrhea, or constipation.
   G. There are urinary complaints such as frequency or feeling of urgency to void.
   H. There are menstrual changes and abnormal uterine bleeding.

III. **The client/caregiver can list risk factors for ovarian cancer.**

   A. Inherited gene mutation
   B. Family history
   C. Age. Most ovarian cancers develop after menopause but can occur earlier.
   D. Childbearing status. Women with at least one pregnancy have a lower risk.
   E. Infertility increases the risk.
   F. Ovarian cysts that form after menopause are more likely cancerous.
   G. Obesity in early adulthood. It is also linked to a more aggressive type of ovarian cancer.

IV. **The client/caregiver can list stages of ovarian cancer.**

   A. Stage I is confined to one or both ovaries.
   B. Stage II has spread to locations in the pelvis such as uterus or fallopian tubes.
   C. Stage III has spread to the lining of the abdomen or to the lymph nodes. This typically is when ovarian cancer is diagnosed.
   D. Stage IV is when the cancer has spread beyond the abdomen.

V. **The client/caregiver can list methods of screening for ovarian cancer.**

   A. Regular pelvic exams
   B. Ultrasound of pelvis
   C. CA 125 blood test
   D. Pelvic CT or MRI
   E. Laparotomy or laparoscopy to obtain samples of abdominal fluid and/or ovary tissue.

VI. **The client/caregiver can list measures to manage and treat ovarian cancer.**

   A. Have surgery.
   B. Have chemotherapy.

(Continued)

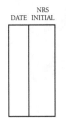

C. Eat protein-rich foods. Eat smaller amounts of food more frequently. Eat nutritionally dense foods.
D. Reduce stress.
E. Be informed and learn what to expect.
F. Build and maintain a support system.

RESOURCES

Clergy

Support groups

Ovarian Cancer National Alliance
www.ovariancancer.org/

The National Women's Health Information Center
www.4woman.gov/

National Cancer Institute
www.cancer.gov/cancerinfo/types/ovarian

REFERENCES

Ackley, B. J., & Ladwig, G. B. (2006). *Nursing diagnosis handbook: A guide to planning care.* St. Louis: Mosby Inc.

Canobbio, M. M. (2006). *Mosby's handbook of patient teaching.* St. Louis: Mosby Inc.

Lutz, C., & Przytulski, K. (2001). *Nutrition and diet therapy.* Philadelphia: F. A. Davis Company.

Timby, B. K., & Smith, N. C. (2003). *Introductory medical-surgical nursing* (8th ed.). Philadelphia: J. B. Lippincott Williams & Wilkins.

3 Leukemia

Patient name: _____

NRS
DATE INITIAL

I. **The client/caregiver can define leukemia.**

   A. It is the rapid production of white blood cells, many of which are immature.
   B. The white blood cells, leukocytes, may invade and damage bone marrow, lymph nodes, spleen, kidneys, and other organs of the body.
   C. The disease can be acute or chronic.
      1. In acute leukemia, symptoms occur suddenly and progress rapidly.
      2. In chronic leukemia, symptoms appear gradually.

II. **The client/caregiver can list factors that increase the risk of leukemia.**

   A. Cancer therapy
   B. Exposure to high levels of radiation and other chemicals
   C. Genetic factors (Down syndrome is associated with increased risk of leukemia)

III. **The client/caregiver can recognize signs and symptoms.**

   A. Fatigue and weakness
   B. Fever and chills
   C. Frequent infections
   D. Signs of bleeding
      1. Bleeding into the skin causing discoloration
      2. Nose bleeds
      3. Small reddish-purple spots on the skin (petechiae)
   E. Loss of appetite or weight
   F. Swollen lymph nodes and enlarged liver and spleen
   G. Shortness of breath when physically active
   H. Excessive sweating (especially at night)

IV. **The client/caregiver can list measures to manage leukemia.**

   A. Obtain adequate rest to decrease anemia. Pace activities with rest periods.

NRS
DATE INITIAL

   B. Prevent bleeding.
      1. Report first signs of bleeding such as bruising, petechiae, bleeding gums, and so forth.
      2. Follow safety measures to avoid cuts and hemorrhage (soft toothbrush, electric razor, etc.).
      3. Avoid aspirin, which may increase bleeding tendency.
      4. Avoid activities that increase risk of injury or trauma.
   C. Prevent infection.
      1. Perform meticulous hygiene.
      2. Avoid large crowds and people with infections.
      3. Increase fluids to decrease possibility of urinary-tract infections.
      4. Provide good mouth care to decrease possibility of mouth sores.
      5. All caretakers should wash hands thoroughly.
      6. Report early signs of infection.
      7. Avoid uncooked eggs, unpeeled fruit, and unwashed vegetables.
      8. Change filters in air conditioners and furnace.
   D. Take medications as ordered.
   E. Obtain adequate nutrition.
      1. Use measures to increase intake (refer to teaching guide "alteration in nutrition: less than body require- ments").
      2. Eat bland, high-calorie, high-protein foods.
      3. Avoid alcohol, hot or spicy foods, and acidic beverage to prevent mouth ulcers.
      4. Discuss resources for delivery or preparation of meals such as Meals on Wheels or home health aide.
   F. Provide comfort measures as needed such as analgesics, position changes, etc.
   G. Drink at least 2 to 3 liters per day of fluids.
   H. Avoid over-the-counter medications unless recommended by physician.

(Continued)

NRS
DATE INITIAL

    I. Keep follow-up appointments with physician.
   J. Wear a Medic Alert bracelet.

V. The client/caregiver can list possible treatments.

A. Chemotherapy
B. Immunotherapy (substances to bolster immune system)
C. Kinase inhibitors or other drug therapies
D. Radiation therapy
E. Bone marrow transplant
F. Stem cell transplant

VI. The client/caregiver can list possible complications.

A. Hemorrhage
B. Stroke or seizures
C. Infection
D. Kidney or liver failure

RESOURCES

The Leukemia and Lymphoma Society
www.leukemia-lymphoma.org

National Marrow Donor Program
www.marrow.org/

Support groups

REFERENCES

Ackley, B. J., & Ladwig, G. B. (2006). *Nursing diagnosis handbook: A guide to planning care.* St. Louis: Mosby Inc.
Canobbio, M. M. (2006). *Mosby's handbook of patient teaching.* St. Louis: Mosby Inc.
Lutz, C., & Przytulski, K. (2001). *Nutrition and diet therapy.* Philadelphia: F. A. Davis Company.
Timby, B. K., & Smith, N. C. (2003). *Introductory medical-surgical nursing* (8th ed.). Philadelphia: J. B. Lippincott Williams & Wilkins.

Lung Cancer

4

Patient name: _____ Admission: _____

NRS
DATE INITIAL

I. **The client/caregiver can list some general facts about lung cancer.**

    A. Lung cancer is the number one cancer killer.
    B. Ninety percent of lung cancer patients are smokers.
    C. Early lung cancer may have no signs or symptoms.
    D. Prognosis improves with early detection.

II. **The client/caregiver can list the two main types of lung cancer.**

    A. Small cell lung cancer spreads early and occurs mostly in smokers. It occurs in 10% to 25% of lung tumors.
    B. Non-small cell lung cancer is more common (accounts for more than 75% of lung cancers). There are four categories of non-small cell lung cancers.
        1. Squamous cell carcinoma forms in cells lining the airways. It is the most common type of cancer in men.
        2. Adenocarcinoma usually begins in the mucous-producing cells. It is the most common type of lung cancer seen in women and in people who have never smoked.
        3. Large cell carcinoma originates in the peripheral part of the lungs.
        4. Bronchoalveolar carcinoma is an uncommon type of cancer and it tends to grow more slowly.

III. **The client/caregiver can list factors that increase the risk of lung cancer.**

    A. Smoking is the greatest risk factor.
    B. Current or former women smokers have a greater risk.
    C. Risk increases with exposure to secondhand smoke.
    D. Risk increases with exposure to asbestos, radioactive dusts, arsenic, and plastics.

E. Black Americans have a higher risk of lung cancer.
F. Hereditary factors increase the risk.

IV. **The client/caregiver can recognize signs and symptoms of lung cancer.**

    A. Persistent cough (smoker's cough)
    B. Blood in sputum
    C. New onset of wheezing in the chest
    D. Chest pain
    E. Fever
    F. Weight loss
    G. Repeated episodes of pneumonia or bronchitis
    H. Shortness of breath
    I. Hoarseness that lasts more than 2 weeks
    J. Arm and shoulder pain

V. **The client/caregiver can list measures for prevention of lung cancer.**

    A. Do not smoke. Quitting can reduce the risk.
    B. Avoid secondhand smoke.
    C. Test your home for radon.
    D. Avoid carcinogens such as vinyl chloride, nickel chromates, and coal products.
    E. Eat a healthy diet that includes five to six servings of fruits and vegetables.
    F. Have routine health care and report any early signs and symptoms.

VI. **The client/caregiver can list possible treatments of lung cancer.**

    A. Treatments depend on the type and stage of cancer. Also, your overall health is a factor to consider when planning treatment.
    B. Small cell lung cancer has usually spread to other organs by the time it is diagnosed. Surgery is not a treatment option in most

(Continued)

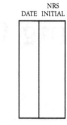

NRS
DATE INITIAL

cases. Chemotherapy and radiation are used.

C. Surgery is usually the treatment for early stage non-small cell lung cancer. Operations used are
   1. Wedge resection removes the section with tumor.
   2. Lobectomy involves removing an entire lobe of one lung.
   3. Pneumonectomy is when an entire lung is removed.

VII. **The client/caregiver can list measures for management of disease.**

A. Increase fluid intake to liquefy secretions.
B. Nutritional measures
   1. Eat a diet that is high in protein and calories.
   2. Eat small, frequent meals rather than three large ones.
   3. Suggest easily digested foods such as soups or broth, rice, toast, baked potatoes, and so forth.
   4. Avoid rich or spicy foods.
C. Do not smoke and avoid secondhand smoke.
D. Regular exercise balanced with adequate rest.
E. Report weight loss, increased coughing, pain, fatigue, or blood in sputum to physician.
F. Reduce stress.
G. Keep follow-up appointments with physician.

VIII. **The client/caregiver can list possible complications.**

A. Atelectasis (collapse of lung)
B. Pneumonia
C. Metastasis (especially small cell tumors) to brain, bones, liver, and so forth

RESOURCES

The National Cancer Institute
800-4-CANCER or 800-422-6237
www.cancer.gov/

American Cancer Society
800-227-2345
www.cancer.gov/

Support groups

Smoking cessation

The Office of the Surgeon General
www.surgeongeneral.gov/tobacco/index.html
www.smokefree.gov/

REFERENCES

Ackley, B. J., & Ladwig, G. B. (2006). *Nursing diagnosis handbook: A guide to planning care.* St. Louis: Mosby Inc.

Canobbio, M. M. (2006). *Mosby's handbook of patient teaching.* St. Louis: Mosby Inc.

Cohen, B. J., & Taylor, J. J. (2005). *Memmler's the human body in health and disease* (10th ed.). Philadelphia: Lippincott Williams & Wilkins.

Lutz, C., & Przytulski, K. (2001). *Nutrition and diet therapy.* Philadelphia: F. A. Davis Company.

Timby, B. K., & Smith, N. C. (2003). *Introductory medical-surgical nursing* (8th ed.). Philadelphia: J. B. Lippincott Williams & Wilkins.

5 | Prostate Cancer

Patient name: _____   **Admission:** _____

NRS
DATE INITIAL

I. The client/caregiver can define the prostate gland.

    A. It squeezes fluid into the urethra during ejaculation to aid in transport and nourishment of the sperm.

    B. It is a small walnut sized gland that surrounds the male urethra at the neck of the bladder.

II. The client/caregiver can list general facts about prostate cancer.

    A. It is a cancer of the prostate gland.

    B. It is the third leading cause of cancer-related deaths in men.

    C. It is detected through digital exam.

    D. Prostate cancers grow slowly and have a high survival rate if detected early.

    E. Most prostate tumors are not cancerous.

III. The client/caregiver can list factors that can increase risk of prostate cancer.

    A. Advanced age

    B. Race (Blacks have increased risk)

    C. Hereditary

    D. Diet high in fat

    E. Occupation—working with cadmium, zinc, rubber, dewaxing process in oil refining

    F. Obesity

    G. Sexually transmitted disease

IV. The client/caregiver can recognize symptoms of prostate cancer, which usually only appears at advanced stages.

    A. Frequent urination, especially at night

    B. Difficulty starting or holding urine

    C. Weak or interrupted urine flow

    D. Pain or burning during urination

    E. Blood in urine

    F. Pain in lower back, upper pelvis, and upper thighs

    G. Weight loss

NRS
DATE INITIAL

V. The client/caregiver can list common diagnostic tests.

    A. Digital exam

    B. Prostatic-specific antigen

    C. Transrectal ultrasound

    D. Needle biopsy with ultrasound probes

    E. Bone scan

VI. The client/caregiver can list stages of prostate cancer.

    A. Stage I—early cancer as seen on microscopic exam of tissue.

    B. Stage II—cancer can be felt, but remains confined to prostate gland.

    C. Stage III—cancer has spread outside the prostate.

    D. Stage IV—cancer has spread to lymph nodes or organs far away from prostate such as bones, lungs, or other organs.

VII. The client/caregiver can state possible treatments.

    A. Surgery

    B. Radiation

        1. External

        2. Implantation

    C. Hormone therapy

VIII. The client/caregiver can list measures for management of disease.

    A. Eat a well-balanced diet with adequate fluid intake.

    B. Exercise daily with planned rest periods.

    C. Take medications as ordered.

    D. Keep follow-up appointments with physician including annual digital exam.

    E. Report signs of decreased output, swelling, hypertension, weight gain, and so forth.

(Continued)

NRS
DATE INITIAL

IX. **The client/caregiver can list possible complications.**

   A. Spread of cancer
   B. Pain
   C. Urinary incontinence
   D. Erectile dysfunction or impotence
   E. Depression

RESOURCES

American Urology Association
www.urologyhealth.org/index.cfm

Prostate Cancer Foundation
www.prostatecancerfoundation.org/

Support groups

Sexual counseling

REFERENCES

Ackley, B. J., & Ladwig, G. B. (2006). *Nursing diagnosis handbook: A guide to planning care.* St. Louis: Mosby Inc.

Canobbio, M. M. (2006). *Mosby's handbook of patient teaching.* St. Louis: Mosby Inc.

Cohen, B. J., & Taylor, J. J. (2005). *Memmler's the human body in health and disease* (10th ed.). Philadelphia: Lippincott Williams & Wilkins.

Timby, B. K., & Smith, N. C. (2003). *Introductory medical-surgical nursing* (8th ed.). Philadelphia: J. B. Lippincott Williams & Wilkins.

6 Skin Cancer

Patient name: _____ **Admission:** _____

NRS
DATE INITIAL

I. **The client/caregiver can state general facts about skin cancer.**

A. Skin cancer usually develops on skin exposed to the sun, but it can also develop on areas of the skin not ordinarily exposed to sunlight.
B. It is the most common form of cancer.
C. Melanoma is the most serious form of skin cancer.
D. Prevention or early detection is essential.
E. One in seven Americans will develop skin cancer each year.
F. More than 1 million new cases of skin cancer will be diagnosed in the United States this year.

II. **The client/caregiver can list factors that increase risk of skin cancer.**

A. Fair skin
B. History of sunburns
C. Excessive sun exposure
D. Living in sunny or high-altitude climates
E. Large number of moles or abnormal moles
F. Precancerous skin lesions (most common on face, lower arms, and hands of fair-skinned people)
G. Family or personal history of skin cancer
H. People with a weakened immune system
I. Fragile or weakened skin such as psoriasis or skin that has been burned or injured
J. Exposure to environmental hazards, chemical, or herbicides
K. Advanced age

III. **The client/caregiver can list three main types of skin cancer.**

A. Basal cell is the most common type of skin cancer and is the easiest to treat.
B. Squamous cell is also easily treated if found early.
C. Melanoma is the most serious. It can develop in normal skin or in an existing mole. It accounts for only 4% of the cases

NRS
DATE INITIAL

of skin cancer but is the cause of 75% of skin cancer deaths.

IV. **The client/caregiver can use the A-B-C-D skin self-exam guide from the American Academy of Dermatology to detect skin cancers.**

A. A is for asymmetrical shape. Note any moles with irregular shapes or that do not match on each side.
B. B is for irregular border. Note any moles that have a notched, scalloped, or indistinct border.
C. C is for change in color. Note any moles that are unusually dark or have variegated or uneven colors.
D. D is for diameter. Note any moles that are larger than one-quarter inch in size or the size of a pencil eraser.

V. **The client/caregiver can list signs and symptoms of the three types of skin cancer.**

A. Basal cell carcinoma (cancer) symptoms are
  1. A pearly or waxy bump on the face, ears, or neck
  2. A flat, flesh colored or brown scar-like lesion on your chest or back
B. Squamous cell carcinoma (cancer) symptoms are
  1. A firm, red nodule on your face, lips, ears, neck, hands, or arms
  2. A flat lesion with a scaly, crusted surface on the face, ears, neck, hands, or arms
C. Melanoma symptoms are
  1. A large brownish spot with darker speckles located anywhere on your body
  2. A simple mole located anywhere on your body that changes in color, size, or feel or that bleeds
  3. A lesion with an irregular border and red, white, blue, or blue-black spots

(Continued)

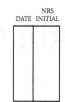

<table>
<tr><td>NRS
DATE INITIAL</td></tr>
</table>

4. A shiny, firm, dome-shaped bump located anywhere on your body

5. Dark lesions, on your palms, soles, fingertips, or toes

6. Dark lesions on mucous membranes lining your mouth, nose, vagina, vulva, or anus

VI. **The client/caregiver can list measures to prevent skin cancer.**

A. Avoid the sun between 10 a.m. and 4 p.m.

B. Wear sunscreen.
1. Use year round.
2. Sunscreen with protection factor of at least 15 is recommended.
3. Do not miss use of sunscreen on lips, ears, and back of hands and neck and tops of feet.
4. Apply sunscreen 20 to 30 minutes before exposure, and reapply every 2 hours or after swimming or exercising.
5. Check with the Food and Drug Administration for list of currently approved sunscreen products.

C. Wear protective clothing including broad brimmed hat, sunglasses, and so forth.

D. Avoid tanning beds.

E. Be alert to medications that can make your skin more sensitive to sunlight.

F. Routine self skin checks should include (using a mirror if necessary):
1. Check face, neck, ears, and scalp.
2. Examine both front and back of legs and feet (even between toes).
3. Check tops and undersides of arms and hands.

4. Examine chest and trunk of body.

5. Check genital areas.

G. If you are older than 40 or have a high risk of developing skin cancer, consult your physician for annual skin exams.

RESOURCES

American Academy of Dermatology
www.aad.org/

National Cancer Institute
www.cancer.gov/

U.S. Food and Drug Administration
www.fda.gov/

REFERENCES

Ackley, B. J., & Ladwig, G. B. (2006). *Nursing diagnosis handbook: A guide to planning care.* St. Louis: Mosby Inc.

American Academy of Dermatology. *2007 Skin cancer fact sheet.* Schaumburg, IL. Available from: *www.aad.org/aad/ Newsroom/2007+Skin+Cancer+Fact+Sheet.htm.*

Canobbio, M. M. (2006). *Mosby's handbook of patient teaching.* St. Louis: Mosby Inc.

Cohen, B. J., & Taylor, J. J. (2005). *Memmler's the human body in health and disease* (10th ed.). Philadelphia: Lippincott Williams & Wilkins.

Hunt, R. (2005). *Introduction to community based nursing.* Philadelphia: Lippincott Williams & Wilkins.

Timby, B. K., & Smith, N. C. (2003). *Introductory medical-surgical nursing* (8th ed.). Philadelphia: J. B. Lippincott Williams & Wilkins.

1 | Anxiety Disorders

Patient name: _____   Admission: _____

<table>
<tr><td>NRS
DATE INITIAL</td><td></td></tr>
</table>

I.   The client/caregiver can define anxiety disorders.

A. Anxiety is an emotional feeling of uneasiness and apprehension. It is a normal reaction to stress and helps a person to cope.

B. When the anxiety level becomes excessive, it can become a disabling disorder.

C. The level of anxiety becomes a problem when it
   - Interferes with adaptive behavior
   - Causes physical symptoms
   - Becomes intolerable to client
   - Interferes with personal, occupational, and social function

D. Anxiety disorders include
   - Panic disorder (with or without agoraphobia)
   - Phobias (agoraphobia, social phobia, and specific phobia)
   - Obsessive-compulsive disorder
   - Generalized anxiety disorder
   - Stress disorders (posttraumatic stress disorder and acute stress disorder)

II.   The client/caregiver can recognize signs and symptoms of anxiety.

A. Signs and symptoms vary in severity and can appear in any combination. They may include
   - Restlessness
   - Feeling of being keyed up or on edge
   - Feeling a lump in your throat
   - Difficulty concentrating
   - Fatigue
   - Irritability
   - Being easily distracted
   - Muscle tension
   - Trouble falling or staying asleep
   - Shortness of breath
   - Stomachache
   - Diarrhea
   - Headache

III.   The client/caregiver can explain the behavioral and physical changes at the four levels of anxiety.

A. Mild anxiety
   1. Reality is intact.
   2. Person feels in control.
   3. Information can be processed accurately.
   4. Muscle tone increases.
   5. Heart rate, blood pressure, and breathing slightly increase.
   6. Perspiration is noticeable.

B. Moderate anxiety
   1. Person is easily distracted.
   2. Concentration is impaired but can redirect attention.
   3. Problem solving becomes difficult.
   4. Person feels irritable and has feelings of inadequacy.
   5. Muscles are tense.
   6. Slight tremor of hands.
   7. There are changes in speech (rate, pitch, and volume changes).
   8. Sleep is disturbed.

C. Severe anxiety
   1. Person's attention span decreases.
   2. Person is unable to concentrate or remain focused.
   3. Learning ability is impaired.
   4. There are feelings of extreme discomfort.
   5. Person has trouble keeping control of emotions.
   6. Person feels incompetent.
   7. Hyperventilation, dizziness, heart palpitations, and hypertension are seen.
   8. Fine motor skills are impaired.
   9. Communication is limited.

D. Panic levels of anxiety
   1. Person exaggerates details.
   2. Perception is distorted.
   3. Person is unable to learn.
   4. Person has fragmented thoughts.

(Continued)

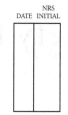

5. Feelings of helplessness are seen.
6. Speech is incoherent.
7. Movements are haphazard.
8. There is shortness of breath, tremors, sweating, and even fainting.

IV. **The client/caregiver can list measures to control anxiety.**

A. Reduce external stimuli (noise, activity, etc.) to promote comfort and communication. Remove to calm, quiet location without extra stimuli.
B. Avoid touching client without asking permission. Position self at least an arm's length to allow client sense of control.
C. Encourage client to seek out supportive person when anxiety level increases to describe how they feel.
D. Assist in identifying the source of anxiety.
E. Establish trust by being available and keeping promises.
F. Stay with client during times of severe anxiety.
G. Remain calm, and speak to client with soft voice, short sentences, and clear messages.
H. Create and follow consistent schedule for routine activities.
I. Discuss present coping methods and evaluate their effectiveness.
J. Introduce and assist client with relaxation techniques.
   1. Slowly count backward from 100.
   2. Breathe slowly and deeply (in through the nose and out through the mouth).
   3. Suggest warm bath or offer back massage.
   4. Progressively relax groups of muscles beginning with toes and moving toward head.
   5. Create and repeat positive statements using "I am" format.
   6. Visualize a pleasant, relaxing, and safe place.
   7. Listen to relaxation tape or music.
   8. Participate in activities that use large muscles, such as walking or biking.

K. Take medication (antianxiety) as ordered.
L. Encourage no use of caffeine, nicotine, alcohol, or stimulating drugs (diet pills).
M. Advise client to talk with physician before discontinuation or addition of any medications.

RESOURCES

Emergency numbers, such as crisis intervention, near the phone

Spiritual support/clergy

Support groups

National Institute of Mental Health
www.nimh.nih.gov/publicat/anxiety

Mental Health: A Report from the Surgeon General
www.surgeongeneral.gov/library/mentalhealth/chapter4/sec 2.html

Anxiety Disorders Association of America
www.adaa.org/

National Institutes of Mental Health—Public Inquiries and Dissemination Branch
866-615-NIMH (6464)
www.nimh.nih.gov

Anxiety Disorders Association of America
240-485-1001
www.adaa.org

Obsessive-Compulsive Foundation, Inc.
203-315-2190
www.ocfoundation.org

REFERENCES

Ackley, B. J., & Ladwig, G. B. (2006). *Nursing diagnosis handbook: A guide to planning care.* St. Louis: Mosby Inc.

Timby, B. K., & Smith, N. C. (2003). *Introductory medical-surgical nursing* (8th ed.). Philadelphia: J. B. Lippincott Williams & Wilkins.

Varcarolis, E. M. (2006). *Manual of psychiatric nursing care plans.* St. Louis: Saunders Elsevier.

Bipolar Disease (Manic Depression)

2

Patient name: _____ **Admission:** _____

I. The client/caregiver can define bipolar disease or manic depression.

A. It is a mental health disorder characterized by mood swings from overly high and irritable to sad and hopeless.
B. The highs and lows can last from a few days to several months.
C. It usually begins in adolescence or early adulthood.

II. The client/caregiver can list factors that increase risk.

A. Familial tendency
B. Affects men and women equally
C. Usually appears before the age of 30 years

III. The client/caregiver can recognize signs and symptoms.

A. Mania
 1. Increased energy, restlessness, and hyperactivity
 2. Irritability and distractibility
 3. Decreased need for sleep
 4. Racing thoughts and loud, rapid speech
 5. Manipulative
 6. Increased sexual drive
 7. Abuse of drugs
 8. Loss of appetite
 9. Inflated self-esteem
 10. Impractical schemes and poor judgment
 11. Denial that anything is wrong
 12. Unrealistic in financial and legal matters
 13. Anger
 14. Distractibility
 15. Hallucinations/delusions
B. Depression
 1. Persistent sad, anxious mood
 2. Feelings of guilt and hopelessness
 3. Decreased energy and fatigue
 4. Loss of appetite

 5. Weight gain or loss
 6. Loss of interest in ordinary activities
 7. Irritability
 8. Thoughts of death or suicide

IV. The client/caregiver can list measures to manage disease.

A. Limit alcohol.
B. Eat a well-balanced diet.
C. Exercise daily with rest periods.
D. Avoid competitive games.
E. Follow measures to decrease insomnia.
 1. Decrease stimulating activity at bedtime.
 2. Avoid caffeine.
 3. Drink warm milk.
 4. Avoid noise and distractions.
F. Keep follow-up appointments as scheduled.
G. Take medication as instructed. There is a need for routine blood tests to evaluate medication.

V. The client/caregiver can list measures for management of disease.

A. Watch closely to prevent client from causing injury to self or others.
B. Define acceptable behaviors to client.
C. Stress the importance of keeping appointments and taking medications to client.
D. Be honest and consistent.
E. Encourage good nutrition.
 1. Offer finger foods to increase ease of eating.
 2. Offer high-calorie, nutritious foods.
 3. Offer foods frequently.
F. Provide quiet atmosphere for manic stage.
G. Ask whether there is a suicide plan when in the depressed stage.
H. Have client hospitalized if severely depressed, suicidal, or at risk for injury.

(Continued)

RESOURCES

Emergency numbers, including therapist's number or clinic number, close to the phone.

SAMHSA's National Mental Health Information Center
http://mentalhealth.samhsa.gov/publications/allpubs/ken 98-0049/default.asp

Depression and Bipolar Support Alliance (formerly National Depressive and Manic-Depressive Association)
800-826-3632
www.dbsalliance.org

Healthy People 2010
www.healthypeople.gov/Document/HTML/Volume2/18 Mental.htm

Psychological counseling

Spiritual counseling

Support groups

REFERENCES

Ackley, B. J., & Ladwig, G. B. (2006). *Nursing diagnosis handbook: A guide to planning care.* St. Louis: Mosby Inc.

Hitchcock, J. E., Schubert, P. E., & Thomas, S. A. (2003). *Community health nursing: Caring in action.* Clifton Park, NY: Thomson Delmar Learning.

Timby, B. K., & Smith, N. C. (2003). *Introductory medical-surgical nursing* (8th ed.). Philadelphia: J. B. Lippincott Williams & Wilkins.

Varcarolis, E. M. (2006). *Manual of psychiatric nursing care plans.* St. Louis: Saunders Elsevier.

3 Depression

Patient name: _____ Admission: _____

NRS DATE INITIAL

I. The client/caregiver can define depression.

A. It is a mood state that is characterized by low mood, sadness, and hopelessness that persists beyond a few weeks.
B. It may be caused by a life event (reactive depression) or occur independent of any life event (major or unipolar depression).
C. It can be chronic or short term.
D. The exact cause of depression in not known. Two neurotransmitters (serotonin and norepinephrine) that allow brain cells to communicate may be implicated.

II. The client/caregiver can list factors that increase risk of depression.

A. National Institute for Mental Health states that 3 to 4 million men are affected by depression. Depression affects twice as many women.
B. People who are separated, divorced, and widowed are more at risk.
C. People who use drugs or alcohol are more at risk.
D. Parents whose children recently left home are more susceptible.
E. People with chronic debilitation and chronic or terminal illnesses are vulnerable.
F. People who think negatively are more at risk.
G. People with a family history of depression are more vulnerable.

III. The client/caregiver can recognize signs and symptoms of depression.

A. Sad mood
B. Appetite changes (increase or decrease)
C. Sleep changes (insomnia or hypersomia)
D. Inability to concentrate
E. Marked decrease in pleasure
F. Apathy (including lack of interest in sex)
G. Guilty feelings
H. Energy changes (restlessness or inactivity)
I. Suicidal thoughts

NRS DATE INITIAL

IV. The client/caregiver can list results of depression.

A. Poor work performance
B. Poor relationships with others
C. Disruption of families
D. Suicide

V. The client/caregiver can list some treatment options for depression.

A. Psychotherapy
B. Medication therapy
C. Electroconvulsive therapy

VI. The caregiver can list measures to assist client in dealing with depression.

A. Encourage client to stay with treatment.
B. If needed, monitor the client's compliance with appointments and use of medication.
C. Encourage client to follow treatment plan and avoid use of alcohol or any substance abuse.
D. Other emotional support includes the following:
   1. Recognize and praise even minor accomplishments.
   2. Encourage client to verbalize emotions.
   3. Be honest and consistent. Do not criticize.
   4. Do not accuse client of "faking" or being "lazy."
   5. Do not ignore remarks about suicide.
E. Encourage client to make decisions for himself or herself.
F. Encourage client to become involved in interests and activities.
G. Encourage independence.
H. Obtain medical attention for prolonged signs of depression.

VII. The client can list self-help measures to cope with depression.

A. Eat a well-balanced diet.
B. Use vitamin and mineral supplements approved by physician.

(Continued)

C. Take medications and keep appointments for therapy.

D. Set realistic goals in consideration of new diagnosis of depression.

E. Break large task into small ones, and do what you can.

F. Try to be with other people. Have someone to confide in. Avoid keeping yourself isolated and alone.

G. Participate in activities that you enjoy or that make you feel better.

H. Do mild exercise or participate in activity.

I. Expect your mood to improve gradually, not instantly.

J. Postpone important decisions until depression has improved.

K. Try to replace negative thinking with positive thinking.

L. Allow family and friends to help you.

VIII. **The caregiver can list measures to prevent suicide.**

A. Ask the client whether he or she has ever considered suicide.

B. Remove any dangerous objects (i.e., knives, guns, and stockpiling pills).

C. Arrange for hospitalization if client is threatening suicide.

D. Assist client to identify one or more alternatives to suicide.

RESOURCES

SAMHSA's National Mental Health Information Center
http://mentalhealth.samhsa.gov/publications/allpubs/ken 98-0049/default.asp

Depression and Bipolar Support Alliance (formerly National Depressive and Manic-Depressive Association)
800-826-3632
www.dbsalliance.org

Healthy People 2010
www.healthypeople.gov/Document/HTML/Volume2/18Mental.htm

Psychological counseling

Spiritual counseling

Crisis intervention hot line

Support groups

REFERENCES

Ackley, B. J., & Ladwig, G. B. (2006). *Nursing diagnosis handbook: A guide to planning care.* St. Louis: Mosby Inc.

Timby, B. K., & Smith, N. C. (2003). *Introductory medical-surgical nursing* (8th ed.). Philadelphia: J. B. Lippincott Williams & Wilkins.

Varcarolis, E. M. (2006). *Manual of psychiatric nursing care plans.* St. Louis: Saunders Elsevier.

4 Schizophrenia

Patient name: _____ **Admission:** _____

I.   **The client/caregiver can define schizophrenia.**

A. It is a psychosis characterized by withdrawal from reality.
B. There is deterioration in mental functioning.
C. The onset is usually before age 45.
D. Symptoms are continuous for 6 months or more.
E. There may be exacerbations and remissions, but the condition is life-long.

II. **The client/caregiver can list five types of schizophrenia.**

A. Disorganized (hallucinations and delusions, incoherent, and inappropriate affect)
B. Catatonic (sudden excitement followed by stupor or posturing)
C. Paranoid (preoccupation with delusion, suspicion, anxiety, and anger)
D. Residual (partial remission of symptoms)
E. Undifferentiated (symptoms of various types)

III. **The client/caregiver can recognize symptoms of schizophrenia from three categories.**

A. Positive symptoms are unusual thoughts or perceptions.
  1. Hallucinations (sensory experiences that others do not perceive), which can be auditory (hear), visual (see), tactile (touch), olfactory (smell), or gustatory (taste).
  2. Delusions (false beliefs that cannot be changed by logical reasoning)
  3. Thought disorders (unusual thought processes)—garbled speech, inventing new words, rhyming, or repeating what others say
  4. Disorders of movement, which can include uncoordinated movements or involuntary movements or mannerisms

B. Negative symptoms show as a loss or decrease in the ability to plan, speak, express emotion, or find pleasure in everyday life.
  1. Flat affect or expression and monotonous voice
  2. Lack of pleasure in everyday life
  3. Diminished ability to plan, initiate, or sustain any activity. Basic hygiene and care are often neglected.
  4. Rarely speaking, even when pressured to interact

C. Cognitive symptoms are problems with attention, types of memory, and executive functions that enable to plan and organize.
  1. Poor "executive functioning" leads to inability to absorb and interpret information.
  2. There is an inability to sustain attention.
  3. There are problems with "working memory" or inability to recall recently learned information.

IV. **The caregiver can list measures in communicating and caring for a person with schizophrenia.**

A. Promote getting and maintaining treatment.
  1. Clients often resist treatment.
  2. Family or friends need to be prepared to take action to keep client safe if crisis occurs.
  3. If client stops therapy or medication, he or she may be unable to care for their basic needs for food, clothing, and shelter.

B. Promote a trusting relationship.
  1. Treat the client with respect and honesty.
  2. Explain carefully what is to be done before it happens.
  3. Speak directly and simply.

(Continued)

NRS
DATE INITIAL

C. Promote self-esteem.
  1. Reinforce the client's strengths and skills.
  2. Encourage client's sense of self-control.
  3. Encourage any interests or talents.
  4. Encourage independence.
D. Promote reality orientation.
  1. Orient the client to time, person, and place as needed.
  2. Avoid confirming delusions and hallucinations, but do not argue with the client.
  3. Attempt to redirect from a hallucination or delusion to a reality situation.
E. Encourage socialization.

V. **The client can list measures to manage disease.**

A. Continue counseling with health professional.
B. Continue medications as instructed.
C. Use community supports and resources.

RESOURCES

National Institute of Mental Health
www.nimh.nih.gov/healthinformation/schizophreniamenu.cfm

National Institute of Mental Health—Public Information and Communications Branch
866-615-NIMH (6464)
www.nimh.nih.gov

Support groups

REFERENCES

Ackley, B. J., & Ladwig, G. B. (2006). *Nursing diagnosis handbook: A guide to planning care*. St. Louis: Mosby Inc.

Hitchcock, J. E., Schubert, P. E., & Thomas, S. A. (2003). *Community health nursing: Caring in action*. Clifton Park, NY: Thomson Delmar Learning.

Timby, B. K., & Smith, N. C. (2003). *Introductory medical-surgical nursing* (8th ed.). Philadelphia: J. B. Lippincott Williams & Wilkins.

Varcarolis, E. M. (2006). *Manual of psychiatric nursing care plans*. St. Louis: Saunders Elsevier.

5 Suicide

Patient name: _____ Admission: _____

I. The client/caregiver can list general facts about suicide.

A. It is the eighth leading cause of death.
B. The suicide rate is increasing rapidly among adolescents.

II. The client/caregiver can list people at greater risk for suicide.

A. There is a history of previous attempts.
B. Men are four times more likely to die from suicide.
C. There is a family history of suicide.
D. There is a history of mistreatment as child.
E. There are feelings of hopelessness.
F. There is a plan for committing suicide.
G. The person is widowed, separated, divorced, or single.
H. There is a job loss or failure.
I. The person has physical health problems.
J. There is drug or alcohol abuse.
K. The person is living alone.
L. There is a recent loss of spouse, child, or pet.
M. The person has a lack of social support system.
N. There is a history of mental disorders, especially depression.

III. The caregiver can list signs and symptoms of impending suicide.

A. Giving things away
B. Refusing food
C. Suddenly improving mood or attitude
D. Feeling depressed and tearful
E. Getting affairs in order
F. Verbalizing death wish
G. Collecting medications (hoarding medications)

IV. The client/caregiver can list measures to identify or decrease risk of suicide.

A. Ask the client whether he or she has a plan for suicide.
B. Remove any dangerous objects (i.e., guns, knives, and razors). Check supply of medication. Do they have more than a 1-week supply and/or hoarding medication?
C. Discuss coping methods that have helped in the past.
D. Discuss other possible coping methods. Help plan for alternative ways to handle anger or frustration.
E. Identify two people to contact when feeling self-destructive.
F. Implement a written no-suicide contract if needed.
G. Encourage the client to take medications as ordered.
H. Encourage the client to keep follow-up appointments.
I. Contact family or friend. Arrange for crisis counseling.
J. Arrange for hospitalization if client is threatening suicide.
K. Stay with the client who is at risk until in a safe environment.
L. Activate contact with self-help groups. Encourage participation in support or therapy group where others have similar experiences or thoughts.
M. Develop skills in problem solving, conflict resolution, and nonviolent handling of disputes.
N. Discuss cultural and religious beliefs that discourage suicide.

(Continued)

RESOURCES

National Center for Disease Control and Prevention Fact Sheet on Suicide

www.cdc.gov/ncipc/factsheets/suifacts.htm

Suicide Awareness Voices of Education

www.save.org/

Clergy

Mental health professional

REFERENCES

Ackley, B. J., & Ladwig, G. B. (2006). *Nursing diagnosis handbook: A guide to planning care.* St. Louis: Mosby Inc.

Hitchcock, J. E., Schubert, P. E., & Thomas, S. A. (2003). *Community health nursing: Caring in action.* Clifton Park, NY: Thomson Delmar Learning.

Timby, B. K., & Smith, N. C. (2003). *Introductory medical-surgical nursing* (8th ed.). Philadelphia: J. B. Lippincott Williams & Wilkins.

Varcarolis, E. M. (2006). *Manual of psychiatric nursing care plans.* St. Louis: Saunders Elsevier.

Attention Deficit Hyperactivity Disorder

6

NRS
DATE INITIAL

I. **The client/caregiver can define attention deficit hyperactivity disorder (ADHD).**

    A. It is a persistent pattern of inattention and/or hyperactivity and impulsivity that is more frequently displayed and more severe than the typical individual.
    B. Condition continues into adulthood.
    C. It seems to run in families.
    D. The three types of ADHD are
        • Predominantly inattentive
        • Predominantly hyperactive/impulsive
        • Combination

II. **The client/caregiver can list symptoms of ADHD.**

    A. Symptoms for inattention
        • Often fails to pay attention to details
        • Often makes careless mistakes
        • Often does not listen when directly spoken to
        • Often does not follow instructions and fails to finish activities, schoolwork, chores, or duties in the workplace
        • Often has difficulty organizing tasks and activities
        • Often avoids or dislikes tasks that require ongoing mental effort or concentration
        • Often loses important things
        • Often is easily distracted by unimportant things
        • Often moves hands and feet nervously or squirms
        • Often leaves seat when staying seated is expected
        • Often feels restless
        • Often cannot be involved in leisure activities quietly
        • Often talks too much or too fast
    B. Symptoms for hyperactivity
        • Often moves hands and feet nervously or squirms
        • Often leaves seat when staying seated is expected

NRS
DATE INITIAL

• Often feels restless
• Often cannot be involved in leisure activities quietly
• Often talks too much or too fast

    C. Symptoms of impulsivity
        • Often blurts out answers before questions are fully asked
        • Often has hard time awaiting turn
        • Often butts in on others' conversations or activities
        • Ongoing, strong feelings of frustration, guilt, or blame

III. **The client/caregiver can list measures to help manage ADHD.**

    A. Medication and behavior therapy are used to treat ADHD in both children and adults.
    B. Basic principles to help children cope with ADHD:
        1. Set specific goals—primarily timed goals.
        2. Provide rewards and consequences.
        3. Consistently use rewards and consequences, but adjust to age and situation.
        4. Reward positive behavior. Positive behavior in reaching goal in timely manner or good behavior, such as paying attention, should always be praised.
        5. Calmly discipline with time-out, distraction, and so forth. Discuss unwanted behavior when calm.
        6. Inform teachers, coaches, and so forth of treatment and plan.
        7. Child will learn skills to monitor their behavior as they mature.
    C. Management and coping skills for people with ADHD of any age are
        1. Arrange daily schedule for activities. Remain consistent.
        2. Cut down on distractions. Loud music, television, and so forth can overstimulate when trying to do homework. At work, develop

(Continued)

NRS
DATE   INITIAL

measures that help you focus, such as closing office door; limit phone calls to specific times. Keeping desk organized and clean.

3. Organize and have specific places to keep items.

4. Break projects into smaller parts to avoid feeling overwhelmed.

5. Use charts, checklists, and so forth to track progress.

6. Make yourself brief notes regarding details, instructions, schedules, and so forth.

7. Limit choices to only two or three options at a time.

8. Find activities that you like and can be successful doing.

9. Use any tools that help you stay organized.

10. Get exercise, and eat a balanced diet. Some medications can alter appetite.

11. Practice relaxation techniques.

IV.   **The client/caregiver can list possible consequences of untreated ADHD.**

A. Children with ADHD have more injuries and falls, resulting in emergency room visits.

B. Adolescents with ADHD are more likely to engage in risky behaviors.
   • Substance abuse
   • Unprotected sexual activity leading to sexually transmitted diseases and teen pregnancy
   • More speeding tickets and involvement in auto accidents

C. Adolescents and young adults are more likely to drop out of school.

D. Adults with ADHD are
   • More likely to suffer from depression and anxiety
   • More likely to be fired from jobs or change jobs frequently
   • More likely to get divorced or failed relationships

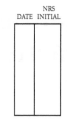

E. People of all ages with ADHD often have poor self-esteem and are told they are lazy, not trying, and so forth because they perform as underachievers. They have ongoing, strong feelings of frustration, guilt, or blame.

RESOURCES
Support groups

ADHD coach

Children and Adults with Attention-Deficit/Hyperactivity Disorder
800-233-4050
www.chadd.org

Attention Deficit Disorder Association
www.add.org

Learning Disabilities Association of America
www.ldaamerica.org

National Center for Learning Disabilities
www.ld.org

National Institute of Mental Health
www.nimh.nih.gov

REFERENCES
Ackley, B. J., & Ladwig, G. B. (2006). *Nursing diagnosis handbook: A guide to planning care.* St. Louis: Mosby Inc.

Hitchcock, J. E., Schubert, P. E., & Thomas, S. A. (2003). *Community health nursing: Caring in action.* Clifton Park, NY: Thomson Delmar Learning.

Muscari, M. E. (2005). *Pediatric nursing.* Philadelphia: Lippincott Williams & Wilkins.

Timby, B. K., & Smith, N. C. (2003). *Introductory medical-surgical nursing* (8th ed.). Philadelphia: J. B. Lippincott Williams & Wilkins.

Varcarolis, E. M. (2006). *Manual of psychiatric nursing care plans.* St. Louis: Saunders Elsevier.

7 Eating Disorders

Patient name: _____ Admission: _____

NRS
DATE INITIAL

I. **The client/caregiver can define eating disorders.**

A. Eating disorders are serious but treatable medical illnesses involving severe disturbances in eating behavior.
B. The two main eating disorders are anorexia nervosa and bulimia nervosa.
C. Denial of the problem is common. Families and friends may become involved to ensure medical help for the person suffering from eating disorders.

II. **The client/caregiver can list factors that increase risk of an eating disorder.**

A. Girls and women are more likely to develop eating disorders.
B. Patients are most common during teens and early 20s.
C. Feelings of insecurity or an overly critical family may increase risk.
D. Patients are more common in people with a close family member suffering from an eating disorder.
E. People with depression, anxiety disorders, and obsessive-compulsive disorder have a higher risk. Some people with bulimia have impulse control issues.
F. People who participate in highly competitive athletic activities have a greater risk.

III. **The client/caregiver can explain anorexia nervosa and its symptoms.**

A. Anorexia nervosa is a condition that results from self imposed starvation.
B. Symptoms of anorexia nervosa are
- Loss of 20% to 40% of usual body weight
- Intense fear of becoming obese
- Preoccupation with food (avoiding food, picking out only few foods to eat,

NRS
DATE INITIAL

weighing food to cut back size portions)
- Body image disturbance
- Misconceptions of physical status
- Intake as low as 500 to 800 calories a day
- Poor muscle tone
- Self-esteem that is directly related to body weight or shape
- After reaching puberty have infrequent or missing menstrual periods
- Repeatedly check body weight
- Use intense and compulsive exercise to maintain low weight
- Excessive hair loss

IV. **The client/caregiver can explain bulimia nervosa and its symptoms.**

A. Bulimia nervosa is when a person binges and purges.
B. Binging is the consumption of large amounts of food in short periods of time. Binging can mean consuming as much as 5,000 to 20,000 calories a day.
C. Purging is the intentional clearing of food from body by
- Vomiting (self-induced or use of Ipecac)
- Abuse of laxatives or diuretics
- Enemas
D. Because of the cycle, they appear to be of normal weight.
E. Symptoms of bulimia nervosa are
- Body image disturbance
- Much of the activity done in secrecy
- Weight determines self-esteem.
- Sneaking food or lying about eating habits
- Eating to relieve stress or depression
- Perfectionism
- Eating when not hungry
- Repeated attempts at dieting or very strict dieting

(Continued)

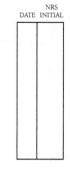

V. **The client/caregiver can list components of treatment.**

  A. Nutrition education
  B. Psychotherapy
  C. Family counseling
  D. Medications

VI. **The client/caregiver can list measures to manage and cope with eating disorders.**

  A. General self-care measures to develop are
    1. Follow a regular schedule for meals.
    2. Stop eating when you are full, but not stuffed.
    3. Eat healthy, well-balanced meals.
    4. Take vitamin and mineral supplements as ordered by physician.
    5. Exercise regularly, but use moderation.
    6. Take medications as ordered.
  B. Coping skills to break the self-destructive behaviors involved with eating disorders.
    1. See your physician, counselor, or health care professional regularly.
    2. Improve self-esteem by getting involved in activities or groups you enjoy, and learn a new skill or hobby.
    3. Get help to improve family dynamics.
    4. Seek out support group or supportive friends.
    5. Be realistic about healthy weight and body image.

VII. **The client/caregiver can list possible complications of eating disorders.**

  A. Heart conditions such as slow pulse, low blood pressure, electrocardiogram (EKG) abnormalities, and congestive heart failure
  B. Kidney stones or kidney failure
  C. Elevated uric acid
  D. Low blood glucose levels
  E. Erosion of enamel on teeth, increased cavities, and bleeding gums
  F. Esophageal perforations or lacerations (from induced vomiting)
  G. Aspiration pneumonia
  H. Death from cardiac arrest or electrolyte imbalance

RESOURCES

National Eating Disorders Association
www.nationaleatingdisorders.org

American Dietetic Association
www.eatright.org

Nemours Foundation/Kids Health for Parents
www.kidshealth.org/parent/emotions/feelings/eating_disorders.html

National Mental Health Information Center
www.mentalhealth.samhsa.gov/publications

REFERENCES

Ackley, B. J., & Ladwig, G. B. (2006). *Nursing diagnosis handbook: A guide to planning care*. St. Louis: Mosby Inc.

Cohen, B. J., & Taylor, J. J. (2005). *Memmler's the human body in health and disease* (10th ed.). Philadelphia: Lippincott Williams & Wilkins.

Lutz, C., & Przytulski, K. (2001). *Nutrition and diet therapy*. Philadelphia: F. A. Davis Company.

Taylor, C., Lillis, C., & LeMone, P. (2005). *Fundamentals of nursing*. Philadelphia: Lippincott, Williams & Wilkins.

Varcarolis, E. M. (2006). *Manual of psychiatric nursing care plans*. St. Louis: Saunders Elsevier.

Part III

Hospice

Teaching Guides

1 Care of the Dying

Patient name: _____ Admission: _____

NRS
DATE INITIAL

I. **The client/caregiver can define hospice.**

   A. Hospice is a coordinated program of palliative services delivered to terminally ill clients and their families.
   B. The client usually has a prognosis of 6 months or less to live.
   C. Palliative care serves to control pain or symptoms without curing.
   D. Hospice stresses quality of life—peace, comfort, and dignity.
   E. Interventions of the hospice team provide for the physical, psychological, social, and spiritual needs of the dying client and their caregivers.
   F. These interventions can take place in variety of settings such as the home, hospice centers, a long-term care facility, or an acute-care facility.

II. **The client/caregiver can state purpose of hospice.**

   A. The focus of hospice is on care not cure.
   B. To provide pain relief and symptom control.
   C. To support a comfortable and humane death.
   D. To provide physical assistance and emotional support for client and caregiver.
   E. To provide an understanding of the meaning of life.
   F. To provide bereavement follow-up and counseling to families and caregivers.

III. **The client/caregiver can recognize signs and symptoms of imminent death.**

   A. Color and temperature changes in hands, arms, feet, and legs
   B. Weak, rapid pulse rate and drop in blood pressure
   C. Increased amount of time sleeping and less responsive to stimuli
   D. Restlessness and/or confusion about time, place, and person

NRS
DATE INITIAL

   E. Difficulty in handling oral secretions and possible lung congestion
   F. Change in breathing patterns and apnea (periods of no breathing)
   G. Little or no urinary output
   H. Loss of bladder and bowel control
   I. Perspiration
   J. Decreased intake of food and liquids (Do not force client to eat or drink.)

IV. **The client/caregiver can list and recognize the five stages of grief.**

   A. Denial
   B. Anger
   C. Bargaining
   D. Depression
   E. Acceptance

V. **The caregiver can promote comfort for the client.**

   A. Give pain medication as needed.
      1. Monitor closely for signs of pain (i.e., restlessness, anxiousness, moaning, irritability, and sweating).
      2. Give the medication preventively or at the first onset of pain.
      3. Provide medication in form most easily taken by client as progression of the disease advances.
   B. Provide a quiet, calm atmosphere. Reduce unnecessary external stimulation to client.
   C. Control temperature of room. Promote comfort and privacy as client desires.
   D. Give Tylenol suppositories if temperature is elevated and the client is unable to swallow.
   E. Provide complementary methods of pain control (i.e., massage, soft music, guided imagery, and therapeutic touch).
   F. Give medications for nausea as needed.
   G. Provide general comfort measures.
      1. Provide daily bath with lubrication of skin. Assess for any redness or breakdown on skin.

(Continued)

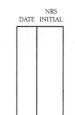

2. Reposition at least every 2 hours.
3. Provide good oral care by frequent cleansing, and keep lips and oral mucosa moist and lubricated.
4. Provide eye care to cleanse, and use of artificial tears as needed.
5. Cleanse perineal areas after any incontinence.
6. Keep client warm and comfortable by adjusting clothing or bedding as needed.
7. Conserve the client's energy, and allow rest periods.

H. Teach and involve family in client care.

VI. **The caregiver provides spiritual and emotional needs of client.**

A. Allow the client to discuss death and any end of life issues.
B. Request pastor or clergy to provide spiritual support.
C. Spend time with client to assure him or her that he or she is not alone.
D. Talk to the client even when nonresponsive because hearing is the last sense to leave.

VII. **The caregiver can provide nutrition/fluids as tolerated.**

A. Give nutritional supplements such as Ensure, Boost, and so forth.
B. Give small, frequent meals.

C. Give ground or pureed food as needed.
D. Do not attempt food or liquids if unable to swallow.
E. Vitamins and antinausea medications may increase appetite.
F. Refer to increased calorie diet suggestions.

RESOURCES

National Hospice and Palliative Care Organization
www.nhpco.org

American Cancer Society
www.cancer.org

American Medical Association Advance Directives

REFERENCES

Ackley, B. J., & Ladwig, G. B. (2006). *Nursing diagnosis handbook: A guide to planning care*. St. Louis: Mosby Inc.

Dunn, H. (2001). *Hard choices for loving people*. Las Cruces, NM: Geriatric Resources.

Hitchcock, J. E., Schubert, P. E., & Thomas, S. A. (2003). *Community health nursing: Caring in action*. Clifton Park, NY: Thomson Delmar Learning.

Hunt, R. (2005). *Introduction to community based nursing*. Philadelphia: Lippincott Williams & Wilkins.

Perry, A., & Potter, P. (2006). *Clinical nursing skills & technique*. St. Louis: Mosby Inc.

Part IV

Procedures and Surgeries

Teaching Guides

1 Chemotherapy

Patient name: _____ Admission: _____

<table>
<tr><td>NRS
DATE INITIAL</td><td></td></tr>
</table>

I. The client/caregiver can define chemotherapy.

A. Chemotherapy (or antineoplastic drugs) is the use of one or more drugs to destroy or slow the growth of malignant tumor cells.

B. Antineoplastic drugs are toxic to normal and abnormal cells.

C. It can be given alone or in combination with surgery or radiation.

D. Chemotherapy can be given in several ways:
- Oral (by mouth)
- Injection (into a muscle, under the skin, or directly into a cancerous area in the skin)
- Topically (applied to the skin)
- Delivered intravenously through needle, or catheter (central venous catheter, peripherally inserted central catheter [PICC])
- Intrathecal—delivered into the spinal fluid
- Intracavitary—delivered in the abdomen, pelvis, or chest

E. Medicines that help speed recovery of white blood cells, called colony-stimulating factors (CSF), are often ordered by the physician during chemotherapy.

II. The client/caregiver can name most common side effects of chemotherapy and measures to prevent or manage them.

A. Infections caused by a low white blood count
1. Wash your hands often such as before you eat, after you use bathroom, or after touching animals.
2. Obtain prompt treatment for any signs of infection.
3. Avoid people with upper-respiratory infections, flu, or chicken pox.
4. Avoid crowds.
5. Stay away from children who recently received "live virus" vaccines.

6. Maintain good nutrition and fluid intake.
7. Avoid cuts and scrapes. Clean and treat cuts/scrapes promptly.
8. Cook and prepare food carefully to prevent bacteria.
9. Take a warm (not hot) bath or shower and pat dry. Use lotions to soften the skin.
10. Do not eat raw fish, seafood, meat, or eggs.
11. Avoid contact with animal litter boxes, bird cages, and fish tanks.

B. Nausea and vomiting
1. Take medication to control nausea before treatment and as needed.
2. Avoid odors that increase nausea.
3. Eat small, frequent meals.
4. Eat foods cold or at room temperature to avoid strong smells.
5. Avoid sweet, fried, or fatty foods.
6. Drink cool, clear, unsweetened fruit juices, such as apple juice. Use light-colored sodas that have lost their fizz. Avoid caffeine.
7. Rest, but sit up at least 2 hours after meals.
8. Breathe deeply and slowly when nauseated.
9. Notify physician if vomiting is severe or lasts over 24 hours.

C. Mouth sores and/or dry mouth
1. Use mouthwash of salt, baking soda, or hydrogen peroxide, avoiding commercial mouthwashes with alcohol that dry mucous membranes.
2. Avoid spicy or acidic foods.
3. Avoid alcohol and use of tobacco products.
4. Perform good oral hygiene using toothettes or glycerin swabs.
5. Obtain routine dental exams.
6. Brush teeth regularly with soft toothbrush and floss.
7. Eat foods cold or at room temperature.

(Continued)

8. Eat soft foods such as
   - Ice cream, milkshakes, yogurt, cottage cheese, and puddings
   - Soft fruits such as bananas or applesauce
   - Baby foods or puree cooked foods
9. Suck on ice chips, popsicles, sugarless hard candy, or sugarless chewing gum. Sorbitol is a sugar substitute that can cause diarrhea. Check labels if you are having problem with diarrhea.
10. Use artificial saliva. Use lip balm or lubricant to lips.
11. Drink plenty of liquids. Cover water bottle.

D. Hair loss (alopecia)
   1. Change hairstyle (usually shorter hairstyles look thicker).
   2. Purchase wig or hairpiece.
   3. Wash hair gently (with mild shampoo), and use a soft bristled hairbrush.
   4. Use only low heat when drying hair.
   5. Avoid permanents and hair coloring.
   6. Use sunscreen, a hat, or a scarf to protect scalp.

E. Susceptibility to bleeding due to low platelet count
   1. Prevent injury or cuts by using an electric razor. Use a soft toothbrush, and avoid going barefooted.
   2. Prevent constipation (may cause rectal bleeding).
   3. Avoid use of aspirin and aspirin products.
   4. Symptoms to report to physician are
      - Reddish or pink urine
      - Black or bloody bowel movements
      - Bleeding from gums or mouth
      - Vaginal bleeding that lasts longer than a regular period
      - Unexpected bruising or small, red spot under the skin
      - Changes in vision

F. Diarrhea
   1. Eat bland, high-carbohydrate, low-fiber foods.
   2. Drink plenty of fluids. Use clear broth, sport drinks, and carbonated drinks that have lost the fizz. Drink slowly, and have drinks at room temperature.
   3. Eat small amounts of food throughout the day.
   4. Eat BRAT diet of bananas, rice, apples, and tea.

5. Take antidiarrheal medicine as ordered.
6. Avoid hot or very cold liquids.
7. Limit milk and milk products if they make diarrhea worse.
8. Avoid coffee, tea with caffeine, and alcohol.
9. Notify physician if diarrhea is severe or lasts several days.

G. Constipation
   1. Eat high-fiber foods (i.e., fresh fruits and vegetables and whole grain breads and cereals).
   2. Increase fluids.
   3. Increase exercise.

H. Fatigue and anemia
   1. Chemotherapy can reduce the bone marrow's ability to produce red blood cells. This results in body tissue not getting enough oxygen (anemia).
   2. Symptoms of anemia are
      - Fatigue (complaints of feeling weak and tired)
      - Dizziness or feeling faint
      - Shortness of breath
      - Feeling your heart "pounding" or beating very fast
   3. Measures to help fatigue and anemia are
      - Plan activities with time to rest.
      - Take naps or breaks during the day.
      - Save energy for the most important activities.
      - Try modified (easier or shorter) versions of activities.
      - Do light exercise if possible.
      - Eat and drink fluids as tolerated.
      - Limit the use of caffeine and alcohol.
      - Accept help from others.
      - Try complementary therapies, such as guided imagery and mediation.
      - Change positions (sitting to standing, etc.) slowly to avoid dizziness or loss of balance.

III. **The client/caregiver can list general health measures when receiving chemotherapy.**

   A. Obtain adequate rest to prevent fatigue.
   B. Eat a high-protein, high-carbohydrate diet.
   C. Drink fluids up to 3000 ml per day.
   D. Keep follow-up appointments with physician and laboratory.
   E. Be informed about disease and treatment.
   F. Seek support groups for information and emotional support.

(Continued)

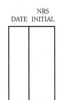

NRS
DATE INITIAL

G. Read the booklet *Taking Time: Support for People with Cancer*, produced by the National Cancer Institute at *www.cancer.gov/cancertopics/takingtime*.

RESOURCES

American Cancer Society
800-227-2345
www.cancer.org/

National Cancer Institute
www.cancer.gov/

Support groups

REFERENCES

Ackley, B. J., & Ladwig, G. B. (2006). *Nursing diagnosis handbook: A guide to planning care*. St. Louis: Mosby Inc.

Canobbio, M. M. (2006). *Mosby's handbook of patient teaching*. St. Louis: Mosby Inc.

Lutz, C., & Przytulski, K. (2001). *Nutrition and diet therapy*. Philadelphia: F. A. Davis Company.

Perry, A., & Potter, P. (2006). *Clinical nursing skills & technique*. St. Louis: Mosby Inc.

National Cancer Institute. *Taking time: Support for people with cancer*. Available at *www.cancer.gov/cancertopics/takingtime*.

Timby, B. K., & Smith, N. C. (2003). *Introductory medical-surgical nursing* (8th ed.). Philadelphia: J. B. Lippincott Williams & Wilkins.

2 Radiation

Patient name: _____ **Admission:** _____

I. The client/caregiver can define radiation.

A. It is the use of ionizing radiation to produce biologic effects to tissues and causing DNA damage. This damage then creates the loss of cellular reproduction.

B. Radiation can be given externally or internally.
1. External radiation is administered by a machine directing rays to the part of the body involved.
2. Internal radiation is given by placing radioactive material within the tissues or body cavity.

C. High-dose radiation can cause sterility. Issues of fertility and sexual function should be addressed.

II. The client/caregiver can list general health measures while receiving radiation.

A. Provide good skin care.
1. Inspect radiation treatment sites daily.
2. Bathe carefully. Avoid using soap and friction over treated area. Do not wash off markings on the skin.
3. Avoid using ointments or creams on the treated area unless prescribed by physician.
4. Avoid extreme temperatures of hot or cold, including
   - Heating pads
   - Ultraviolet light
   - Whirlpool bath
   - Sauna or steam baths
   - Direct sunlight
5. Protect skin from sunlight or wind exposure.
6. Wear soft nonrestrictive clothing.
7. If receiving treatment to head
   - Avoid use of harsh shampoo.
   - Avoid hair coloring or permanents.
   - Avoid use of curling irons and hair dryers.

B. Promote good nutrition.
1. Eat a well-balanced diet with a variety of foods. Use frequent smaller meals.

2. Weigh daily for early detection of weight loss.
3. Avoid eating several hours before and after treatment to prevent nausea.
4. Encourage fluid intake of up to 3000 ml/day.

C. Obtain adequate rest to prevent fatigue.

D. Prevent bleeding.
1. Report early signs of bruises, bleeding gums, and so forth.
2. Follow safety measures to prevent injuries.
3. Avoid aspirin.

E. Prevent infection.
1. Avoid crowds or persons with respiratory infection.
2. Report any early sign of infection.

F. Notify physician of side effects from radiation.

G. Keep follow-up appointments with physician.

III. The client/caregiver can list possible complications or side effects.

A. Side effects are seen early in the skin, mucous membranes, and hair follicles. Later side effects are noted in the vascular system and muscles.

B. General effects are fatigue and loss of appetite.

C. Alopecia (loss of hair) can occur.

D. Skin has local redness and inflammation. There can be dry or moist shedding of epidermis layer of skin.

E. Changes can occur in the mucous membranes such as inflammation, dryness, or change and/or loss of taste.

F. Nausea or vomiting is possible.

G. Diarrhea can occur.

H. Cystitis (inflammation of bladder) can occur.

I. Pneumonitis (inflammation of the lungs) is possible.

J. There could be depression of bone marrow function, resulting in anemia.

(Continued)

RESOURCES

American Cancer Society
800-227-2345
www.cancer.org/

National Cancer Institute
www.cancer.gov/cancertopics/factsheet/Therapy/radiation

Cancer Information Service
800-4-CANCER (800-422-6237)
www.cancer.gov

LiveHelp, National Cancer Institute's live online assistance
https://cissecure.nci.nih.gov/livehelp/welcome.asp

Support groups

Counseling

REFERENCE

Ackley, B. J., & Ladwig, G. B. (2006). *Nursing diagnosis handbook: A guide to planning care.* St. Louis: Mosby Inc.

Canobbio, M. M. (2006). *Mosby's handbook of patient teaching.* St. Louis: Mosby Inc.

Lutz, C., & Przytulski, K. (2001). *Nutrition and diet therapy.* Philadelphia: F. A. Davis Company.

Perry, A., & Potter, P. (2006). *Clinical nursing skills & technique.* St. Louis: Mosby Inc.

Timby, B. K., & Smith, N. C. (2003). *Introductory medical-surgical nursing* (8th ed.). Philadelphia: J. B. Lippincott Williams & Wilkins.

Colostomy Care

3

Patient name: _____

Admission: _____

NRS
DATE INITIAL

NRS
DATE INITIAL

I. **The client/caregiver can define colostomy.**

   A. A colostomy is a surgical opening between the large intestine and the surface of the abdomen.
   B. A small portion of the intestine is sewed to the surface of the abdomen creating a "stoma."
   C. The purpose of the colostomy is to bypass the diseased rectum and colon to rid the body of solid wastes.
   D. The large intestine consists of the ascending, transverse, and descending portions.
   E. Its primary purpose is to absorb water and store feces.

II. **The client/caregiver can list three types of colostomies.**

   A. Ascending colostomy has a stoma that is located on the right side of the abdomen. The output that drains is in liquid form.
   B. Transverse colostomy has a stoma that is located in the upper abdomen toward the middle or right side. The output that drains is loose or soft.
   C. Descending or sigmoid colostomy has a stoma that is located on the lower left side of the abdomen. The output that drains is firm.

III. **The client/caregiver can list different types of colostomy pouches.**

   A. An open-ended pouch is open at the bottom to drain output. The open end of this pouch is usually closed with a plastic clamp. This type of pouch is used by people with an ascending or transverse colostomies.
   B. Closed-ended pouch is removed and thrown away when the pouch is filled. This type of pouch is usually used by people with a descending or sigmoid colostomy.

   C. A one-piece pouch has the pouch and the adhesive skin barrier as one piece. When the pouch requires changing, the new pouch must be reattached to the skin.
   D. The two-piece pouch has two parts, including the adhesive flange and the pouch. The adhesive part remains when the pouch is cleaned or replaced.

IV. **The client/caregiver can demonstrate emptying the pouch.**

   A. Empty when one third full.
   B. Sit on toilet or place on chair with the pouch opening placed in the toilet.
   C. Put toilet paper on the surface of the toilet water to avoid splashing.
   D. Remove clamp and let contents empty into toilet.
   E. Squeeze the remaining contents out of the pouch.
   F. While holding up the end of the pouch, pour a cup of water into pouch, swish, and empty. Do not get the stoma or adhesive seal wet.
   G. Use toilet paper to clean around opening of pouch and clamp pouch shut.

V. **The client/caregiver can demonstrate procedure of changing the pouching system.**

   A. Change pouch every 5 to 7 days or as needed.
   B. Assemble all of the equipment.
   C. Hold skin taut, and peel off the pouch being worn.
   D. Wash the skin thoroughly with soap and water, rinse, and pat dry.
   E. Inspect the stoma for any change in size or color.
   F. Inspect the skin for signs of irritation and apply skin barrier.
   G. Apply pouch over the stoma, being sure it is the appropriate size and fits closely around the stoma.

(Continued)

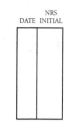

VI. **The client/caregiver can list dietary measures for management of colostomy.**

A. Eat a healthy balanced diet. Eat slowly and chew well.

B. Avoid the use of straws to reduce gas.

C. Foods that may help to control odor and gas in some people are fresh parsley, yogurt, and buttermilk.

D. Drink 8 to 10 glasses of water or liquids each day. Healthy choices are water, juices, and milk. Limit the intake of caffeine and soda.

E. Foods that may cause gas and odor are
- Broccoli, cabbage, cucumbers, Brussels sprouts, or cauliflower
- Beans, eggs, and fish
- Cheese, onions, garlic, or alcohol

VII. **The client/caregiver can list general measures for management of colostomy.**

A. Avoid contact sports and weight lifting.

B. Avoid tight, constrictive clothing.

C. Bathing, showering, and swimming can be done with appliance on.

D. Keep extra colostomy supplies on hand.

E. Report to physician any change in size or color of stoma, persistent diarrhea or severe constipation, frank bleeding from stoma, purulent drainage or pain at stoma, and fever.

F. Provide information concerning sexual activity, such as
1. Resume sexual activity when stoma is healed.
2. Empty pouch before intercourse.
3. Get counseling if needed.

RESOURCES

United Ostomy Associations of America, Inc.
www.uoaa.org

Wound, Ostomy, Continence Nurses
www.wocn.org

REFERENCES

Ackley, B. J., & Ladwig, G. B. (2006). *Nursing diagnosis handbook: A guide to planning care*. St. Louis: Mosby Inc.

Canobbio, M. M. (2006). *Mosby's handbook of patient teaching*. St. Louis: Mosby Inc.

Perry, A., & Potter, P. (2006). *Clinical nursing skills & technique*. St. Louis: Mosby Inc.

Timby, B. K., & Smith, N. C. (2003). *Introductory medical-surgical nursing* (8th ed.). Philadelphia: J. B. Lippincott Williams & Wilkins.

Ileostomy Care

Patient name: _____   **Admission:** _____

NRS DATE INITIAL	

I. The client/caregiver can define ileostomy.

A. An ileostomy is a surgical opening between the ileum and the abdominal wall.

B. A small portion of the intestine is sewed to the surface of the abdomen to create a "stoma."

C. The purpose of an ileostomy is to bypass a diseased colon and rid the body of wastes.

II. The client/caregiver can describe the basic anatomy and physiology of the small intestine.

A. The small intestine is approximately 18 feet long and is divided into three sections.

B. The ileum is the last section of the small intestine and is connected to the large intestine at the ileocecal valve.

C. Digestive enzymes are secreted and fluid is absorbed in the small intestine.

III. The client/caregiver can demonstrate emptying a pouch.

A. Empty when one third full.

B. Sit on toilet or place on chair with the pouch opening placed in the toilet.

C. Put toilet paper on the surface of the toilet water to avoid splashing.

D. Remove clamp and let contents empty into toilet.

E. Squeeze the remaining contents out of the pouch.

F. While holding up the end of the pouch, pour a cup of water into pouch, swish, and empty. Do not get the stoma or adhesive seal wet.

G. Use toilet paper to clean around opening of pouch and clamp pouch shut.

IV. The client/caregiver can demonstrate procedure of changing the pouching system.

A. Change pouch every 5 to 7 days or as needed.

B. Assemble all of the equipment.

C. Hold skin taut, and peel off the pouch being worn.

D. Wash the skin thoroughly with soap and water, rinse, and pat dry.

E. Inspect the stoma for any change in size or color.

F. Inspect the skin for signs of irritation and apply skin barrier.

G. Apply pouch over the stoma, being sure that it is the appropriate size and fits closely around the stoma.

V. The client/caretaker can list dietary measures for management of ileostomy.

A. Chew food slowly and completely for better digestion.

B. Drink at least six to eight glasses of fluids per day.

C. Avoid foods that may cause blockage such as celery, corn, lettuce, popcorn, nuts, coleslaw, and seeds.

D. Decrease fiber in diet if stools are excessively loose.

E. Limit or avoid foods such as eggs, fish, onions, and cabbage, which can increase odor.

F. Eat foods such as spinach, parsley, yogurt, or buttermilk, which can decrease odor.

VI. The client/caregiver can list general measures for management of an ileostomy.

A. Avoid laxatives, enteric-coated pills, and timed-release pills.

B. Avoid stress and smoking.

C. Assess for skin irritation caused by enzymes in stools, and provide skin care.

D. Avoid contact sports and weight lifting.

E. Avoid tight, constrictive clothing.

F. Keep extra ileostomy supplies on hand.

G. Wear a Medic Alert bracelet.

H. Report to physician any signs of bleeding, persistent diarrhea, change in size or color of stoma, and continued skin irritation.

(Continued)

NRS DATE	INITIAL	
		VII. **The client/caregiver is aware of possible complications.**

VII. **The client/caregiver is aware of possible complications.**

A. Dehydration
B. Bowel obstruction
C. Electrolyte imbalance

RESOURCES

United Ostomy Associations of America, Inc.
www.uoaa.org

Wound, Ostomy, Continence Nurses
www.wocn.org

REFERENCES

Ackley, B. J., & Ladwig, G. B. (2006). *Nursing diagnosis handbook: A guide to planning care.* St. Louis: Mosby Inc.

Canobbio, M. M. (2006). *Mosby's handbook of patient teaching.* St. Louis: Mosby Inc.

Perry, A., & Potter, P. (2006). *Clinical nursing skills & technique.* St. Louis: Mosby Inc.

Timby, B. K., & Smith, N. C. (2003). *Introductory medical-surgical nursing* (8th ed.). Philadelphia: J. B. Lippincott Williams & Wilkins.

5 Hemodialysis

Patient name: _____

Admission: _____

I. **The client/caregiver can define hemodialysis.**

A. It is a process that mimics the functions of the kidney, removing wastes and other impurities and excessive fluid from the body.

B. The blood is removed from the body and put into a dialyzer to filter it and is then returned to the body.

C. The procedure usually lasts approximately 3 to 6 hours and is usually required three times per week.

II. **The client/caregiver can list various types of vascular access for hemodialysis.**

A. An external shunt may be placed in the wrist or forearm to connect an adjacent artery and vein.

B. An internal fistula may be placed in the wrist or forearm to connect an adjacent artery and vein.

C. An artificial graft is an additional segment added to client's own vessel to connect the artery and vein.

D. For temporary hemodialysis, a catheter may be inserted into the subclavian vein at shoulder or into the femoral vein at the groin.

III. **The client/caregiver can list measures to follow when receiving dialysis.**

A. Follow the diet as prescribed, usually low protein, low sodium, high carbohydrate, high fat, and low potassium.

B. Restrict fluid as prescribed.

C. Weigh as recommended.

D. Avoid infection.

E. Obtain adequate rest and exercise.

F. Take medications as prescribed.

G. Wear Medic Alert bracelet.

H. Keep follow-up appointments with physician and dialysis.

I. Report any light-headedness, dizziness, nausea and vomiting, sweating, headache, weakness, lethargy, muscle weakness or cramps, and irregular pulses.

IV. **The client/caregiver can adequately care for access blood route.**

A. Never allow anyone to take blood pressure, draw blood, or give injections on the arm being used for dialysis.

B. Avoid trauma to site.

C. Avoid constrictive clothing on affected arm.

D. Avoid heavy lifting.

E. Cleanse cannula as instructed and apply a dry, sterile dressing.

F. Palpate the site for a vibration (thrill), which indicates blood circulation or listen with a stethoscope for a rushing sound (bruit).

G. Report any swelling or pain over site or absence of thrill or bruit to physician.

H. Report any signs of infection (i.e., redness, tenderness, and warmth).

I. Report any signs of lack of circulation, i.e., numbness, tingling, or coolness in extremity.

J. Report any bleeding.

V. **The client/caregiver is aware of possible complications.**

A. Infection

B. High or low blood pressure

C. Heart arrhythmias

D. Hemorrhage and anemia

E. Air embolus

F. Restless leg syndrome

G. Hepatitis B

H. Muscle cramps

I. Hypovolemia and shock

J. Disequilibrium syndrome

(Continued)

RESOURCES

American Association of Kidney Patients
www.aakp.org

American Kidney Fund
www.kidneyfund.org

National Kidney Foundation
www.kidney.org

Dietitian

Support groups

Counseling

REFERENCES

Ackley, B. J., & Ladwig, G. B. (2006). *Nursing diagnosis handbook: A guide to planning care.* St. Louis: Mosby Inc.

Canobbio, M. M. (2006). *Mosby's handbook of patient teaching.* St. Louis: Mosby Inc.

Perry, A., & Potter, P. (2006). *Clinical nursing skills & technique.* St. Louis: Mosby Inc.

Timby, B. K., & Smith, N. C. (2003). *Introductory medical-surgical nursing* (8th ed.). Philadelphia: J. B. Lippincott Williams & Wilkins.

6

Peritoneal Dialysis

Patient name: _____   Admission: _____

I.   **The client/caregiver can define peritoneal dialysis.**

   A. It is a process that mimics the function of the kidney.
   B. A dialysis solution is put into the membrane of the abdomen to remove wastes and other impurities and excess fluid from the body.

II. **The client/caregiver can list various types of peritoneal dialysis.**

   A. Intermittent peritoneal dialysis
      1. The process is performed by a machine, usually in the hospital at night while sleeping.
      2. It is done three to five times a week in 8- to 10-hour sessions.
      3. The abdomen is empty between dialyses.
   B. Continuous ambulatory peritoneal dialysis
      1. A bag of dialysate solution is instilled into the abdomen, which takes about 10 minutes.
      2. This solution is left in place for 4 to 8 hours and then drained.
      3. This procedure is repeated four to five times daily.
   C. Continuous cycling peritoneal dialysis
      1. This procedure is done at night by connecting a tubing from a machine to the abdomen.
      2. The machine performs approximately three to seven exchanges during the night.
      3. The peritoneal fluid is left in the abdomen during the day.

III. **The client/caregiver can describe the basic procedure.**

   A. Peritoneal dialysis is done by inserting a catheter through the abdominal wall.
   B. The dialysis solution is allowed to flow into the abdomen between the abdominal

wall and the visceral wall, which covers the abdominal organs.
   C. The solution is allowed to stay in the abdomen for a set amount of time.
   D. The peritoneum acts as a membrane, allowing diffusion and osmosis to occur to remove toxic wastes and excess fluid from the body.
      1. Diffusion is the movement of a solution of higher concentration to a solution of lower concentration.
      2. Osmosis is the passage of fluid through a membrane from a solution of lower concentration to a solution of higher concentration.
   E. The fluid is then drained from the abdomen.

IV. **The client/caregiver can list precautions to follow when doing the procedure.**

   A. Wash your hands every time you need to handle your catheter.
   B. Store supplies in a cool, clean, dry place.
   C. Warm the fluid before beginning procedure.
   D. Maintain sterile technique when opening and closing catheter connections.
   E. Notify physician if pain occurs.
   F. Inspect each bag of solution for signs of contamination before use.

V.   **The client/caregiver can list measures to follow between dialysis treatments.**

   A. Follow the diet as instructed by physician, usually low in protein, sodium, and potassium.
   B. Restrict fluids as instructed.
   C. Obtain adequate rest and exercise.
   D. Take temperature for early detection of infection.
   E. Weigh daily at the same time each day.
   F. Wear a Medic Alert bracelet.

(Continued)

NRS
DATE INITIAL

G. Keep follow-up appointment with physician.

H. Avoid using over-the-counter medication without approval from physician.

I. Report any increased abdominal girth, distention, pain, absence of bowel movements, and fever.

VI. **The client/caregiver can list measures for care of exit site of the dialysis catheter.**

A. Assess for signs and symptoms of infection.

B. Apply antiseptic and dry sterile dressing as instructed.

C. Keep sterile cap in place.

D. Report any signs of infection at site (i.e., redness, swelling, tenderness, and drainage).

VII. **The client/caregiver is aware of possible complications of peritoneal dialysis.**

A. Infection, the most common problem (peritonitis)

B. Dehydration

C. Hernias

D. Constipation

E. Respiratory difficulty

F. Catheter-related complications

G. Dialysis complications

VIII. **The client/caregiver can list specific symptoms of infection, which need to be reported promptly.**

A. Signs and symptoms of infection to report are
  • Fever
  • Nausea or vomiting

NRS
DATE INITIAL

• Redness or pain around the catheter
• Unusual color or cloudiness in used dialysis solution
• A catheter cuff that has been pushed out

RESOURCES

American Association of Kidney Patients
www.aakp.org

American Kidney Fund
www.kidneyfund.org

National Kidney Foundation
www.kidney.org

Dietitian

Support groups

Counseling

REFERENCES
Ackley, B. J., & Ladwig, G. B. (2006). *Nursing diagnosis handbook: A guide to planning care.* St. Louis: Mosby Inc.

Canobbio, M. M. (2006). *Mosby's handbook of patient teaching.* St. Louis: Mosby Inc.

Perry, A., & Potter, P. (2006). *Clinical nursing skills & technique.* St. Louis: Mosby Inc.

Timby, B. K., & Smith, N. C. (2003). *Introductory medical-surgical nursing* (8th ed.). Philadelphia: J. B. Lippincott Williams & Wilkins.

7   Nasogastric

Patient name: _____   **Admission:** _____

NRS
DATE INITIAL

I. **The client/caregiver can define nasogastric tube feedings.**

A. When swallowing is severely impaired, a nasogastric tube may be inserted.

B. The nasogastric tube is inserted through the nose and it reaches to the stomach. This will bypass the mouth, throat, and esophagus.

C. The client can receive complete nutrition without eating/swallowing.

D. It can be given continuously or intermittently.

E. The nasogastric tube is commonly used when the swallowing/eating problem is expected to last less than a month.

II. **The client/caregiver can demonstrate the nasogastric tube feeding procedure.**

A. Gather all equipment.

B. Wash hands.

C. Put client in an upright position.

D. Aspirate stomach contents to check for residual and then return aspirated contents to stomach. (Hold feeding if residual is greater than 50 to 100 ml and notify physician.)

E. Check position of tube.
   1. Using a syringe, inject 10 ml of air into the tube, and listen with a stethoscope over the stomach to hear a whoosh of air.

F. Pour room-temperature feeding solution into bag and prime tubing by filling with formula to prevent air from going into stomach.

G. Connect to preprogrammed pump and attach to the nasogastric tube. Set the pump for amount required and rate for flow.

H. If pump is unavailable, attach the feeding bag tube to the nasogastric tube and open clamp to allow solution to flow.

NRS
DATE INITIAL

I. Use drip rate as ordered by physician if ordered continuously.

J. Allow approximately 20 to 30 minutes for each feeding if feedings are intermittent. Avoid rapid infusion to avoid nausea and vomiting.

K. Assess tolerance of feeding. Stop feedings and report to physician for symptoms such as
   • Coughing
   • Choking
   • Gagging
   • Vomiting

L. Follow feeding by flushing with 50 to 150 cc of water.

M. Keep client in an upright position for at least 15 to 30 minutes after the feeding.

III. **The client/caregiver can list measures to prevent complications.**

A. Wash hands well, and keep working area very clean to prevent infection.

B. Weigh regularly to prevent weight loss.

C. Keep head of bed elevated at least 30 degrees.

D. Refrigerate opened cans of feeding solutions, and discard after 24 hours to prevent spoilage.

E. Formula must not hang for more than 8 hours.

F. Check position of tube before each feeding or administration of medications.

G. Flush tube as ordered to prevent clogging.

H. Monitor blood sugar if diabetic, and report to physician.

I. Cleanse nose and apply a water-based jelly to prevent skin breakdown.

J. Provide mouth care.

K. Check that the tube is secure to face, and avoid tension on the tube during feedings.

L. Wear Medic Alert bracelet to inform others of medical information.

(Continued)

NRS
DATE INITIAL

M. Report any intolerance of feeding solution to physician (i.e., nausea, vomiting, cramping, diarrhea, and abdominal distention).

N. Keep follow-up appointments with physician and laboratory.

IV.   **The client/caregiver can list possible complications.**

A. Infection
B. Aspiration pneumonia
C. Clogging of the tubing
D. Respiratory distress
E. Diarrhea, nausea, or vomiting
F. Inadequate nutrition

RESOURCES

Medical supply companies

Dietician

REFERENCES

Ackley, B. J., & Ladwig, G. B. (2006). *Nursing diagnosis handbook: A guide to planning care.* St. Louis: Mosby Inc.

Canobbio, M. M. (2006). *Mosby's handbook of patient teaching.* St. Louis: Mosby Inc.

Lutz, C., & Przytulski, K. (2001). *Nutrition and diet therapy.* Philadelphia: F. A. Davis Company.

Perry, A., & Potter, P. (2006). *Clinical nursing skills & technique.* St. Louis: Mosby Inc.

Timby, B. K., & Smith, N. C. (2003). *Introductory medical-surgical nursing* (8th ed.). Philadelphia: J. B. Lippincott Williams & Wilkins.

8 Gastrostomy

Patient name: _____

Admission: _____

I. **The client/caregiver can define a gastrostomy.**

A. It is a catheter inserted surgically through the abdomen into the stomach for the purpose of feeding the client.

B. It is used when a client is unable to swallow for a long period of time and in order to provide complete nutrition.

C. They are larger in diameter than most nasogastric tubes. This could result in less chance of the tube becoming blocked.

D. The feeding can be given continuously or intermittently.

II. **The client/caregiver can demonstrate a gastrostomy feeding procedure.**

A. Gather all equipment.

B. Wash hands well.

C. Put client in an upright position.

D. Aspirate stomach contents to check residual and then return aspirated contents to stomach. (Hold feeding if residual is greater than 50 to 100 ml and notify physician.)

E. Check feeding solution for expiration date.

F. Warm feeding solution to room temperature.

G. Remove clamp and attach bulb syringe to end of gastrostomy tube.

H. If giving bolus feeding

1. Pour room temperature feeding solution into syringe and adjust height of syringe to increase or decrease rate of flow, allowing approximately 20 to 30 minutes to infuse.

I. If using pump or continuous feeding

1. Pour room-temperature feeding solution into bag and prime tubing by filling with formula to prevent air from going into stomach.

2. Connect to pump and attach to gastrostomy tube.

3. Set the pump for quantity to be infused and at what rate.

J. Flush tube after feeding with approximately 30 ml of water or as ordered.

K. Clamp tube securely.

L. Client should remain in an upright position at least 15 to 30 minutes after a meal.

III. **The client/caregiver can list measures for skin care around tube.**

A. Keep skin around tubing clean and dry.

B. Apply dressing or ointments as ordered.

C. Report any signs of wound infection (i.e., fever, redness, drainage, odor, and tenderness).

IV. **The client/caregiver can list measures to prevent complication.**

A. Wash hands well and keep work area very clean to prevent infection.

B. Weigh regularly to detect any weight loss.

C. Keep head of bed elevated at least 30 degrees to prevent aspiration.

D. Refrigerate opened cans of feeding solution and discard after 24 hours to prevent spoilage.

E. Hang only the amount of feeding that will infuse in 4 hours to prevent spoilage and accidental excess infusion.

F. Use a delivery pump for a continuous feeding to assure a correct rate of flow.

G. Infuse slowly at rate ordered by physician to decrease nausea.

H. Flush tube as ordered to prevent clogging.

I. Have client sit in an upright position after eating to prevent aspiration.

J. Assess and monitor blood sugar if diabetic, and report to physician.

K. Wear Medic Alert bracelet to inform others of medical information.

L. Report to physician any intolerance to feedings (i.e., nausea, vomiting, cramping, diarrhea, and abdominal distention).

M. Keep follow-up appointments with physician and laboratory.

(Continued)

NRS	
DATE	INITIAL

V. **The client/caregiver can list possible complications.**

   A. Tube obstruction
   B. Aspiration pneumonia
   C. Diarrhea, nausea, or vomiting
   E. Local skin infection
   F. Inadvertent removal of the tube

RESOURCES

Medical equipment companies

Counseling

REFERENCES

Ackley, B. J., & Ladwig, G. B. (2006). *Nursing diagnosis handbook: A guide to planning care.* St. Louis: Mosby Inc.

Canobbio, M. M. (2006). *Mosby's handbook of patient teaching.* St. Louis: Mosby Inc.

Lutz, C., & Przytulski, K. (2001). *Nutrition and diet therapy.* Philadelphia: F. A. Davis Company.

Perry, A., & Potter, P. (2006). *Clinical nursing skills & technique.* St. Louis: Mosby Inc.

Timby, B. K., & Smith, N. C. (2003). *Introductory medical-surgical nursing* (8th ed.). Philadelphia: J. B. Lippincott Williams & Wilkins.

9 Foley Catheter Care

Patient name: _____ **Admission:** _____

NRS
DATE INITIAL

NRS
DATE INITIAL

I. **The client/caregiver can define Foley catheter.**

   A. It is a catheter inserted through the urethra into the bladder to drain the urine.
   B. It is usually inserted because of
      • Incontinence (inability to hold urine)
      • A neurogenic bladder
      • Bladder or prostate surgery
      • Obstruction causing an inability to release urine
   C. An indwelling Foley catheter is held in place (in the bladder) by a small balloon filled with water.

II. **The client/caregiver can perform catheter care procedure.**

   A. Wash hands well before and after touching the catheter.
   B. Use mild soap and water to wash the area around the catheter and perineal area.
   C. Wash the catheter by cleaning gently from the meatus outward
   D. For males, retract foreskin 0.5 to 1 inch to cleanse, being sure to replace it when finished.
   E. Do not use powders or lotions after cleaning.
   F. Procedure should be done at least daily and after each bowel movement.
   G. Indwelling catheters should be changed only as necessary. Changing the catheter more frequently only increases chance of infection developing.

III. **The client/caregiver can perform care of catheter bags and catheter tubing.**

   A. Maintain good drainage by checking frequently for kinks or loops in the tubing.
   B. Secure catheter tubing to leg to prevent pulling or tension on catheter.
   C. Change anchoring sites by alternating sites daily. Use the inner thighs for women and the upper thighs for men.

   D. Keep drainage bag below level of the bladder at all times to prevent infection.
   E. Empty bag at least every 8 hours or when drainage bag is just over half full.
   F. If catheter and tubing are disconnected, wipe the end of both with antiseptic solution before reconnecting them.
   G. Drainage bags may be reused after careful cleansing.
      1. Rinse inside of bag with soapy water and then rinse with clear water.
      2. Fill the bag with one part vinegar to four parts water and soak for 30 minutes.
      3. Empty the bag, and let it air dry.
      4. Store in clean, dust-free place.

IV. **The client/caregiver can demonstrate how to empty a drainage bag.**

   A. Free the drain tip from holder on drainage bag. Loosen the clamp and drain urine.
   B. Let the urine drain into the toilet or measuring container while being careful not to let the tip touch anything.
   C. Reclamp the tube and clean tip before replacing in holder.

V. **The client/caregiver can demonstrate how and when to use a leg drainage bag.**

   A. Leg collection bags are usually used during the day.
   B. They usually only hold about 500 ml of urine.
   C. The leg bag is attached to the leg with straps. Use cloth or Velcro straps to avoid possible irritation from rubber straps.
   D. A drainage valve or cap is secured at the bottom opening of the bag.
   E. Use the same precautions when changing or draining the leg bag as when using the large drainage bag.

(Continued)

VI. **The client/caregiver can discuss general measures to prevent problems while using a urinary catheter.**

A. Monitor and record urine output for amount and color of urine.

B. Stress increased intake of clear fluids (10 to 15 glasses per day). Unless prohibited by physician, try drinking cranberry, plum, and prune juices along with water, as they help increase the acidity and prevent infection.

C. Keep intake of caffeine and alcohol to limited amount.

D. Showering and bathing may be done as ordered by physician.

E. Review signs, symptoms, or problems to report promptly, such as
- A lack of urine output longer than 4 hours
- Persistent leakage around catheter
- Pain, swelling, or tenderness around catheter
- A break in the catheter or if the catheter falls out
- Fever or chills

F. A latex-free catheter may be needed if client has latex allergy.

VII. **The client/caregiver is aware of possible complications.**

A. Urinary-tract infection: cloudy urine, foul odor, fever, and pain in bladder area.

B. Blocked catheter: lack of urine draining into catheter and firm, distended abdomen.

RESOURCES

Medical supply companies

Visiting nurse

REFERENCES

Ackley, B. J., & Ladwig, G. B. (2006). *Nursing diagnosis handbook: A guide to planning care.* St. Louis: Mosby Inc.

Canobbio, M. M. (2006). *Mosby's handbook of patient teaching.* St. Louis: Mosby Inc.

Taylor, C., Lillis, C., & LeMone, P. (2005). *Fundamentals of nursing.* Philadelphia: Lippincott, Williams & Wilkins.

Timby, B. K., & Smith, N. C. (2003). *Introductory medical-surgical nursing* (8th ed.). Philadelphia: J. B. Lippincott Williams & Wilkins.

10   Suprapubic Catheter Care

Patient name: _____   Admission: _____

NRS
DATE INITIAL

I. **The client/caregiver can define a suprapu-bic catheter.**

A. It is a tubing surgically inserted into the bladder directly through the lower abdomen.

B. It is performed to divert the flow of urine from the urethra.

II. **The client/caregiver can demonstrate care of insertion site or stoma.**

A. With new stoma site, cleanse with Betadine solution, and apply sterile drain dressing (slit in one side of dressing) as ordered.

B. Any crusting or exudates around stoma may be cleaned with cotton-tip applicator and hydrogen peroxide and carefully rinsed with water.

C. A healed stoma may be cleansed with mild soap and water daily.

D. A suprapubic catheter may be taped to the abdomen if necessary.

E. If the catheter accidentally drops out, cover with clean gauze, and secure with tape. Notify physician or nurse promptly.

III. **The client/caregiver can perform care of catheter bags and catheter tubing.**

A. Maintain good drainage by checking frequently for kinks or loops in the tubing.

B. Secure catheter tubing to leg to prevent pulling or tension on catheter.

C. Change anchoring sites by alternating sites daily. Use the inner thighs for women and the upper thighs for men.

D. Keep drainage bag below level of the bladder at all times to prevent infection.

E. Empty bag at least every 8 hours or when drainage bag is just over half full.

F. If catheter and tubing are disconnected, wipe the end of both with antiseptic solution before reconnecting them.

NRS
DATE INITIAL

G. Drainage bags may be reused after careful cleansing.

1. Rinse inside of bag with soapy water and then rinse with clear water.

2. Fill the bag with one part vinegar to four parts water, and soak for 30 minutes.

3. Empty bag, and let it air dry.

4. Store bag in clean, dust-free place.

IV. **The client/caregiver can demonstrate how to empty a drainage bag.**

A. Free the drain tip from holder on drainage bag. Loosen the clamp and drain urine.

B. Let the urine drain into the toilet or measuring container while being careful not to let the tip touch anything.

C. Reclamp the tube and clean tip before replacing in holder.

V. **The client/caregiver can demonstrate how and when to use a leg drainage bag.**

A. Leg collection bags are usually used during the day.

B. They usually only hold about 500 ml of urine.

C. The leg bag is attached to the leg with straps. Use cloth or Velcro straps to avoid possible irritation from rubber straps.

D. Keep a drainage valve or cap secured at the bottom opening of the bag.

E. Use the same precautions when changing or draining the leg bag as when using the large drainage bag.

VI. **The client/caregiver can discuss general measures to prevent problems while using a urinary catheter.**

A. Monitor and record urine output for amount and color of urine.

B. Stress increased intake of clear fluids (10 to 15 glasses per day). Unless prohibited by physician, try drinking cranberry, plum, and prune juices along with water, as they help increase the acidity and prevent infection.

(Continued)

NRS
DATE INITIAL

C. Keep intake of caffeine and alcohol to limited amount.

D. Showering and bathing may be done as ordered by physician.

E. Review signs, symptoms, or problems to report promptly, such as
  • Lack of urine output longer than 4 hours
  • Persistent leakage around catheter
  • Pain, swelling, or tenderness around catheter
  • Break in the catheter or if catheter falls out
  • Fever or chills

F. Latex-free catheter may be needed if client has latex allergy.

VII. The client/caregiver is aware of possible complications.

A. Urinary-tract infection: cloudy urine, foul odor, fever, or pain in bladder area.

NRS
DATE INITIAL

B. Blocked catheter: lack of urine draining into catheter and firm, distended abdomen.

RESOURCES

Medical supply companies

Visiting nurse

REFERENCES

Ackley, B. J., & Ladwig, G. B. (2006). *Nursing diagnosis handbook: A guide to planning care.* St. Louis: Mosby Inc.

Canobbio, M. M. (2006). *Mosby's handbook of patient teaching.* St. Louis: Mosby Inc.

Taylor, C., Lillis, C., & LeMone, P. (2005). *Fundamentals of nursing.* Philadelphia: Lippincott, Williams & Wilkins.

Timby, B. K., & Smith, N. C. (2003). *Introductory medical-surgical nursing* (8th ed.). Philadelphia: J. B. Lippincott Williams & Wilkins.

11 Oxygen Therapy

Patient name: _____ Admission: _____

NRS
DATE INITIAL

I. **The client/caregiver can define oxygen therapy.**

A. Oxygen therapy is needed when a condition interferes with adequate oxygen supply to the tissues of the body. The delivery of oxygen to the tissues of the body helps ensure normal metabolism.

B. Sources of therapeutic oxygen can come from
1. A liquid oxygen container (stores oxygen at very cold temperatures)
2. Oxygen tank (stores oxygen under pressure)
3. Portable tanks that are available with liquid and gas oxygen
4. A portable air oxygen concentrator (removes components of the air and stores and concentrates remaining oxygen)

C. Oxygen can be delivered via
• Nasal cannula
• Simple mask
• Specialty masks such as partial rebreather mask, nonrebreather mask, or venturi mask
• Nasal catheter
• Transtracheal catheter

II. **The client/caregiver can recognize signs and symptoms of lack of oxygen.**

A. Restlessness or anxiety
B. Tiredness, drowsiness, and trouble waking up
C. Persistent headache
D. Slurred speech
E. Confusion and difficulty in concentrating
F. Bluish fingernails or lips

III. **The client/caregiver can list measures for skin care.**

A. Nostrils, earlobes, and bridge of nose may be padded with commercially made foam pieces or gauze to prevent skin breakdown.

NRS
DATE INITIAL

B. Teach client how to remove and reposition oxygen equipment to aid in bathing, eating, etc.
C. If nostrils become irritated, apply a soluble gel like K-Y gel—never a petroleum-based lubricant because of fire safety.

IV. **The client/caregiver can list safety tips necessary for oxygen therapy.**

A. No smoking or open flames within 10 feet of oxygen source. Place "No Smoking" signs to warn visitors.
B. Keep oxygen away from open flames, heat, gas stoves, hot pipes, radiators, kerosene heater, and so forth. Check all electrical equipment used in the same room for faulty or frayed cords.
C. Equip the home with an all-purpose fire extinguisher and smoke alarm.
D. Keep oxygen at least 5 feet away from electric outlets and electrical equipment, and avoid use of electric blankets and heating pads close to oxygen.
E. Avoid the use of flammable products such as body lotion, face creams, and rubbing alcohol.
F. Avoid the use of aerosol sprays.
G. Keep oxygen in an upright position, and secure tank in holder.
H. Report to physician any signs of persistent headache, slurred speech, confusion, drowsiness, increased shortness of breath, vomiting, and so forth.
I. Keep car windows partly open while using oxygen.
J. Keep emergency numbers next to phone. Notify local fire department and utility companies of the use of oxygen.
K. If using a concentrator, have a back-up oxygen tank in case of power failure. Allow adequate air flow around oxygen concentrator—avoid placing directly against the wall.

(Continued)

<table>
<tr><td>NRS
DATE INITIAL</td></tr>
</table>

V. **The client/caregiver can list general care measures to provide oxygen therapy.**

A. Stress the need to follow the prescribed oxygen flow rate.

B. Encourage fluids up to 2500 ml per day unless contraindicated.

C. If using humidification with oxygen therapy, use distilled or sterile water. Do not allow the water to enter the oxygen flow tubing.

D. To check whether oxygen is flowing through tube, place the cannula in water and check for bubbling. Always shake off water before placing in nose.

E. Reorder oxygen 2 to 3 days before needing a new tank.

F. Use portable tanks when going out of home to increase mobility.

G. Never adjust oxygen rate without permission from physician.

H. Administer oxygen exactly as prescribed by a physician.

I. Keep follow-up appointments with physician.

RESOURCES
American Lung Association

Respiratory therapist

Medical supply company

REFERENCES
Ackley, B. J., & Ladwig, G. B. (2006). *Nursing diagnosis handbook: A guide to planning care.* St. Louis: Mosby Inc.

Canobbio, M. M. (2006). *Mosby's handbook of patient teaching.* St. Louis: Mosby Inc.

Cohen, B. J., & Taylor, J. J. (2005). *Memmler's the human body in health and disease* (10th ed.). Philadelphia: Lippincott Williams & Wilkins.

Taylor, C., Lillis, C., & LeMone, P. (2005). *Fundamentals of nursing.* Philadelphia: Lippincott, Williams & Wilkins.

Timby, B. K., & Smith, N. C. (2003). *Introductory medical-surgical nursing* (8th ed.). Philadelphia: J. B. Lippincott Williams & Wilkins.

12   Oral and Nasal Suctioning

Patient name: _____   **Admission:** _____

<table>
<tr><td>NRS
DATE INITIAL</td><td></td><td>NRS
DATE INITIAL</td><td></td></tr>
</table>

I.   The client/caregiver can state the purpose of oral or nasal suctioning.

  A. To mechanically remove secretions from client's airway via the nose (nasopharynx), mouth (oropharynx), or trachea

  B. To maintain an open and patent airway

II.   The caregiver can discuss/demonstrate how to prepare for suctioning.

  A. Show proper hand washing before and after suctioning.

  B. Explain purpose of the procedure, and include the method to be used.

  C. Gather equipment, including suctioning machine, suction catheters, sterile saline solution, and disposable gloves.

  D. Review signs and symptoms that indicate need for suctioning, such as
- Congested-sounding cough
- Coarse wheezing that can be heard by client or caregiver
- Visible secretions

  E. Discuss that suctioning can be repeated as needed, but it is important to try deep breaths and to allow 20 to 30 seconds between suctioning attempts.

III.   The client/caregiver can demonstrate how to suction.

  A. Position client.
1. The client should be in semi-Fowler's position.
2. The unconscious client should be placed in the lateral position facing you.

  B. Turn on suction machine and adjust to appropriate pressure level.

  C. Open the suction catheter kit, and pour saline touching only outside surface.

  D. Put on sterile gloves. The dominant hand that handles the catheter must remain sterile.

  E. Attach catheter to suction tubing and moisten catheter with saline.

  F. Place finger over Y tube to check suction.

  G. Gently insert catheter with the suction off.

  H. Place catheter along the base of nostril to trachea for nasopharynx suctioning.

  I. Insert catheter along side of the mouth towards trachea for oropharynx suctioning.

  J. Do not suction until catheter is fully inserted.

  K. Apply suction and gently rotate catheter as it is withdrawn limiting suctioning to 10 to 15 seconds.

  L. Flush tubing with sterile water after suctioning.

  M. Apply oxygen or instruct client to take deep slow breaths after suctioning.

  N. Note the characteristics of sputum and client's response to suctioning.

  O. Use each catheter only once.

  P. Offer oral care and clean suction equipment.

IV.   The client/caregiver can state measures to care for equipment.

  A. Keep adequate supplies on hand.

  B. Empty collection bottle after each suctioning.

V.   The client/caregiver can list general care measures.

  A. Signs and symptoms that should be reported to physician or nurse are
- Restlessness, anxiety, confusion, or difficulty concentrating
- Bluish fingernails or lips
- Palpitations
- Fever
- Changes in color, consistency, amount, and odor of secretions

  B. Keep follow-up appointments with physician.

  C. Take medications as ordered.

(Continued)

RESOURCES

Home health agency

Medical supply company

Respiratory therapist

REFERENCES

Ackley, B. J., & Ladwig, G. B. (2006). *Nursing diagnosis handbook: A guide to planning care.* St. Louis: Mosby Inc.

Canobbio, M. M. (2006). *Mosby's handbook of patient teaching.* St. Louis: Mosby Inc.

Taylor, C., Lillis, C., & LeMone, P. (2005). *Fundamentals of nursing.* Philadelphia: Lippincott, Williams & Wilkins.

Timby, B. K., & Smith, N. C. (2003). *Introductory medical-surgical nursing* (8th ed.). Philadelphia: J. B. Lippincott Williams & Wilkins.

13 Tracheostomy Care

Patient name: _____ **Admission:** _____

I. The client/caregiver can define a tracheostomy.

  A. It is insertion of a tube into the trachea by making a surgical incision.

  B. The opening is called a "stoma."

  C. It can be permanent or temporary.

II. The client/caregiver can list indications for the use of a tracheostomy tube.

  A. Tumor occluding the airway

  B. Upper airway obstruction from a foreign body, edema, or mucus

  C. Radial neck resection surgery or laryngectomy

  D. Inability to maintain patent airway

  E. To provide a method of mechanical ventilation

III. The client/caregiver can describe a tracheostomy tube.

  A. The tracheostomy tube can be semiflexible plastic, rigid plastic, or metal.

  B. The tracheostomy tube consists of
    1. Outer cannula
    2. Inner cannula
    3. Obturator (used for initial placement and then removed)

  C. The tube may be cuffed or uncuffed.

  D. The tube is held in place by Velcro strips fastened around the neck. Usually sterile gauze pads (drain or precut by manufacture) are placed between skin and edges of tracheostomy cuff. Avoid cutting a gauze pad because fragments of gauze may enter the stoma.

IV. The client/caregiver can demonstrate cleaning the inner cannula.

  A. Wash hands. Put on clean gloves and remove soiled gauze dressing. Discard dressing inside of removed gloves.

  B. Wash hands and open tracheostomy cleaning kit without contamination.

  C. Put on sterile gloves.

  D. Add sterile normal saline in one side of the sterile kit basin and equal parts hydrogen peroxide and saline in the other side.

  E. If kit does not include sterile saline and peroxide, have assistant pour correct solutions.

  F. Unlock inner cannula and turn counterclockwise. Remove and place in peroxide and saline solution to soak.

  G. Clean inside and outside the outer cannula with brush or pipe cleaner.

  H. Rinse cleaned cannula in normal saline, and remove excess liquid by tapping against the basin.

  I. Replace the inner cannula and turn clockwise until it clicks into place and dots on both cannula match.

  J. Cleanse around stoma with Q-tips dipped into hydrogen peroxide.

  K. Then rinse with normal saline soaked Q-tip.

  L. Replace drain (precut) gauze under the sides of the outer cannula.

  M. Check ties for fit and to evaluate whether it needs to be changed due to soiling.

  N. After cleanup, place pressure call bell, tap bell, or whatever method is used for client to signal for assistance.

V. The client/caregiver can demonstrate changing tracheostomy ties.

  A. Always have two people for this procedure so that one person can hold the tube firmly in place while the other person changes the ties.

  B. Use the Velcro strips provided in tracheostomy care kit.

  C. Allow enough space for little finger to fit between strip and the client's skin.

VI. The client/caregiver is aware of need for skin care.

  A. Assess for signs and symptoms of infection (i.e., fever, redness, and irritation).

(Continued)

NRS
DATE INITIAL

B. Cleanse skin frequently, and place a dry gauze around stoma.

VII. **The client/caregiver can state procedure to follow if trach tube accidentally falls out.**

A. Remove the inner cannula from the dislodged tube.
B. Insert the obturator into the outer cannula, and reinsert the tube.
C. Remove the obturator and insert the inner cannula.

VIII. **The client/caregiver can list general precautions.**

A. Do not allow smoking in the same room.
B. Avoid aerosol sprays and dust that may enter trach.
C. Provide adequate humidification.
D. Keep a suction machine at the bedside at all times.
E. Perform suctioning as needed, but avoid oversuctioning because it may increase secretions.
F. Tape obturator to head of bed, and keep an extra tracheostomy set and hemostat at the bedside.
G. Prevent infection with good oral hygiene; avoid persons with respiratory infections. Use good hand-washing procedures.
H. Avoid getting any water into the stoma.
I. Use other communication techniques if speaking is impaired (call bell, sign language, pictures, etc.).

NRS
DATE INITIAL

J. Cover the stoma loosely if going out into very cold weather.
K. Drink at least 3000 ml of water per day unless contraindicated.
L. Avoid smoking.
M. Wear Medic Alert bracelet.
N. Keep follow-up appointments with physician.

RESOURCES

American Head and Neck Society
www.headandneckcancer.org/patienteducation/docs/ tracheostomy.php

Speech therapist

Support groups

Medical supply company

REFERENCES

Ackley, B. J., & Ladwig, G. B. (2006). *Nursing diagnosis handbook: A guide to planning care.* St. Louis: Mosby Inc.
Canobbio, M. M. (2006). *Mosby's handbook of patient teaching.* St. Louis: Mosby Inc.
Taylor, C., Lillis, C., & LeMone, P. (2005). *Fundamentals of nursing.* Philadelphia: Lippincott, Williams & Wilkins.
Timby, B. K., & Smith, N. C. (2003). *Introductory medical-surgical nursing* (8th ed.). Philadelphia: J. B. Lippincott Williams & Wilkins.

14 Central Venous Access Device

Patient name: _____ Admission: _____

NRS
DATE INITIAL

NRS
DATE INITIAL

I. **The client/caregiver can describe a tunneled central venous catheter.**

A. These devices can be used to administer
1. Various IV fluids
2. Medications
3. Blood products
4. Nutritional solutions
B. They can also provide means for hemodynamic monitoring and taking blood samples.
C. They are usually introduced into the subclavian or internal jugular vein and ending in the superior vena cava.
D. All central venous access devices (CVADs) require radiographic confirmation of position before therapy is begun.
E. Types of CVADs include the following:
1. Peripherally inserted central catheters (PICCs). Check additional information.
2. Nontunneled percutaneous central venous catheters
3. Tunneled central venous catheters. Check additional information.
4. Implanted ports. Check additional information.

II. **The client/caregiver can list advantages of this type of catheter.**

A. Allows monitoring of central venous pressure.
B. Permits aspiration of blood samples.
C. It allows administration of large amounts of IV fluids in case of an emergency.
D. It reduces the number of venipunctures needed to maintain access.
E. It can handle the volume of fluids when the solutions need to be diluted as in chemotherapy or total parenteral nutrition solutions.

III. **The client/caregiver can list possible risks or complications of using CVADs.**

A. Pneumothorax
B. Sepsis

C. Thrombus (clot) formation
D. Vessel and/or adjacent organ perforation

IV. **The client/caregiver can demonstrate proper procedure for dressing change.**

A. Wash hands thoroughly before procedure. Use mask for self and client per policy. If client is not using mask, have him or her turn head away from site.
B. Put on clean gloves. Carefully remove old dressing and dispose into disposal bag. Leave in place the tape that anchors catheter in place. Remove gloves and wash hands again.
C. Open package, and create sterile field.
D. Put on sterile gloves.
E. Carefully remove tape and support catheter with one hand while cleaning.
F. Cleanse area with an alcohol swab by beginning at the exit site and cleansing in a circular motion going out away from the catheter approximately 2 inches, never returning to the exit site with the same applicator. Allow skin to dry.
G. Use povidone-iodine solution to cleanse using same technique. Allow skin to dry.
H. Make a loop in the tubing and secure to prevent tension or tugging at insertion site. Apply an occlusive dressing as instructed. Make note of dressing date and time of change.
I. Dispose of soiled dressings, remove gloves, and wash hands.

V. **The client/caregiver can demonstrate the procedure of catheter cap change.**

A. Assemble equipment.
B. Wash hands.
C. Open package, keeping it sterile. Put on clean gloves.
D. Clamp catheter.
E. Stabilize hub, and remove old cap.
F. Cleanse the connection area of cap and catheter with alcohol.

(Continued)

NRS
DATE INITIAL

G. Screw on the new cap.

H. Change catheter caps one to two times per week or as ordered by physician.

VI. **The client/caregiver can list general measures for catheter.**

A. Sharps and any equipment contaminated by blood are disposed of in puncture-resistant containers with lids.

B. Stress the importance of good hand hygiene and aseptic technique.

C. Keep catheter clamped as ordered.

D. Daily inspect skin for any signs of infection such as redness, drainage, swelling, or tenderness, and report to nurse.

E. Use transparent or sterile gauze dressing to cover catheter site.

F. Clean injection ports with approved antiseptic agents before accessing system.

NRS
DATE INITIAL

G. Keep emergency numbers next to telephone.

H. Wear Medic Alert identification.

REFERENCES

Canobbio, M. M. (2006). *Mosby's handbook of patient teaching.* St. Louis: Mosby Inc.

Centers for Disease Control and Prevention. *Guidelines for the prevention of catheter-related infections.* MMWR 51(No. RR-10):1-26-2002.

Perry, A., & Potter, P. (2006). *Clinical nursing skills & technique.* St. Louis: Mosby Inc.

Portable RN: The all-in-one nursing reference. (2002). Springhouse: Lippincott, Williams & Wilkins.

Taylor, C., Lillis, C., & LeMone, P. (2005). *Fundamentals of nursing.* Philadelphia: Lippincott, Williams & Wilkins.

Timby, B. K. (2005). *Fundamental nursing skills and concepts.* Philadelphia: J. B. Lippincott Williams & Wilkins.

15   Implanted (Infusion) Port

Patient name: _____   Admission: _____

NRS
DATE   INITIAL

I. **The client/caregiver can define implanted port access device.**

   A. It is a self-sealing injection port in a plastic or metal case, placed in subcutaneous tissue below the collarbone.

   B. It has a metal base and a rubber top usually about 1 inch in diameter and a small, flexible catheter that goes to the bloodstream via the subclavian or jugular vein.

   C. No external parts are visible.

   D. The implanted port can be used for the same purpose as other CVADs.

II. **The client/caregiver can demonstrate flushing procedure, which is usually done monthly or after each use.**

   A. Wash hands well. Use masks for self and client per policy.

   B. Gather equipment (Huber needle, alcohol swabs, heparin, povidone-iodine swabs).

   C. Create sterile field.

   D. Assess site for redness, swelling, tenderness, drainage, or bleeding.

   E. Locate port by feeling bump on upper chest.

   F. Clean injection site with three antimicrobial swabs by moving in a horizontal pattern, secondly a vertical pattern and finally in circular pattern moving outward. Allow to dry.

   G. Apply sterile gloves.

   H. Attach end of sterile extension tubing to syringe and attach correct size Huber needle to the other end. Fill tubing with saline solution.

NRS
DATE   INITIAL

   I. Palpate port with nondominant hand.

   J. With dominant hand holding wings or hub, insert Huber needle through skin at a 90-degree angle.

   K. Check for signs of correct needle placement by aspiration of blood.

   L. If good blood return, flush tubing with saline. Observe for swelling.

   M. Stop infusion if unusual resistance is felt or swelling noted, and notify physician.

   N. If continuous infusion is not needed, flush with 3 ml of heparin solution.

III. **The client caregiver can list precautions necessary with a port.**

   A. Protect skin over port.

   B. Assess and report any signs of infection.
      1. Redness, pain, or swelling
      2. Drainage
      3. Fever
      4. Shortness of breath

REFERENCES

Canobbio, M. M. (2006). *Mosby's handbook of patient teaching.* St. Louis: Mosby Inc.

Centers for Disease Control and Prevention. *Guidelines for the prevention of catheter-related infections.* MMWR 51(No. RR-10):1-26-2002.

Perry, A., & Potter, P. (2006). *Clinical nursing skills & technique.* St. Louis: Mosby Inc.

Portable RN: The all-in-one nursing reference. (2002). Springhouse: Lippincott, Williams & Wilkins.

Taylor, C., Lillis, C., & LeMone, P. (2005). *Fundamentals of nursing.* Philadelphia: Lippincott, Williams & Wilkins.

Timby, B. K. (2005). *Fundamental nursing skills and concepts.* Philadelphia: J. B. Lippincott Williams & Wilkins.

16 Peripherally Inserted Central Line

■ Patient name: _____   Admission: _____

NRS
DATE INITIAL

I.   **The client/caregiver can describe a peripherally inserted central line.**

   A. A catheter is inserted into a vein at or above the antecubital space of the arm, and the tip extends into the distal superior vena cava.

   B. Insertion requires verification of placement by x-ray.

   C. A specially trained nurse or physician must do insertion and removal of PICC.

II. **The client/caregiver can list precautions for use of PICC line.**

   A. Do not take blood pressure on that arm.

   B. Avoid any trauma to that arm.

III. **The client/caregiver can demonstrate care of PICC.**

   A. Use a sterile technique when changing dressing. The use of a mask for client and person changing dressing is often required.

   B. Dressing should be changed 24 hours after insertion and at least weekly (check physician or agency policy for specific instructions).

   C. As needed, change dressing if loose or soiled.

   D. Keep the external part of the catheter coiled under the dressing.

   E. Injection caps should be changed every three to seven days or per policy/physician order.

NRS
DATE INITIAL

   F. Catheter should be flushed with heparin solution per policy or as ordered by physician.

IV. **The client/caregiver can list possible complications of PICC line and what to do.**

   A. Malposition of PICC lines may occur, as evidenced by increased length of external portion of catheter or difficulty with infusion.
      1. Notify nurse.

   B. Bleeding may occur 24 hours after insertion.
      1. Notify nurse.

   C. Phlebitis may occur between insertion site and top.
      1. Apply warm compresses.
      2. Notify nurse.

REFERENCES

Canobbio, M. M. (2006). *Mosby's handbook of patient teaching.* St. Louis: Mosby Inc.

Centers for Disease Control and Prevention. *Guidelines for the prevention of catheter-related infections.* MMWR 51(No. RR-10):1-26-2002.

Perry, A., & Potter, P. (2006). *Clinical nursing skills & technique.* St. Louis: Mosby Inc.

Portable RN: The all-in-one nursing reference. (2002). Springhouse: Lippincott, Williams & Wilkins.

Taylor, C., Lillis, C., & LeMone, P. (2005). *Fundamentals of nursing.* Philadelphia: Lippincott, Williams & Wilkins.

Timby, B. K. (2005). *Fundamental nursing skills and concepts.* Philadelphia: J. B. Lippincott Williams & Wilkins.

17 Total Parenteral Nutrition

Patient name: _____ Admission: _____

I. **The client/caregiver can define total parenteral nutrition or hyperalimentation.**

  A. It is a hypertonic solution consisting of dextrose, amino acids, lipids, and select electrolytes and minerals. It is given through a central line to provide all nutrients for the body.

  B. The solution is a sterile mixture that is prepared by a pharmacist.

  C. The client will need to be monitored by ongoing assessments and laboratory testing.

II. **The client/caregiver can list possible reasons for receiving total parental nutrition therapy.**

  A. Reduced intake of calories because of
    1. Inability to absorb or digest food (i.e., severe vomiting or diarrhea, obstruction, severe burns, trauma, and cancer)

  B. Prolonged alteration in gastrointestinal function because of
    1. Disease, requiring the bowel or other organs to rest (pancreatitis, severe inflammatory bowel disease, etc.)

  C. Weight loss of 10% or more of usual body weight

  D. Reduction in values for
    • Prealbumin
    • Serum albumin
    • Total lymphocyte count
    • Total iron-binding capacity

  E. Intolerance to food or enteral feedings

III. **The client/caregiver can demonstrate how to care for TPN solution.**

  A. Keep TPN solution in refrigerator.

  B. Take next bag of solution from the refrigerator 4 to 6 hours before using, and allow solution to reach room temperature before using.

  C. Keep supplies in a clean, dry place.

  D. Keep solution away from children.

  E. Check solution bag before use.
    1. Solution should be clear and free of floating material. If lipids are added, the solution may appear milky but free of floating material.
    2. Make sure that the bag has no leaks or damage.
    3. Make sure that the bag is labeled with contents and expiration date.

IV. **The client/caregiver can demonstrate the administration of the solution.**

  A. Clean work area. Wash hands. Assemble equipment.

  B. Read the label carefully to be sure that it is exactly what the physician prescribed.

  C. Inspect solution and warm solution to room temperature.

  D. Prepare solution and tubing as instructed.

  E. Set the pump to infuse solution at the rate ordered by physician.

  F. Flush the catheter as ordered when solution is finished.

V. **The client/caregiver can list general care measures to prevent complications.**

  A. Prevent infection by using strict technique as instructed.

  B. Inspect catheter insertion site daily for signs of redness, warmth, swelling, or drainage.

  C. Monitor for fluid overload by checking for any swelling in arms, legs, hands, and so forth.

  D. Weigh at the same time every day.

  E. Check urine for glucose and acetone as ordered.

  F. Provide good oral care frequently.

  G. Change dressing as ordered.

  H. Flush catheter as ordered.

  I. Take temperature as ordered.

(Continued)

J. Use your solution exactly as directed.

K. Have contact numbers for physician, pharmacist, nurse, and any other health care provider available to call if problems or questions occur.

L. It is important to keep all appointments with your doctor and the laboratory.

VI. **The client/caregiver can list signs and symptoms of complications when receiving TPN.**

A. Report these side effects if they are severe or do not go away:
- Mouth sores
- Poor night vision
- Skin changes

B. Call physician or health care provider if any of the following symptoms occur:
- Fever or chills
- Stomach pain
- Difficulty breathing
- Rapid weight gain or loss
- Increased urination
- Upset stomach or vomiting
- Confusion or memory loss
- Muscle weakness, twitching, or cramps
- Swelling of hands, feet, or legs
- Extreme thirst
- Fatigue

- Changes in heartbeat
- Tingling in the hands or feet
- Convulsion or seizures

C. Call if there is a catheter occlusion or partial occlusion: lack of flow or decreased flow of solution.

RESOURCES

Home health agency

Medical equipment company

REFERENCES

Ackley, B. J., & Ladwig, G. B. (2006). *Nursing diagnosis handbook: A guide to planning care*. St. Louis: Mosby Inc.

Canobbio, M. M. (2006). *Mosby's handbook of patient teaching*. St. Louis: Mosby Inc.

Lutz, C., & Przytulski, K. (2001). *Nutrition and diet therapy*. Philadelphia: F. A. Davis Company.

Perry, A., & Potter, P. (2006). *Clinical nursing skills & technique*. St. Louis: Mosby Inc.

Taylor, C., Lillis, C., & LeMone, P. (2005). *Fundamentals of nursing*. Philadelphia: Lippincott, Williams & Wilkins.

Timby, B. K., & Smith, N. C. (2003). *Introductory medical-surgical nursing* (8th ed.). Philadelphia: J. B. Lippincott Williams & Wilkins.

18 Cardiac Ambulatory Monitoring

Patient name: _____ Admission: _____

NRS
DATE INITIAL

NRS
DATE INITIAL

I. The client/caregiver can define an ambulatory electrocardiogram or a cardiac event recorder.

  A. It is a small, portable device that records electrical activity of the heart for up to 24 hours.
  B. It is a continuous recording of heart rate and rhythm during normal activity, rest, and sleep.

II. The client/caregiver can describe the advantages of this method of a cardiac monitor.

  A. It can be used for the client that might have major health risks that contraindicate a stress electrocardiogram.
  B. It can help associate abnormal rhythms to the client's complaint or symptoms.
  C. It also helps in evaluation of a client's progress in cardiac rehabilitation.

III. The client/caregiver can describe the procedure for a Holter monitor.

  A. Chest leads will be attached to body and then connected to monitor.
  B. The monitor is then attached to a belt or shoulder strap and will be worn for a specific amount of time.
  C. The client will be instructed to keep a log or diary, which will include
    1. Time and type of activity during testing
    2. Documentation if any medication was taken
    3. Documentation of any symptoms such as palpitations, chest pain, and dizziness.
  D. At the end of the test period, the monitor will be returned and the results plus diary entries will be evaluated.
  E. The client will return to physician for report and instructions.

IV. The client/caregiver will list measures to aid in accurate test results using the Holter monitor.

  A. Avoid shower, tub bath, or swimming during testing.
  B. A sponge bath is allowed, but avoid getting the device wet.
  C. Avoid magnets, metal detectors, electric blankets, or high-voltage areas.
  D. Avoid oily or greasy skin creams or lotions where the self-sticking electrodes will be applied.
  E. Keep appointments with physician for follow-up.
  F. Have list of telephone numbers to call, if having problems or questions with test.

V. The client/caregiver can explain how to use an event monitor or event recorder.

  A. This device is worn for a longer period of time.
  B. It can be removed during showers or bathing.
  C. The electrodes are attached the same way to the chest and monitor.
  D. This device has a button to depress when having symptoms that will start recording the activity. It usually can store three events.
  E. This information can be sent immediately via the phone. If the results indicate an emergency situation, you will be instructed to call 911 or go to the emergency room.

VI. The client/caregiver will list measures to aid accurate test results using an event monitor.

  A. Avoid magnets, metal detectors, electric blankets, or high-voltage areas.
  B. Avoid oily or greasy skin creams or lotions where the self-sticking electrodes will be applied.

(Continued)

C. Keep appointments with physician for follow-up.

D. Have a list of telephone numbers to call, if having problems or questions with test.

REFERENCES

Canobbio, M. M. (2006). *Mosby's handbook of patient teaching*. St. Louis: Mosby Inc.

Lutz, C., & Przytulski, K. (2001). *Nutrition and diet therapy*. Philadelphia: F. A. Davis Company.

Perry, A., & Potter, P. (2006). *Clinical nursing skills & technique*. St. Louis: Mosby Inc.

Taylor, C., Lillis, C., & LeMone, P. (2005). *Fundamentals of nursing*. Philadelphia: Lippincott, Williams & Wilkins.

Timby, B. K., & Smith, N. C. (2003). *Introductory medical-surgical nursing* (8th ed.). Philadelphia: J. B. Lippincott Williams & Wilkins.

1   Amputation (Lower-Extremity)

Patient name: _____   **Admission:** _____

NRS
DATE INITIAL

I.   The client/caregiver can list measures to promote comfort.

   A.   Pain medications as ordered
   B.   Compression dressing to stump as instructed
   C.   Massage therapy when allowed
   D.   Relaxation methods

II.   The client/caregiver can state measures for postoperative care of the residual limb.

   A.   Daily hygiene to prevent infection and skin breakdown. Cleanse residual limb daily with soap and water. Dry well, and expose to air for 20 minutes.
   B.   Inspect skin daily. If needed, use a hand-held mirror to check the site.
   C.   Signs of infection to report to physician or nurse are
      • Fever or chills
      • Increased discomfort of the extremity
      • Redness, swelling around incision
      • Drainage increase or foul odor of drainage from incision line
   D.   Avoid use of powder, creams, or lotion on incision site.
   E.   Apply compression dressing as instructed to prevent swelling and aid in molding the shape of the residual limb.
   F.   Review concept of phantom pain in the missing limb.

III.   The client/caregiver can state measures to manage use of prosthesis limb.

   A.   Explain the use of elastic sleeve or sock after molding is complete.
      • Change and wash daily.
      • Assure smooth fit and avoid wrinkles.
   B.   Wash the socket of the prosthesis with mild soap and water. Dry completely before use.
   C.   Follow complete instructions from prosthetist and have contact numbers in the event of problems.
   D.   Discontinue use of prosthesis if skin becomes irritated, and contact physician.
   E.   See a prosthetist if experiencing any problems with prosthesis.

NRS
DATE INITIAL

   F.   Monitor for signs of bleeding, irritation, pressure areas, or infection.

IV.   The client follows exercises and activity as prescribed.

   A.   Attends rehabilitation program for
      • Physical and occupational therapy
      • Conditioning
      • Residual limb exercises
      • Exercise to unaffected joints and extremities
   B.   Evaluate the need for assistive devices for bathing, toileting, or dressing.
   C.   Review safe transfer techniques and the use of mobility aids, such as cane, walker, crutches, and so forth.
   D.   Evaluate the home environment for safety.

V.   The client/caregiver can list possible complications of amputation.

   A.   Wound infection
   B.   Skin breakdown from prosthesis irritation
   C.   Phantom pain
   D.   Contracture of the limb
   E.   Abduction deformity

RESOURCES

National Amputation Foundation
212-767-0596
www.nationalamputation.org/

Physical and occupational therapy

Support groups

Clergy/counseling

Vocational counseling

REFERENCES

Ackley, B. J., & Ladwig, G. B. (2006). *Nursing diagnosis handbook: A guide to planning care.* St. Louis: Mosby Inc.

Canobbio, M. M. (2006). *Mosby's handbook of patient teaching.* St. Louis: Mosby Inc.

Perry, A., & Potter, P. (2006). *Clinical nursing skills & technique.* St. Louis: Mosby Inc.

Timby, B. K., & Smith, N. C. (2003). *Introductory medical-surgical nursing* (8th ed.). Philadelphia: J. B. Lippincott Williams & Wilkins.

2 Cataract Removal

Patient name: _____   **Admission:** _____

<table>
<tr><td>DATE</td><td>NRS
INITIAL</td></tr>
</table>

I. **The client/caregiver can define cataracts and cataract surgery.**

   A. A cataract is the clouding of the lens and lens capsule of the eye, which is usually clear.
   B. The cataract causes the pupil of the eye to appear gray or white instead of black.
   C. The development of cataracts is usually associated with aging.
   D. Other causes for cataract formation can be
   • Congenital disease
   • Trauma
   • Toxins
   • Intraocular inflammation
   • Chronic diseases such as diabetes

II. **The client/caregiver can describe the types of cataract surgery.**

   A. Intracapsular is the surgical removal of the entire lens and surrounding capsule. This is the most common type of cataract removal surgery.
   B. Extracapsular is the surgical removal of the anterior portion of the lens and capsule. The posterior capsule is left intact.
   C. Phaco emulsion is the use of ultrasonic vibrations to break lens into particles that can be removed by suction. This is the preferred method for clients younger than 30 years.
   D. Lens implantation is the insertion of an intraocular lens implant after cataract removal.

III. **The client/caregiver can recognize signs and symptoms of cataracts.**

   A. Painless, gradual blurred vision
   B. Poor reading vision
   C. Gray or white opacity over pupil
   D. Decreased peripheral vision
   E. Photophobia, glare (especially at night)

IV. **The client/caregiver can list postoperative instructions.**

   A. Wear eye patch over eye as ordered and eye shield at night when sleeping as ordered.

<table>
<tr><td>DATE</td><td>NRS
INITIAL</td></tr>
</table>

   B. Discuss the use of postoperative eye drops/medications as ordered.
   C. If wearing patch, warn that depth perception will be lost.
   D. Give pain medications as ordered.
   E. Discuss with physician any medication to be administered (as needed) for nausea.
   F. Avoid straining at stool.
   G. Avoid vomiting.
   H. Wear dark glasses if eyes are sensitive to bright sunlight.
   I. Report symptoms of possible complications (i.e., visual changes, pain, increased redness or drainage, or persistent headaches).
   J. Keep follow-up appointment with physician.

V. **The client/caregiver can adequately instill eye drops as prescribed.**

   A. Wash hands before and after installation.
   B. Instill drops onto inner lower eyelid.
   C. Do not touch eye with the eyedropper.

VI. **The client/caregiver can list possible complications.**

   A. Hemorrhage
   B. Corneal edema or scarring
   C. Infection
   D. Retinal detachment

REFERENCES

Ackley, B. J., & Ladwig, G. B. (2006). *Nursing diagnosis handbook: A guide to planning care*. St. Louis: Mosby Inc.

Canobbio, M. M. (2006). *Mosby's handbook of patient teaching*. St. Louis: Mosby Inc.

Perry, A., & Potter, P. (2006). *Clinical nursing skills & technique*. St. Louis: Mosby Inc.

Timby, B. K., & Smith, N. C. (2003). *Introductory medical-surgical nursing* (8th ed.). Philadelphia: J. B. Lippincott Williams & Wilkins.

3 Hip Replacement Teaching Guide

Patient name: _____ **Admission:** _____

NRS
DATE INITIAL

I. **The client/caregiver can list indications for hip replacement and repair.**

   A. Arthritis-osteoarthritis or rheumatoid arthritis
   B. Benign and malignant bone tumors
   C. Severe hip trauma
   D. Congenital hip disease

II. **The client/caregiver can list factors that increase risk of hip fracture.**

   A. Advanced age
   B. Osteoporosis
   C. Prolonged immobility
   D. Poor nutrition

III. **The client/caregiver can recognize signs and symptoms of hip fracture.**

   A. Shortening of affected extremity
   B. Severe pain and tenderness
   C. External rotation
   D. Inability to bear weight

IV. **The client/caregiver can define surgical methods to repair or replace a hip fracture.**

   A. Fracture of the femoral neck of the hip is repaired.
      1. Internal fixation. If the bone is still properly aligned after fracture, a metal screw can be inserted to hold the fractures together until healed.
      2. Hemiarthroplasty. If the ends of the broken bones are damaged and not aligned, the head and neck of the femur will be replaced by a metal prosthesis.
      3. Total hip replacement. This replaces the upper femur and socket with a prosthesis. This is often used when prior damage from arthritis or prior fracture has occurred.
   B. Intertrochanteric region fractures have a metal compression screw placed across the fracture and are attached to a plate

NRS
DATE INITIAL

running down the side of the femur with a second screw. This compresses the edges, and they heal together.

V. **The client/caregiver can follow general postoperative orders.**

   A. Follow activity and weight-bearing instructions exactly as ordered by physician.
   B. Follow precautions to prevent injury to hip.
      1. Avoid flexion of hip beyond 90 degrees.
      2. Avoid bending at the waist. Use adaptive devices such as long-handled shoe horn and so forth.
      3. Never cross legs or ankles while standing, sitting, or lying.
      4. When sitting keep knees below the hips. Keep feet 6 inches apart when sitting.
      5. Bear weight on affected leg only as ordered.
      6. Use toilet elevator on toilet seat to ease transfers.
      7. Use pillow between legs to sleep for the first 8 weeks after surgery.
      8. Avoid sleeping on operative side.
      9. Lie on your stomach for 15 minutes every day.
      10. Follow progressive exercises as ordered.
      11. Do not drive until approved by physician.
      12. Use chairs with arms for aid in rising. Avoid low stools or reclining chairs.
   C. Wear elastic stockings as ordered to prevent embolism.
   D. Eliminate safety hazards in the home.
   E. Use ordered assistive devices (walker, cane, crutches) as instructed.
   F. Provide care for incision as instructed.
      1. Cleanse the wound as instructed, and keep a dry sterile dressing over the incision as ordered.

(Continued)

NRS
DATE INITIAL

2. Report any signs of infection such as fever, redness, odor, painful swelling, and drainage.
G. Nutrition recommendations are
   1. Have a diet high in protein, fiber, and vitamins to promote healing and prevent constipation.
   2. Increase fluids to help prevent constipation.
   3. Limit caffeine and alcohol intake.
H. Keep follow-up appointments with physician and therapist.
I. Explore the possible need for extended care or rehabilitation services.

VI. **The client/caregiver is aware of possible complications.**

   A. Infection
   B. Dislocated prosthesis
   C. Loosening of implant
   D. Thrombophlebitis
   E. Embolus (blood clot that travels to lung or brain)
   F. Neurovascular dysfunction

RESOURCES

Skilled nursing facility or assisted living

Outpatient or home physical and/or occupational therapy

Durable medical equipment companies for adaptive or assistive aids

REFERENCES

Ackley, B. J., & Ladwig, G. B. (2006). *Nursing diagnosis handbook: A guide to planning care.* St. Louis: Mosby Inc.

Canobbio, M. M. (2006). *Mosby's handbook of patient teaching.* St. Louis: Mosby Inc.

Taylor, C., Lillis, C., & LeMone, P. (2005). *Fundamentals of nursing.* Philadelphia: Lippincott, Williams & Wilkins.

Timby, B. K., & Smith, N. C. (2003). *Introductory medical-surgical nursing* (8th ed.). Philadelphia: J. B. Lippincott Williams & Wilkins.

Hystrectomy

Patient name: _____ **Admission:** _____

NRS
DATE INITIAL

I. **The client/caregiver can define hysterectomy.**

  A. A total hysterectomy is the removal of the uterus and cervix (may be performed through the abdomen or the vagina).

  B. A panhysterectomy is the removal of the uterus, fallopian tubes, cervix, and ovaries.

  C. Removal of the uterus results in cessation of menstruation.

II. **The client/caregiver can list indications for hysterectomy.**

  A. Reasons or indications for hysterectomy could be
- Uterine fibroids
- Endometriosis not responding to medication or surgery
- Uterine prolapse
- Cancer of the uterus, cervix, or ovaries
- Vaginal bleeding that persists despite treatment

III. **The client/caregiver understands postoperative instructions.**

  A. Perform abdominal muscle-strengthening exercises.

  B. Provide care of abdominal incision by washing with soap and water.

  C. Avoid vigorous activities and heavy lifting until permission is given by the surgeon.

  D. Avoid constipation with stool softeners, increased fluids, diets high in fiber.

  E. Avoid constrictive clothing.

  F. Avoid sitting for prolonged periods.

  G. Avoid tub baths or sexual activity until permission is given by surgeon.

  H. Report heavy vaginal bleeding, fever, foul odor, pain, purulent drainage, and so forth.

  I. Take medications as ordered.

NRS
DATE INITIAL

  J. Provide perineal care.
1. Wash with soap and water.
2. Wipe from front to back.
3. Change pad frequently.
4. May use sitz baths or ice packs as ordered.

  K. Keep follow-up appointments.

IV. **The client/caregiver is aware of possible postoperative complications.**

  A. Symptoms, such as hot flashes, headache, nervousness, palpitations, fatigue, and depression

  B. Wound dehiscence (especially if client is obese)

  C. Thrombophlebitis

  D. Infection

  E. Urinary tract infection

  F. Pneumonia

  G. Constipation

  H. Urinary retention

RESOURCES

American College of Obstetricians and Gynecologists Resource Center
www.acog.org

National Women's Health Information Center
800-994-9662

REFERENCES

Ackley, B. J., & Ladwig, G. B. (2006). *Nursing diagnosis handbook: A guide to planning care*. St. Louis: Mosby Inc.

Canobbio, M. M. (2006). *Mosby's handbook of patient teaching*. St. Louis: Mosby Inc.

Perry, A., & Potter, P. (2006). *Clinical nursing skills & technique*. St. Louis: Mosby Inc.

Timby, B. K., & Smith, N. C. (2003). *Introductory medical-surgical nursing* (8th ed.). Philadelphia: J. B. Lippincott Williams & Wilkins.

5 Breast Surgeries: Mastectomy, Lumpectomy, and Sentinel Lymph Node Mapping

Patient name: _____   Admission: _____

NRS DATE INITIAL	

I. The client/caregiver can define the types of breast surgery used in the treatment of breast cancer.

  A. Lumpectomy is a wide incision and removal of tumor, including a margin of healthy tissue.
  B. Partial mastectomy is excision of tumor with wider margin of healthy tissue.
  C. Modified radical mastectomy is the removal of breast and axillary lymph nodes.
  D. Radical mastectomy is the removal of breast, underlying muscles, and axillary lymph nodes.
  E. Breast reconstruction is surgery to rebuild a breast's shape after a mastectomy.

II. The client/caregiver can list factors that increase the risk of breast cancer.

  A. Positive family history of breast cancer
  B. Onset of menstruation before age 12
  C. Late age at menopause (after 55)
  D. No children or first pregnancy after 30 years old
  E. Fibrocystic breast changes
  F. Previous history of breast cancer
  G. Personal history of other cancers

III. The client can follow exercises as ordered and also incorporate full range of motion into daily activities.

  A. Wall climbing (client sits next to the wall and moves both hands up the wall until pain occurs)
  B. Pendulum arm swinging (client bends at the waist and swings arms from side to side without bending the elbows)
  C. Rope pulling (client hangs a rope over the door and pulls one at a time, which alternately raises the arms)
  D. Elbow spread (client locks hands behind the neck and then gradually brings elbows together)

IV. The client/caregiver can describe postprocedure instructions to follow at home.

  A. Assess incision daily.
  B. Keep area clean and dry.
  C. Call physician if signs and symptoms of infection occur.
    1. Increased redness
    2. Increased pain
    3. Swelling
    4. Yellow, thick drainage from incision
    5. Fever over 100°F
    6. Increased drainage or bleeding

V. The client/caregiver can list measures to protect arm and to prevent injury to arm.

  A. Avoid constrictive clothing, jewelry, or wristwatch.
  B. Avoid blood pressure, venipunctures, or injections.
  C. Avoid carrying heavy objects on the affected arm.
  D. Avoid burns, cuts, scratches, or trauma to affected arm.
  E. Avoid sunburn.
  F. Avoid the use of deodorants or antiperspirants if incision reaches axilla area.
  G. Avoid burns, cuts, scratches, or trauma to affected arm.
  H. Avoid strong detergents and other chemicals.
  I. Use a thimble when sewing.
  J. Wear heavy garden gloves when gardening.
  K. Wear heavy thermal gloves when reaching in oven.
  L. Use hand lotion to prevent skin dryness.
  M. Elevate arm frequently to prevent swelling.

VI. The client/caregiver can list measures to prevent recurrent cancer.

  A. Continue to do breast self-exams (give "breast self-exam" teaching guide).

(Continued)

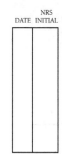

B. Have regular medical checkups and keep follow-up appointments with physician.

VII. **The client/caregiver can list possible complications.**

   A. Lymphedema (an accumulation of fluid) in arm
   B. Infection

RESOURCES

Cancer Response Information
800-227-2345

"Reach for Recovery" Program
- Provides opportunity to talk to another person who has had a mastectomy.
- Provides brochures to show exercises, breast prosthesis information, and so forth.
- Provides a free temporary fluff prosthesis until the client is ready for weighted prosthesis.

Sources for breast prosthesis

Support groups

Counseling

REFERENCES

Ackley, B. J., & Ladwig, G. B. (2006). *Nursing diagnosis handbook: A guide to planning care*. St. Louis: Mosby Inc.

Canobbio, M. M. (2006). *Mosby's handbook of patient teaching*. St. Louis: Mosby Inc.

Perry, A., & Potter, P. (2006). *Clinical nursing skills & technique*. St. Louis: Mosby Inc.

Taylor, C., Lillis, C., & LeMone, P. (2005). *Fundamentals of nursing*. Philadelphia: Lippincott, Williams & Wilkins.

Timby, B. K., & Smith, N. C. (2003). *Introductory medical-surgical nursing* (8th ed.). Philadelphia: J. B. Lippincott Williams & Wilkins.

6 Pacemaker Insertion

Patient name: _____ Admission: _____

NRS
DATE INITIAL

I. The client/caregiver can define a pacemaker.

A. It provides an artificial electrical stimulus to the heart muscle to control or maintain a regular rhythm heartbeat.
B. It consists of a battery-powered pulse generator and a catheter electrode that is inserted into the right side of the heart or ventricle.
C. A pacemaker can be temporary (external) or permanent (internal).

II. The client/caregiver can list and describe two types of pacemakers.

A. A demand-rate pacemaker generates an electrical stimulus only if the heart rate falls below a preset level.
B. A fixed-rate pacemaker is set at a certain rate and constantly creates electrical stimuli regardless of the heart's rhythm.

III. The client/caregiver can list measures for pacemaker management.

A. Monitor the pulse at rest as instructed by physician, and report rate if less than set amount.
B. Report fatigue, shortness of breath, palpitations, dizziness, chest pain, and so forth.
C. Assess wound and report signs and symptoms of infection (i.e., redness, tenderness, drainage, and fever).
D. Avoid any type of trauma to pulse generator.
 1. Avoid constrictive clothing.
 2. Avoid bumping pulse generator.
 3. Avoid contact sports.
E. Follow postoperative activity as ordered.
 1. Resume driving, sexual relations, exercise, and so forth as ordered by physician.

NRS
DATE INITIAL

 2. Most activities can be resumed in 4 to 6 weeks.
 3. Perform range of motion exercises as instructed to affected shoulder.

IV. The client/caregiver can explain special instructions for pacemaker care.

A. Show pacemaker card at airport security checks.
B. Inform any health care provider (i.e., dentist, technicians, and physician) of pacemaker.
C. Carry a pacemaker identity card that includes
 1. Pacemaker model and leads
 2. Pacemaker settings
 3. Date of insertion, name of surgeon, and hospital with contact telephone numbers
D. Follow precautions around electricity and strong magnetic fields.
 1. Avoid areas of high voltage such as power plants, radio transmitters, large industrial magnets, and certain antitheft alarm systems.
 2. Ground home appliances.
 3. Avoid magnetic resonance imagining.
 4. Avoid resting cellular telephone on chest over site of generator.
E. Wear Medic Alert bracelet.

V. The client/caregiver can state need for follow-up care.

A. Keep follow-up appointments with physician and with pacemaker clinic evaluations.
B. Keep appointment for battery checks, which may be done at the hospital or at home via telephone system.
C. Change battery as needed (most last 5 to 10 years).

(Continued)

NRS	
DATE	INITIAL

VI. **The client/caregiver is aware of signs and symptoms of possible complications.**

    A. Infection
    B. Pacemaker malfunction
    C. Bleeding
    D. Cardiac dysrhythmias

RESOURCES

The American Heart Association
800-242-8721
www.aha.org
Manufacturer of the pacemaker

REFERENCES

Ackley, B. J., & Ladwig, G. B. (2006). *Nursing diagnosis handbook: A guide to planning care.* St. Louis: Mosby Inc.

Canobbio, M. M. (2006). *Mosby's handbook of patient teaching.* St. Louis: Mosby Inc.

Perry, A., & Potter, P. (2006). *Clinical nursing skills & technique.* St. Louis: Mosby Inc.

Taylor, C., Lillis, C., & LeMone, P. (2005). *Fundamentals of nursing.* Philadelphia: Lippincott, Williams & Wilkins.

Part V

Therapeutic Nutrition

Teaching Guides

1 Basic Nutrient Requirements

Patient name: _____ Admission: _____

I. **The client/caregiver can define and list the nutrients that are needed by the body.**

A. Nutrients are chemical substances supplied by food that the body needs for growth, maintenance, and repair.

B. There are six nutrients.
1. Carbohydrates
2. Proteins
3. Fats
4. Minerals
5. Vitamins
6. Water

C. Macronutrients are carbohydrates, proteins, and fats. They all help produce energy and have calories.

D. Micronutrients are minerals, vitamins, and water. They are still very important but do not have any calories.

II. **The client/caregiver can state purpose and food sources of each nutrient.**

A. Fats provide energy and body heat, provide organ protection, are for absorption and digestion of fat-soluble vitamins, carry essential fatty acids, are for satiety and flavor to foods. Food sources include milk, meats, and butter.

B. Proteins provide building tissue and energy; they provide water balance to regulate hormones and enzymes for immunity. Food sources of complete protein include meat, poultry, eggs, and cheese. Food sources of incomplete protein include grains, vegetables, nuts, and seeds.

C. Carbohydrates provide energy and help to spare body protein. Food sources include breads, vegetables, fruit, and milk.

D. Water is essential for almost every body process, including digestion, absorption, circulation, and excretion. It helps maintain a normal body temperature, carries wastes out of the body, and transports nutrients throughout the body. It prevents constipation.

III. **The client/caregiver can state purpose and food sources of vitamins.**

A. Vitamin A
1. It is necessary for maintenance of skin, hair, gums, bones, and teeth.
2. It promotes good vision, helps prevent infections, and acts as an antioxidant.
3. Food sources include liver, kidney, milk, cream, butter, egg yolk, fortified milk and dairy products, carrots, sweet potatoes, tomatoes, pumpkins, apricots, fish liver oils, beets, cantaloupe, garlic, and spinach.

B. Vitamin B1 (thiamine)
1. It is necessary for growth and energy.
2. It improves mental attitude.
3. It improves functioning of nervous system, heart, and muscles.
4. Food sources include lean pork, beef, liver, whole grains, beans, peas, wheat germ, brewers yeast, eggs, fish, brown rice, soy beans, nuts, and oatmeal.

C. Vitamin B2 (riboflavin)
1. It is necessary for metabolism of protein, fats, and carbohydrates.
2. Helps build and maintain body tissues, growth, and reproduction.
3. It releases energy to cells.
4. It protects skin and eyes from disorders.
5. Food sources include milk, liver, eggs, grains, green leafy vegetables, legumes, yogurt, cheese, meat, fish, and poultry.

D. Vitamin B3 (niacin)
1. It is necessary for nervous system, and healthy skin.
2. It aids digestion and helps lower cholesterol.
3. It is used in fat, carbohydrate, and protein metabolism.
4. Food sources include meat, peanuts, peas, beans, sunflower seeds, beef, broccoli, eggs, fish, milk, potatoes, and carrots.

(Continued)

E. Vitamin B5 (pantothenic acid)
1. It is necessary for coping with physical and mental stress and production of antibodies.
2. It helps convert carbohydrates, fats, and protein into energy.
3. It aids in digestion.
4. Food sources include liver, kidney, whole grain, legumes, eggs, peanuts, sunflower seeds, beef, and fresh vegetables.

F. Vitamin B6 (pyridoxine)
1. It is necessary for production of red blood cells.
2. It aids in normal function of nervous system.
3. It helps maintain most body functions.
4. It aids in protein and carbohydrate metabolism.
5. Food sources include whole grains, seeds, liver, kidney, eggs, oatmeal, walnuts, pork, wheat germ, bananas, potatoes, brewers yeast, chicken, fish, brown rice, cabbage, cantaloupe, and carrots.

G. Vitamin B12 (cobalamin)
1. It is necessary for development of vital nerve structures.
2. It prevents pernicious anemia.
3. It aids in cell formation and digestion.
4. Food sources include liver, kidney, sardines, lean meat, milk, cheese, beef, blue cheese, clams, eggs, beef, and herring.

H. Vitamin C
1. It is necessary to combat stress and improves immunity and helps resist infections.
2. It acts as an antioxidant.
3. It is needed for amino acid metabolism and synthesis of hormones.
4. It is needed for wound healing, adrenal gland function, iron absorption, and folic acid conversion.
5. Food sources include citrus fruits, melons, kiwi, strawberries, peppers, tomatoes, cantaloupe, oranges, potatoes, cabbage, and broccoli.

I. Vitamin D (calciferol)
1. It is necessary for normal growth and development.
2. It helps calcium and phosphorous absorption and use for healthy teeth and bones.

3. Food sources include cereal, fortified milk, sardines, tuna, cod liver oil, and egg yolk.
4. A major source is sunshine.

J. Vitamin E
1. It is necessary for metabolism of fats and repair of tissue.
2. It helps protect from toxins.
3. It acts as an antioxidant.
4. Food sources include milk, eggs, fish, cereals, green leafy vegetables, vegetable oils, whole grains and wheat germ, brown rice, liver, sweet potatoes, poultry, and nuts.

K. Vitamin K
1. It is necessary for normal blood clotting and normal liver function.
2. Food sources include leafy vegetables, milk, meats, eggs, cereals, broccoli, cauliflower, oatmeal, liver, spinach, strawberries, tomatoes, liver, and wheat bran.

IV. **The client/caregiver can state purpose and food sources of minerals.**

A. Calcium
1. It is necessary for healthy bones and teeth, muscle, and nerve function.
2. Food sources are milk and milk products, sardines, oysters, salmon, broccoli, cabbage, oats, turnips, and mustard greens.

B. Chromium
1. It is necessary for metabolism of glucose and synthesis of fatty acids and cholesterol.
2. Food sources include cereal, whole grains, brewers yeast, wheat germ, chicken, clams, brown rice, cheese, meat, liver, mushrooms, and potatoes.

C. Iodine
1. It is necessary for function of thyroid gland and for physical and mental development.
2. Food sources include seafood and iodized salt.

D. Iron
1. It is necessary for production of hemoglobin; it increases resistance to stress and disease and helps in energy production.

(Continued)

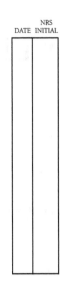

2. Food sources include meat, poultry, fish, eggs, whole grains, leafy vegetables, potatoes, dates, peaches, pears, and iron-fortified foods.
   E. Magnesium
   1. It is necessary for bones, nerves, muscle, and teeth, transmission of nerve impulses; it activates enzymes and aids in the release of energy.
   2. Food sources include all unprocessed foods, whole grain cereals, seeds, legumes, nuts, green vegetables, bananas, milk, cheese, and meat.
   F. Manganese
   1. It is necessary for skeletal development, nerves, and brain.
   2. Food sources include whole grains, leafy vegetables, cereals, peas, nuts, seeds, avocado, milk, tea, and coffee.
   G. Phosphorous
   1. It is necessary for repair of cells and energy production; it builds bones and teeth and promotes nerve function.
   2. Food sources include milk, meat, poultry, fish, cereal, nuts, and legumes.
   H. Potassium
   1. It is necessary for nerves, muscles, and heart; it regulates the body's fluid balance.
   2. Food sources include buttermilk, garlic, nuts, meats, brown rice, legumes, whole grains, apricots, avocados, bananas, and potatoes.

   I. Zinc
   1. It is necessary for healing and development of new cells; it aids in digestion and metabolism, male fertility, and brain development and improves immunity and prostate function.
   2. Food sources include seafood, oysters, liver, meat, milk, cheese, whole grains, pecans, pumpkin seeds, eggs, and lima beans.
   J. Selenium
   1. It acts as an antioxidant and works with vitamin E for some functions.
   2. Food sources include seafood, liver, kidney, and other meats.

REFERENCES

Lutz, C., & Przytulski, K. (2001). *Nutrition and diet therapy.* Philadelphia: F. A. Davis Company.

Lutz, C., & Przytulski, K. (2004). *Nutri notes: Nutrition & diet therapy pocket guide.* Philadelphia: F. A. Davis Company.

Nutrition made incredibly easy. (2003). Philadelphia: Lippincott Williams & Wilkins.

Perry, A., & Potter, P. (2006). *Clinical nursing skills & technique.* St. Louis: Mosby Inc.

Taylor, C., Lillis, C., & LeMone, P. (2005). *Fundamentals of nursing.* Philadelphia: Lippincott, Williams & Wilkins.

Timby, B. K., & Smith, N. C. (2003). *Introductory medical-surgical nursing* (8th ed.). Philadelphia: J. B. Lippincott Williams & Wilkins.

2 Clear Liquid Diet

Patient name: _____   **Admission:** _____

I. **The client/caregiver can define the clear liquid diet.**

  A. The clear liquid diet provides fluid without stimulating extensive digestive processes.
  B. It is inadequate in all essential nutrients; intended for short-term use only.
  C. This diet will yield approximately 700 to 1,000 kcal when served at frequent intervals.

II. **The client/caregiver can list purpose of clear liquid diet.**

  A. It is used whenever an acute illness or surgery causes intolerance for foods.
  B. It is used to temporarily restrict undigested material in the gastrointestinal foods.

III. **The client/caregiver can state what foods are allowed.**

  A. Carbonated beverages and fruit-flavored soft drinks
  B. Regular or decaffeinated coffee and tea

  C. Clear, flavored gelatin, fruit ices, and frozen ice pops
  D. Cranberry, apple, and grape juices
  E. Lightly seasoned clear broth or consommé (fat free)

REFERENCES

Lutz, C., & Przytulski, K. (2001). *Nutrition and diet therapy.* Philadelphia: F. A. Davis Company.

Nutrition made incredibly easy. (2003). Philadelphia: Lippincott Williams & Wilkins.

Perry, A., & Potter, P. (2006). *Clinical nursing skills & technique.* St. Louis: Mosby Inc.

Taylor, C., Lillis, C., & LeMone, P. (2005). *Fundamentals of nursing.* Philadelphia: Lippincott, Williams & Wilkins.

Timby, B. K., & Smith, N. C. (2003). *Introductory medical-surgical nursing* (8th ed.). Philadelphia: J. B. Lippincott Williams & Wilkins.

3 Full Liquid Diet

Patient name: _____ Admission: _____

NRS
DATE INITIAL

I. **The client/caregiver can define the full liquid diet.**

   A. It consists of foods that are liquid at body temperature, including gels and frozen liquids.
   B. This diet provides nutrition that is easy to consume and digest with little stimulation to the gastrointestinal tract.

II. **The client/caregiver can list purpose of full liquid diet.**

   A. It is used for transitional diet after clear liquid.
   B. It is used after oral surgery or plastic surgery of the face or neck.
   C. It is used when a chewing or swallowing dysfunction is present.
   D. Modify the diet if the client has established or temporary lactose intolerance.

NRS
DATE INITIAL

III. **The client/caregiver can list foods allowed on a full liquid diet.**

   A. Carbonated beverages
   B. Regular or decaffeinated coffee and tea
   C. Soft drinks and cocoa
   D. Cooked refined cereal, farina, cream of rice, or strained cereals and custard, plain gelatin, ice cream, sherbet, pudding, yogurt (all without nuts, fruits, or preserves)
   E. Eggnog, milk shakes, and other milk drinks
   F. Butter, margarine, and cream
   G. Fruit and vegetable juices, including one serving of citrus fruit juice daily
   H. Broth, bouillon, consommé, and strained cream soup

4   Full Liquid Blenderized Diet

Patient name: _____   **Admission:** _____

I.   **The client/caregiver can define a full liquid blenderized diet.**

   A.   It is a diet consisting of a variety of liquids and semisolid foods that have been thinned to a consistency that can be consumed through a straw or sipped from a cup.
   B.   This diet can provide more energy and nutrients than the full liquid diet.

II.   **The client/caregiver can list the purpose of full liquid blenderized diet.**

   A.   It is used to provide oral nourishment in a form that requires no chewing.
   B.   It is used with client after oral, face, or neck surgery or trauma.
   C.   It is used with clients who have oral esophageal disorders or neuromuscular problems.
   D.   It is used with clients who have received radiation or chemotherapy and have eating problems.

III.   **The client/caregiver can list foods used in a full liquid blenderized diet.**

   A.   Milk, eggnog, milk shakes, and milk drinks
   B.   All beverages, including coffee and tea
   C.   Yogurt without seeds or fruit and thinned for straw feeding
   D.   Farina, cream of rice, grits, strained oatmeal, or cream of wheat mixed with equal parts whole milk. Iron-fortified cereals are recommended
   E.   Mashed white potato, thinned with soup or broth, vegetable juices, and vegetable purees, thinned with soup
   F.   Fruit juice or pureed fruit thinned with fruit juice, strained if necessary; citrus juices less tolerated
   G.   Pureed meats and poultry thinned with broth
   H.   Broth and strained cream soups
   I.   Ice cream, sherbet, custards, puddings, and fruit juices thinned
   J.   Salt, pepper, herbs, lemon juice, and other seasonings as tolerated

5   Pureed Diet

Patient name: _____   **Admission:** _____

I.   **The client/caregiver can define a pureed diet.**

   A.   This diet is soft in texture and mechanically nonirritating.

II.   **The client/caregiver can list purpose of pureed diet.**

   A.   It is used for clients with problems in chewing or swallowing.

   B.   It is used for clients with esophageal inflammation or varices.

III.   **The client/caregiver can list foods allowed on a pureed diet.**

   A.   All cooked cereals and strained oatmeal and milk-soaked or well-moistened dry cereal

   B.   Doughnuts, pancakes, waffles, French toast, and bread prepared in a slurry.

   C.   Mashed white or sweet potatoes; pureed, mashed, and/or strained thickened vegetables; tomato and vegetable juice

   D.   Applesauce, pureed thickened fruits, and fruit juices

   E.   Pureed to strained meats, poultry, fish, cheese sauce, and eggs

   F.   Butter, margarine, cream, gravy, and mayonnaise

   G.   All smooth cream or broth-based soups with pureed ingredients

   H.   Custard, pudding, ice cream, sherbet, gelatin, cakes, cobblers, and pies pureed to smooth and moist consistency, as well as soft cookies and plain cakes prepared in a slurry

6   Mechanical Soft (Dental) Diet

Patient name: _____   **Admission:** _____

NRS
DATE INITIAL

I.   **The client/caregiver can define the mechanical soft diet.**

A. This diet is a modification of the regular diet. All foods that are easily chewed are included in this diet.

II. **The client/caregiver can list purpose of mechanical soft diet.**

A. It is used for client who has difficulty in chewing or swallowing.
B. It is used for clients with missing or damaged teeth.
C. It is used for clients after temporomandilar joint surgery.
D. It is used in transition as ordered for dysphagia rehabilitation.

NRS
DATE INITIAL

III. **The client/caregiver can list foods NOT allowed on a mechanical soft diet.**

A. Breads with nuts, raisins, or thick crusts
B. Granola-type cereals or cereals with raisins or nuts
C. Raw or cooked vegetables with tough skins or seeds, raw vegetables, and fried vegetables
D. Fruits with tough skin
E. Tough, fibrous meats or meats with casings such as sausage
F. Fried eggs
G. Soups with tough meats or vegetables
H. Desserts containing nuts and coarse dried or tough fruits
I. Desserts or pastries baked to a hard consistency

7 Dysphagia Diets

Patient name: _____ **Admission:** _____

<table>
<tr><td>NRS
DATE INITIAL</td><td></td><td>NRS
DATE INITIAL</td></tr>
</table>

I. **The client/caregiver can define dysphagia diet.**

A. Dysphagia is defined as difficulty in swallowing. The most common causes of this are from disease of the nervous system and muscles.

B. The consistency of the diet is modified according to the client's tolerance. After physical and clinical assessments are done, the physician will give a specific order regarding the consistency of foods and liquids.

C. The client with dysphagia has difficulty in moving food/liquid from the front to the back of the mouth and then into the esophagus.

II. **The client/caregiver can list purpose of dysphagia diet.**

A. Dysphagia diets are designed to meet oral nutrient needs safely.

B. Dysphagia diets reduce the risk of aspiration and pneumonia.

C. The type and severity of dysphagia will determine the level of diet ordered.

III. **The client/caregiver can list the types of dysphagia diets.**

A. Dysphagia pureed diet has foods that have a moist, smooth consistency without pulp or small food particles. Sticky foods such as melted cheese or peanut butter are omitted. Thin liquids should be thickened to required level.

B. Dysphagia mechanically altered have foods that are moist, soft, and simple to chew and can be controlled in the mouth before entering the esophagus. Moistened meats, cooked and mashed vegetables, and fruits are allowed. Thickened liquids are still required.

C. Dysphagia advanced is similar to mechanical soft diet. Meats are soft and bite sized.

D. Regular liquids may be tolerated. Avoid foods that are hard, sticky, or crunchy. A regular diet indicates the client can chew and swallow regular food and liquids safely. Liquids used in this diet can range from thick to thin.

IV. **The client/caregiver can list specific diet consideration when meal planning for dysphagia.**

A. Diet orders from the physician should include the consistency level of both the diet and liquids.

B. Thickened liquids and foods can be accomplished by using commercial thickening products and/or the mechanical altering and combinations of foods.

C. The client/caregiver must be able to explain the type of dysphagia diet ordered by physician.

D. The client/caregiver will know how to prepare the food and liquids to appropriate consistency.

E. Prevention issues when dealing with clients using dysphagia diets include
   1. The client must be sitting in an upright position and should be supervised.
   2. Any instructions from a speech therapist should be posted.
   3. The client/caregiver should be able to recognize signs of eating difficulty or risk for aspiration. Watch for any coughing, gagging, drooling, or holding food in mouth.
   4. The client/caregiver should be able to monitor for symptoms of a "silent aspiration" by checking for changes in temperature and respirations.

(Continued)

RESOURCES

American Dietetic Association
www.eatright.org

National Institutes of Health
www.nih.gov

Registered dietitian

REFERENCES

American Dietetic Association. (2003). *National dysphagia diet: Standardization for optimal care.* Chicago: American Dietetic Association.

Lutz, C., & Przytulski, K. (2001). *Nutrition and diet therapy.* Philadelphia: F. A. Davis Company.

Nutrition made incredibly easy. (2003). Philadelphia: Lippincott Williams & Wilkins.

Perry, A., & Potter, P. (2006). *Clinical nursing skills & technique.* St. Louis: Mosby Inc.

Taylor, C., Lillis, C., & LeMone, P. (2005). *Fundamentals of nursing.* Philadelphia: Lippincott, Williams & Wilkins.

Timby, B. K., & Smith, N. C. (2003). *Introductory medical-surgical nursing* (8th ed.). Philadelphia: J. B. Lippincott Williams & Wilkins.

8   Cholesterol-Lowering Diets

Patient name: _____   Admission: _____

NRS
DATE INITIAL

I. **The client/caregiver can define cholesterol.**

A. Cholesterol is a soft, fat-like substance in the bloodstream of the body. It is produced by the liver, and we ingest large amounts by eating meat and dairy products.

B. Too much cholesterol directly increases the risk of heart disease.

C. A lipid profile is the test often used to evaluate risks for coronary heart disease (the 2001 guidelines from the National Cholesterol Education Panel recommended that all lipid tests be performed after fasting and should measure all four cholesterol components: total cholesterol, high-density lipoproteins, low-density lipoproteins, and triglycerides).

D. A lipid profile includes high-density lipoproteins, low-density lipoproteins, very-low-density lipoprotein, and triglycerides.

E. High-density lipoproteins help to carry away or remove excess cholesterol from the blood stream. Normal values are 45 to 55 mg/dl or higher.

F. Low-density lipoproteins are most responsible for plaque formation that clogs arteries and creates atherosclerotic plaques. Normal values are between 60 to 180 mg/dl. This can vary with the client's risk for heart disease.

G. Triglycerides are fats in the body. They are frequently elevated in clients with obesity, cardiac disease, and diabetes. Triglyceride levels should be less than 150 mg/dl.

H. A goal for total cholesterol should be below 200 mg/dl.

II. **The client/caregiver can list nutritional information to decrease serum cholesterol levels.**

A. Limit milk to skim milk, 1% milk, or cultured buttermilk, and use nonfat or low-fat yogurt or cottage cheese.

B. Limit breads made without whole milk, eggs, or butter.

NRS
DATE INITIAL

C. Do not prepare vegetables with butter, cream, or cheese sauce.

D. Use lean meats with fat trimmed and poultry without skin.

E. Cut down on saturated fats.

F. Use only two egg yolks per week. Use egg whites or egg substitute.

G. Use monounsaturated oils and low-fat dressings. Preferred oils are peanut, olive, and canola oils.

H. Use low-fat frozen desserts or frozen fruit ices, angel-food cake, and low-fat cookies and snacks.

I. Use nonfat beverages, carbonated drinks, juices, tea, and coffee.

J. A diet rich in fiber (20 to 30 grams per day) may also help to reduce cholesterol levels.

K. Limit cholesterol dietary intake to 300 mg or less daily.

III. **The client/caregiver can list additional ways to lower cholesterol and triglyceride levels.**

A. Avoid alcohol.

B. Cook by boiling, baking, or roasting instead of frying.

C. Increase activity level.

D. Achieve and maintain a healthy weight.

E. Avoid trans-fatty acids and hydrogenated oils used in margarines, commercially prepared cookies, cakes, and so forth.

F. Limit sugar intake.

G. Read labels to determine sources of saturated fats and cholesterol.

H. Consult with registered dietitian.

I. Medication therapy as prescribed by physician.

RESOURCES

American Heart Association
www.americanheart.org

(Continued)

National Cholesterol Education Program
www.nhlbi.nih.gov/about/ncep/

National Heart, Lung, and Blood Institute
www.nhlbi.nih.gov

National Institutes of Health
www.nih.gov

The Office of the Surgeon General
www.surgeongeneral.gov/sgoffice

American Diabetes Association
www.diabetes.org

My Pyramid—United States Department of Agriculture
www.mypyramid.gov

REFERENCES

Lutz, C., & Przytulski, K. (2001). *Nutrition and diet therapy.* Philadelphia: F. A. Davis Company.

Lutz, C., & Przytulski, K. (2004). *Nutri notes: Nutrition & diet therapy pocket guide.* Philadelphia: F. A. Davis Company.

Nutrition made incredibly easy. (2003). Philadelphia: Lippincott Williams & Wilkins.

Perry, A., & Potter, P. (2006). *Clinical nursing skills & technique.* St. Louis: Mosby Inc.

Taylor, C., Lillis, C., & LeMone, P. (2005). *Fundamentals of nursing.* Philadelphia: Lippincott, Williams & Wilkins.

Timby, B. K., & Smith, N. C. (2003). *Introductory medical-surgical nursing* (8th ed.). Philadelphia: J. B. Lippincott Williams & Wilkins.

9 Reduced-Fat Diets

Patient name: _____ Admission: _____

I. **The client/caregiver can define the role of dietary fat in disease.**

A. Fats provide energy, help in the absorption of fat-soluble vitamins, supply fatty acids, lubricate body tissues, help regulate temperature, and provide protection for some of the most vital organs in our bodies.

B. A healthy level of dietary fat also gives flavor to our foods and provides a feeling of fullness during meal intake.

C. High levels of fat contribute to many chronic diseases. High-fat diets greatly increase the risk of cardiovascular disease, obesity, and some types of cancer.

II. **The client/caregiver can list the current dietary recommendations for a reduced-fat diet.**

A. The American Heart Association, Surgeon General, American Cancer Society, and the American Diabetes Association agree on the following:
1. Have diets that are low in saturated fat and cholesterol and moderate in total fat.
2. Limit fat to 35% or less of the total daily calorie intake.
3. Limit saturated fat to less than 10% of total daily calorie intake.
4. Limit cholesterol to 300 mg or less daily.

III. **The client/caregiver can list major sources of dietary fat.**

A. Beef, butter (or margarine), salad dressings (including mayonnaise), cheese, and milk are the top five sources of saturated fat in the average diet.

IV. **The client/caregiver can list ways to reduce dietary fat in the diet.**

A. Fruits—avoid avocado, coconut, and olives. Most other fruits are low in fat.

B. Vegetables—eat and prepare vegetables wisely. Avoid fried, creamed vegetables. Avoid cheeses and dressings high in fat on vegetables.

C. Dairy products—select low-fat or fat-free milk, yogurt, and cheese products. Drink two to three servings of low-fat milk and milk products daily.

D. Proteins
1. Use plant sources of protein such as beans and nuts.
2. Use lean meats and trim any excess fat.
3. Remove skin from poultry. Avoid breading or sauces.
4. Eat two to three servings of lean fish, poultry, lean meats, or other protein sources daily.
5. Limit intake of organ meats like liver.
6. Limit shellfish (crab, lobster, etc.) due to high cholesterol levels.

E. Read nutrition fact labels carefully when shopping.
1. Use low-fat or fat-free salad dressings.
2. Choose vegetable oils lower in saturated fats such as canola oil.
3. Season foods with lemon juice, or spices and herbs with label of low fat/low sodium.

F. Cooking and serving foods
1. Use fats and oils sparingly when cooking or serving foods.
2. Use low-fat sauces on rice, pasta, and potatoes.
3. If using some of the commercial fat replacers, be alert for gastrointestinal side effects (cramps and diarrhea).
4. Avoid frying foods. Instead, bake, boil, or broil them.

(Continued)

RESOURCES

American Heart Association
www.americanheart.org

National Heart, Lung, and Blood Institute
www.nhlbi.nih.gov

National Institutes of Health
www.nih.gov

The Office of the Surgeon General
www.surgeongeneral.gov/sgoffice

American Diabetes Association
www.diabetes.org

My Pyramid—United States Department of Agriculture
www.mypyramid.gov

REFERENCES

Lutz, C., & Przytulski, K. (2001). *Nutrition and diet therapy.* Philadelphia: F. A. Davis Company.

Lutz, C., & Przytulski, K. (2004). *Nutri notes: Nutrition & diet therapy pocket guide.* Philadelphia: F. A. Davis Company.

Nutrition made incredibly easy. (2003). Philadelphia: Lippincott Williams & Wilkins.

Perry, A., & Potter, P. (2006). *Clinical nursing skills & technique.* St. Louis: Mosby Inc.

Taylor, C., Lillis, C., & LeMone, P. (2005). *Fundamentals of nursing.* Philadelphia: Lippincott, Williams & Wilkins.

Timby, B. K., & Smith, N. C. (2003). *Introductory medical-surgical nursing* (8th ed.). Philadelphia: J. B. Lippincott Williams & Wilkins.

10 Sodium-Restricted Diets

Patient name: _____ **Admission:** _____

NRS
DATE INITIAL

I. **The client/caregiver will explain the role of sodium.**

   A. Most dietary sodium is added to foods during cooking and processing.

   B. Sodium is absorbed by the intestines and excreted primarily by the kidneys.

   C. Increased levels of sodium in the body promote water retention and swelling.

II. **The client/caregiver can explain when it is important to monitor sodium intake and sodium retention.**

   A. Sodium is monitored to evaluate fluid-electrolyte balance of the body.

   B. Cardiovascular disease and kidney disease will affect the body's use of sodium.

   C. Sodium level testing is also used to monitor effects of diuretic drug therapy.

   D. Diuretics are frequently used in treatment of hypertension.

III. **The client/caregiver can describe important concepts in a sodium-restricted diet.**

   A. One teaspoon of table/cooking salt contains 2300 mg of sodium. The recommended amount of sodium for a healthy adult not on any sodium restrictions is 2400 mg of sodium daily.

   B. Restricted-sodium diets are often classified as
     1. No added salt—usually recognized as a 4-g sodium diet.
     2. A low-sodium or restricted-sodium diet is usually a 2-g sodium (2-g Na) or 1-g sodium (1-g Na).

   C. Unseen sodium is in
     1. Over-the-counter medications such as antacids and laxatives
     2. Commercial beverages and bottled drinking water
     3. Toothpaste and mouthwash—do not swallow
     4. Processed foods, which yield the largest amount of sodium

NRS
DATE INITIAL

IV. **The client/caregiver can list ways to reduce dietary sodium intake.**

   A. Read labels. Sodium will be listed as amount and as percentage.

   B. Use food products with reduced sodium or no added salt.

   C. Use herbs, spices, lemon juice, and so forth instead of salt when cooking.

   D. Rinse foods such as tuna to remove some of the sodium.

   E. Remove salt from table, and avoid adding salt to prepared food.

   F. Avoid condiments such as soy and teriyaki sauce and monosodium glutamate. Limit the usual condiments, such as mustard and ketchup.

   G. Eat fresh foods rather than canned or convenience foods.

   H. Limit cured foods such as bacon, ham, and hot dogs.

   I. Avoid foods packed in brine or pickled, such as sauerkraut, olives, and pickles.

   J. Before using a "salt substitute," check with physician because many of these products have potassium instead of sodium. Salt substitutes are only for use at the table. If cooked, they may taste bitter.

   K. Use unsalted butter or margarine.

   L. Use low-sodium luncheon meats, cheeses, and peanut butter.

   M. Avoid organ meats, clams, lobster, crab, oysters, scallops, shrimp, and other shellfish.

   N. Read labels on ready-to-serve or convenience foods for sodium content.

   O. Information about the Dietary Approaches to Stop Hypertension diet can be obtained at www.dash.bwh.harvard.edu. This diet plan promotes a diet rich in fruits, vegetables, and low-fat dairy foods and the use of fewer snacks and sugars.

(Continued)

RESOURCES

American Heart Association
www.americanheart.org

National Heart, Lung, and Blood Institute
www.nhlbi.nih.gov

National Institutes of Health
www.nih.gov

The Office of the Surgeon General
www.surgeongeneral.gov/sgoffice

American Diabetes Association
www.diabetes.org

My Pyramid—United States Department of Agriculture
www.mypyramid.gov

REFERENCES

Lutz, C., & Przytulski, K. (2001). *Nutrition and diet therapy.* Philadelphia: F. A. Davis Company.

Lutz, C., & Przytulski, K. (2004). *Nutri notes: Nutrition & diet therapy pocket guide.* Philadelphia: F. A. Davis Company.

Nutrition made incredibly easy. (2003). Philadelphia: Lippincott Williams & Wilkins.

Perry, A., & Potter, P. (2006). *Clinical nursing skills & technique.* St. Louis: Mosby Inc.

Taylor, C., Lillis, C., & LeMone, P. (2005). *Fundamentals of nursing.* Philadelphia: Lippincott, Williams & Wilkins.

Timby, B. K., & Smith, N. C. (2003). *Introductory medical-surgical nursing* (8th ed.). Philadelphia: J. B. Lippincott Williams & Wilkins.

11   High-Fiber Diets

Patient name: _____   Admission: _____

NRS
DATE INITIAL

I.   **The client/caregiver can describe benefits of an increased fiber diet.**

A. Fiber cannot be digested. It goes through the large intestine without being absorbed and helps create bulk and formation of stool. This helps in preventing and/or relieving constipation.

B. High-fiber diets may help lower cholesterol levels.

C. High-fiber diets may also decrease risks of certain cancers.

D. High-fiber diets may contribute to weight loss due its ability to create a feeling of fullness when included in meal.

E. Some fibers help slow glucose absorption.

F. The average adult is advised to take in 20 to 35 g of fiber per day. The typical intake is about half of that amount.

NRS
DATE INITIAL

II.   **The client/caregiver can list ways to increase fiber in diet.**

A. Eat five servings of fruits and vegetables a day.

B. Choose whole fruits and vegetables over juice when possible.

C. Eat foods with whole grains instead of refined grains.

D. Read food labels carefully. Choose cereals and breads that have at least 5 g of fiber per serving.

E. Include beans in diet and meal planning.

F. Drink adequate amounts of water or fluids: six to eight glasses per day.

12

Weight Loss Diets
(Low-Calorie Diet)

Patient name: _____   Admission: _____

NRS
DATE   INITIAL

NRS
DATE   INITIAL

I.   **The client/caregiver can state importance of a low-calorie diet to reduce body weight and maintain a healthy percentage of fat mass versus lean mass.**

A. To promote physical health and decrease risks for diabetes and cardiovascular disease
B. To promote positive self-esteem
C. To reduce body weight by 10% at a rate of 1 to 2 pounds per week
D. To recognize three components of weight loss: diet therapy, increased physical activity, and behavioral therapy.

II. **The client/caregiver can list ways to limit caloric intake.**

A. Drink skim milk and use low-fat dairy products.
B. Eat low-calorie snacks such as celery and carrots.
C. Prepare foods by steaming, broiling, or baking.
D. Use nonstick cooking spray, and trim all visible fat before cooking.
E. Eat sensible portions of food.
F. Eat carbohydrates that are high in fiber to promote a sense of fullness.
G. Substitute polyunsaturated fats (vegetable oils) for saturated fats (lard, butter, and shortening).
H. Use lean meat or skinless poultry.
I. Eat plenty of fruits and vegetables.
J. Eat a well-balanced diet from all food groups.

III. **The client/caregiver can list foods to limit or avoid to decrease calories.**

A. Avoid concentrated sweets (empty calories) such as sugar, candy, honey, pies, cakes, cookies, and regular sodas.
B. Avoid alcohol.
C. Avoid fried foods.

D. Avoid foods high in fat, cholesterol, and sodium.
E. Avoid foods in cream or cheese sauce.

IV. **The client/caregiver can list behavior techniques to limit caloric intake.**

A. Keep a food diary that lists all food intake. Keep an exercise diary also.
B. Plan ahead for daily food intake. This includes a packed lunch and eating out.
C. Drink a glass of water before each meal. Drink sips between bits of food.
D. Eat slowly, taking small bites. Swallow food before putting more food on the utensil or taking next bit.
E. Use small plates to make the portions appear larger.
F. Eat only at the table.
G. Measure food portions.
H. Do not skip meals.
I. Plan for occasional treats.
J. Plan menus and shopping list for the week to prevent impulse buying.
K. Do not keep high-calorie foods in the house.
L. Reward yourself for weight loss, but not with food.
M. Order smaller portions when dining out. Ask for container for half of the food for later use.

V. **The client/caregiver can list general rules when choosing a diet plan.**

A. Consult physician for diet and exercise plan.
B. Avoid fad diets and rapid weight-reduction plans.
C. Set realistic goals, and plan to lose only 1 to 2 pounds per week.
D. Eat a well-balanced diet and a variety of foods to promote good nutrition.
E. Avoid fasting, which slows the metabolic rate.

(Continued)

NRS
DATE INITIAL

F. Plan a practical diet that you can follow for the rest of your life.
G. Read food labels on all packaged items.
H. Incorporate an exercise program.

Weight-loss clinics

Low-calorie cookbooks

Nutritionist

REFERENCES

Lutz, C., & Przytulski, K. (2001). *Nutrition and diet therapy.* Philadelphia: F. A. Davis Company.

Lutz, C., & Przytulski, K. (2004). *Nutri notes: Nutrition & diet therapy pocket guide.* Philadelphia: F. A. Davis Company.

Nutrition made incredibly easy. (2003). Philadelphia: Lippincott Williams & Wilkins.

Perry, A., & Potter, P. (2006). *Clinical nursing skills & technique.* St. Louis: Mosby Inc.

Taylor, C., Lillis, C., & LeMone, P. (2005). *Fundamentals of nursing.* Philadelphia: Lippincott, Williams & Wilkins.

Timby, B. K., & Smith, N. C. (2003). *Introductory medical-surgical nursing* (8th ed.). Philadelphia: J. B. Lippincott Williams & Wilkins.

RESOURCES

National Institutes of Health
www.nih.gov

The Office of the Surgeon General
www.surgeongeneral.gov/sgoffice

My Pyramid—United States Department of Agriculture
www.mypyramid.gov

Health clubs

13   High-Calorie Diet

Patient name: _____ Admission: _____

NRS
DATE INITIAL

I.   **The client/caregiver can list diseases or conditions that may impair nutritional status requiring a high-calorie diet.**

   A. Increased metabolic rate from diseases such as cancer or HIV
   B. Trauma resulting in severe wounds or burns can also increase the need for calories and proteins

II. **The client/caregiver can list foods to increase calories in the diet.**

   A. Add wheat germ to meat loaf, pancakes, and so forth.
   B. Add eggs to soups, ground meats, casseroles, and so forth.
   C. Add powdered milk to scrambled eggs, soups, gravies, ground meats, casseroles, puddings, and so forth.
   D. Add baby food to casseroles.
   E. Use milk or half-and-half instead of water when making soups or sauces.
   F. Add cheese or diced meat to foods whenever possible.
   G. Add sour cream or yogurt to vegetables.
   H. Add raisins, nuts, dates, and brown sugar to hot or cold cereals.
   I. Add sauces to vegetables.
   J. Drink high-calorie beverages with fruit, milk, buttermilk, or yogurt.
   K. Add melted butter to foods.
   L. Add ice cream and whipped cream to desserts.
   M. Eat high-calorie snacks such as nuts, dried fruit, popcorn with butter, crackers and cheese, and ice cream.
   N. Eat mayonnaise, oil, and salad dressing.
   O. Serve gravy over meat.
   P. Eat creamed or thick soups.
   Q. Enrich milk by adding 1 cup of nonfat milk with whole milk and add flavorings (i.e., fresh or frozen fruit, ice cream, or syrups).
   R. Spread butter on toast while it is hot.

NRS
DATE INITIAL

III. **The client/caregiver can list nutritional supplements available.**

   A. Carnation Instant Breakfast
   B. Milkshakes with powdered egg substitute, ice cream, or protein powder
   C. Supplements such as Ensure, Sustacal, Pulmocare, Meritene, Isocal, and Boost

IV. **The client/caregiver can list calorie-dense foods (foods that are high in calories per square inch and low in bulk).**

   A. Peanut butter has 90 calories per tablespoon (add to toast, celery, crackers, etc.).
   B. Cream cheese has 52 calories per tablespoon (add to celery, crackers, etc.).
   C. Honey has 64 calories per tablespoon (add to bread, cereal, etc.).
   D. Butter has 100 calories per tablespoon (add to soups, vegetables, mashed potatoes, cooked cereals, rice, etc.).
   E. Whipping cream has 60 calories per tablespoon (add to pies, fruit, puddings, hot chocolate, Jell-O, etc.).
   F. Roasted chopped peanuts have 52 calories per tablespoon (add to ice cream, desserts, salads, etc.).

V.   **The client/caregiver can list general measures to increase calories and promote weight gain.**

   A. Eat small, frequent meals.
   B. Keep high-calorie snacks within sight.
   C. Eat foods high in unsaturated fat. Fats have nine calories per gram while carbohydrates and proteins have four calories per gram.
   D. Avoid empty calories such as chips, candy, and carbonated beverages.
   E. Avoid low-calorie soups, salads, and beverages at the beginning of the meal, which tend to diminish the appetite.

(Continued)

| NRS |
| DATE | INITIAL |
| | |

F. Set realistic goals for weight gain daily. Weight gain of 1 pound per week may be suggested.

G. Do not skip breakfast.

RESOURCES

Registered dietitian

My Pyramid—United States Department of Agriculture
www.mypyramid.gov

REFERENCES

Lutz, C., & Przytulski, K. (2001). *Nutrition and diet therapy.* Philadelphia: F. A. Davis Company.

Lutz, C., & Przytulski, K. (2004). *Nutri notes: Nutrition & diet therapy pocket guide.* Philadelphia: F. A. Davis Company.

Nutrition made incredibly easy. (2003). Philadelphia: Lippincott Williams & Wilkins.

Perry, A., & Potter, P. (2006). *Clinical nursing skills & technique.* St. Louis: Mosby Inc.

Taylor, C., Lillis, C., & LeMone, P. (2005). *Fundamentals of nursing.* Philadelphia: Lippincott, Williams & Wilkins.

Timby, B. K., & Smith, N. C. (2003). *Introductory medical-surgical nursing* (8th ed.). Philadelphia: J. B. Lippincott Williams & Wilkins.

14   High-Protein Diet

Patient name: _____   **Admission:** _____

NRS
DATE INITIAL

I.   **The client/caregiver can state benefits of a high-protein diet.**

   A.   Essential to growth and maintenance of body tissues
   B.   Essential in maintenance of water balance
   C.   Essential in formation of antibodies to resist disease
   D.   Essential in formation of body secretions, such as hormones, enzymes, and milk
   E.   Source of energy if intake of carbohydrates and fat is deficient

II.   **The client/caregiver can list conditions requiring increased protein.**

   A.   Rapid growth periods
   B.   Pregnancy
   C.   Lactation
   D.   Convalescence
   E.   Fever and infections
   F.   Pressure ulcers and wounds
   G.   Severe stress
   H.   Burns
   I.   Diseases such as cancer, AIDS, hyperthyroidism, malabsorption syndrome, celiac disease, inflammatory bowel disease, and renal failure

III.   **The client/caregiver can list foods high in protein.**

   A.   Meat
   B.   Milk
   C.   Cheese
   D.   Eggs
   E.   Fish
   F.   Nuts
   G.   Peanut butter
   H.   Legumes (dried peas and beans)
   I.   Fish

IV.   **The client/caregiver can list measures to increase protein in diet.**

   A.   Add nonfat dry milk to regular milk.

NRS
DATE INITIAL

   B.   Add milk powder to hot or cold cereals, scrambled eggs, soups, gravies, ground meats, and casseroles.
   C.   Use milk or half-and-half instead of water.
   D.   Add diced or ground meat to soups and casseroles.
   E.   Add grated cheese to sauces, vegetables, soups, and casseroles.
   F.   Make desserts with eggs, such as sponge cake, egg custard, bread, or rice pudding.
   G.   Drink instant breakfast products.
   H.   Drink milkshakes with powdered eggs or egg substitute.

V.   **The client/caregiver can list signs and symptoms of protein deficiency.**

   A.   Weight loss
   B.   Decreased resistance to disease
   C.   Impaired healing of wounds
   D.   Weakness and fatigue
   E.   Dry, brittle hair
   F.   Mental depression

RESOURCE

My Pyramid—United States Department of Agriculture
www.mypyramid.gov

REFERENCES

Lutz, C., & Przytulski, K. (2001). *Nutrition and diet therapy.* Philadelphia: F. A. Davis Company.

Lutz, C., & Przytulski, K. (2004). *Nutri notes: Nutrition & diet therapy pocket guide.* Philadelphia: F. A. Davis Company.

Nutrition made incredibly easy. (2003). Philadelphia: Lippincott Williams & Wilkins.

Perry, A., & Potter, P. (2006). *Clinical nursing skills & technique.* St. Louis: Mosby Inc.

Taylor, C., Lillis, C., & LeMone, P. (2005). *Fundamentals of nursing.* Philadelphia: Lippincott, Williams & Wilkins.

Timby, B. K., & Smith, N. C. (2003). *Introductory medical-surgical nursing* (8th ed.). Philadelphia: J. B. Lippincott Williams & Wilkins.

15 Low-Potassium Diet

Patient name: _____ Admission: _____

NRS
DATE INITIAL

I. **The client/caregiver can list causes of high potassium (hypercalcemia) and need for reduced-potassium diets.**

A. Renal (kidney) disease and failure
B. Diabetic acidosis
C. Severe dehydration
D. Excessive cell destruction resulting from traumas such as burns or crushing injuries
E. Excessive potassium intake (intravenous potassium or potassium supplements)
F. Massive and severe infections
G. Potassium-sparing diuretics
H. Overuse of salt substitutes (contains potassium instead of sodium)

II. **The client/caregiver can list signs and symptoms of high potassium.**

A. Diarrhea or nausea
B. Muscle weakness followed by flaccid paralysis beginning in the legs
C. Sensation of numbness and tingling (paresthesias)
D. Changes in the heart rhythm
E. Cardiac fibrillation and arrest

III. **The client/caregiver can list high-potassium foods to avoid.**

A. Vegetables—bamboo shoots, beet greens, baked potato (with skin), fresh sweet potato, and cooked spinach
B. Fruits—avocado, bananas, fresh orange or mango, nectarines, papayas, and dried prunes
C. Others—bran cereals and bran products, chocolate, cocoa, molasses, salt substitute, low-sodium broth, low-sodium baking powder, low-sodium baking soda, and nuts

NRS
DATE INITIAL

IV. **The client/caregiver can list low potassium foods and beverages to use when potassium is restricted.**

A. Low-potassium foods are hard, clear candy, nondairy toppings, jams and jellies, jelly beans, lollipops, marshmallows, lifesavers, chewing gum, and cornstarch.
B. Low-potassium beverages are carbonated beverages, lemonade, cranberry juice, popsicles, Hawaiian punch, Kool-aid.

RESOURCE

My Pyramid—United States Department of Agriculture
www.mypyramid.gov

REFERENCES

Lutz, C., & Przytulski, K. (2001). *Nutrition and diet therapy.* Philadelphia: F. A. Davis Company.

Lutz, C., & Przytulski, K. (2004). *Nutri notes: Nutrition & diet therapy pocket guide.* Philadelphia: F. A. Davis Company.

Nutrition made incredibly easy. (2003). Philadelphia: Lippincott Williams & Wilkins.

Perry, A., & Potter, P. (2006). *Clinical nursing skills & technique.* St. Louis: Mosby Inc.

Taylor, C., Lillis, C., & LeMone, P. (2005). *Fundamentals of nursing.* Philadelphia: Lippincott, Williams & Wilkins.

Timby, B. K., & Smith, N. C. (2003). *Introductory medical-surgical nursing* (8th ed.). Philadelphia: J. B. Lippincott Williams & Wilkins.

16 High-Potassium Diet

Patient name: _____

Admission: _____

NRS
DATE INITIAL

I. **The client/caregiver can list causes of low potassium levels (hypokalemia) and need for increased potassium diets.**

   A. Inadequate diet—protein/calorie malnutrition
   B. Diuretics and other medications
   C. Vomiting, diarrhea, draining fistula, prolonged suctioning, and so forth
   D. Cellular trauma such as burns
   E. Large doses of corticosteroids
   F. Prolonged administration of intravenous fluids without electrolytes
   G. Laxative abuse

II. **The client/caregiver can list signs and symptoms of low potassium.**

   A. Muscle weakness and leg cramps
   B. Fatigue, weakness, and loss of appetite
   C. Nausea and vomiting
   D. Severe losses, which can lead to respiratory arrest
   E. Irregular heart rhythm (dysrhythmias) and cardiac arrest

III. **The client/caregiver can list foods high in potassium.**

   A. Vegetables—potatoes, tomatoes and tomato products, green leafy vegetables, spinach, carrots, and corn

NRS
DATE INITIAL

   B. Fruits—bananas, citrus fruits, melon, raisins, prunes, and cantaloupe
   C. Meats—veal, beef, pork, turkey, and chicken
   D. Whole grains
   E. Milk, yogurt, and ice cream
   F. Others—black beans, lentils, coffee, peanut butter, nuts, and molasses

RESOURCE

My Pyramid—United States Department of Agriculture
www.mypyramid.gov

REFERENCES

Lutz, C., & Przytulski, K. (2001). *Nutrition and diet therapy.* Philadelphia: F. A. Davis Company.

Lutz, C., & Przytulski, K. (2004). *Nutri notes: Nutrition & diet therapy pocket guide.* Philadelphia: F. A. Davis Company.

Nutrition made incredibly easy. (2003). Philadelphia: Lippincott Williams & Wilkins.

Perry, A., & Potter, P. (2006). *Clinical nursing skills & technique.* St. Louis: Mosby Inc.

Taylor, C., Lillis, C., & LeMone, P. (2005). *Fundamentals of nursing.* Philadelphia: Lippincott, Williams & Wilkins.

Timby, B. K., & Smith, N. C. (2003). *Introductory medical-surgical nursing* (8th ed.). Philadelphia: J. B. Lippincott Williams & Wilkins.

17   Lactose-Controlled Diet

Patient name: _____   Admission: _____

NRS
DATE INITIAL

I. **The client/caregiver can define lactose intolerance.**

    A. It is the inability to digest significant amounts of lactose.

    B. Lactose is the main sugar in milk.

    C. It is the result of a shortage in the enzyme lactase.

    D. The problem is more common in the following ethnic groups.
- African Americans
- Native Americans
- Asian Americans

II. **The client/caregiver can list signs and symptoms of lactose intolerance.**

    A. Symptoms appearing about 30 minutes to 2 hours after taking in foods with lactose are
- Abdominal bloating
- Gas or flatulence
- Abdominal cramps
- Diarrhea
- Nausea

III. **The client/caregiver can list measures to manage this problem.**

    A. Lactase enzymes can be taken orally to help digest lactose. They are manufactured in liquid and a chewable tablet.

    B. Some commercial foods (such as lactose-free milk) come already treated with this enzyme.

    C. Avoidance or limiting the use of milk and dairy products.

    D. Ensure alternative source of calcium if unable to tolerate milk and milk products.

IV. **The client/caregiver can list prepared foods that may contain lactose and may need to** be avoided if client has very low tolerance to lactose.

    A. Foods that may contain lactose are
- Breads and baked goods
- Processed breakfast cereals and breakfast drinks
- Instant potatoes, soups, and so forth that may contain dry milk/solids
- Salad dressings
- Mixes for pancakes, biscuits, or cookies
- Powdered coffee creamers, whipped toppings, and so forth

V. **The client/caregiver can list sources of calcium that contain no lactose.**

    A. Sources of dietary calcium for lactose intolerant clients are
- Broccoli
- Collard or turnip greens
- Kale
- Raw oysters
- Salmon with bones (canned)
- Sardines
- Molasses
- Tofu

REFERENCES

Cohen, B. J., & Taylor, J. J. (2005). *Memmler's the human body in health and disease* (10th ed.). Philadelphia: Lippincott Williams & Wilkins.

Lutz, C., & Przytulski, K. (2001). *Nutrition and diet therapy.* Philadelphia: F. A. Davis Company.

Nutrition made incredibly easy. (2003). Philadelphia: Lippincott Williams & Wilkins.

Perry, A., & Potter, P. (2006). *Clinical nursing skills & technique.* St. Louis: Mosby Inc.

Taylor, C., Lillis, C., & LeMone, P. (2005). *Fundamentals of nursing.* Philadelphia: Lippincott, Williams & Wilkins.

Timby, B. K., & Smith, N. C. (2003). *Introductory medical-surgical nursing* (8th ed.). Philadelphia: J. B. Lippincott Williams & Wilkins.

18   Low-Residue Diet

Patient name: _____   **Admission:** _____

NRS
DATE INITIAL

I. **The client/caregiver can define a low residue diet and its uses.**

  A. It is a diet restricted with residue and fiber. Residue is the solid material in the large intestine after the major digestion process.

  B. Foods on a low-residue diet should be easily absorbed and digested (primarily in the small intestines).

  C. It can be used
    1. As part of a bowel preparation prior to surgery
    2. For treatment of severe diarrhea
    3. As part of the progression of diets after bowel surgery
    4. In acute phases of inflammatory bowel disease

  D. Low-residue diets should not be used long term.

II. **The client/caregiver can list recommendations in each food group to use with a low-residue diet.**

  A. Foods to use with low residue diet
    1. Breads and cereals—white bread, refined cereals (such as cream of wheat), crackers without whole grains or seeds, rice, noodles, and so forth
    2. Fruits—juices without pulp, ripe bananas, strained fruits, cooked or canned apples, peaches, or pears
    3. Vegetables—juice without pulp, lettuce, cooked or canned asparagus, beets, carrots, pumpkin, acorn squash, seedless tomatoes, and white or sweet potatoes without skins
    4. Meat, poultry, fish, eggs—lean tender meat without grease, ground or well-

cooked beef, lamb, ham, veal, pork, poultry, fish, and eggs (except fried eggs)
    5. Milk and milk products—limited as per order from physician

III. **The client/caregiver can list foods to avoid or to decrease while on a low-residue diet.**

  A. Foods to decrease or avoid using on a low-residue diet
    1. Whole-grain breads, breads with seeds, nuts or bran, whole grain rice, or pasta
    2. Fruits—prunes and prune juice and dried fruits
    3. Vegetables—dried peas and beans, potato skins or chips, and fried potatoes
    4. Meats—tough, fried or spiced meats, and fried eggs

REFERENCES

Lutz, C., & Przytulski, K. (2001). *Nutrition and diet therapy.* Philadelphia: F. A. Davis Company.

Lutz, C., & Przytulski, K. (2004). *Nutri notes: Nutrition & diet therapy pocket guide.* Philadelphia: F. A. Davis Company.

Nutrition made incredibly easy. (2003). Philadelphia: Lippincott Williams & Wilkins.

Perry, A., & Potter, P. (2006). *Clinical nursing skills & technique.* St. Louis: Mosby Inc.

Taylor, C., Lillis, C., & LeMone, P. (2005). *Fundamentals of nursing.* Philadelphia: Lippincott, Williams & Wilkins.

Timby, B. K., & Smith, N. C. (2003). *Introductory medical-surgical nursing* (8th ed.). Philadelphia: J. B. Lippincott Williams & Wilkins.

19   Gastroesophageal Reflux Disease (GERD) Diet

Patient name: _____   Admission: _____

NRS DATE INITIAL		

I. The client/caregiver can explain GERD.

   A. It is symptoms and/or tissue damage of the esophagus from repeated exposure to the acid contents of the stomach. Complaints are of persistent heartburn or a burning sensation in the upper chest or abdomen areas.

II. The client/caregiver can list measures to prevent or manage symptoms of GERD.

   A. Dietary modifications are the following:
     1. Decrease total fat intake.
     2. Avoid large meals.
     3. Decrease total caloric intake if needed to reach healthy weight.
     4. Avoid chocolate.
     5. Avoid coffee (regular or decaffeinated) if produces symptoms.
     6. Avoid other irritants such as alcohol, mint, carbonated beverages, citrus juice, or tomato products.
   B. Other measures to treat GERD are the following:
     1. Maintain upright posture during and after eating.
     2. Do not smoke.
     3. Avoid wearing clothing that is tight in the abdominal area.
     4. Avoid eating within 3 hours before bedtime.

NRS DATE INITIAL		

     5. If overweight, lose weight.
     6. Sleep on left side.
     7. Chew a non-mint gum, which will increase saliva and decrease acid in esophagus.
     8. Elevate the head of your bed 4 to 6 inches by placing bricks or blocks of wood under the headboard.

RESOURCE

The American College of Gastroenterology
www.acg.gi.org/

REFERENCES

Lutz, C., & Przytulski, K. (2001). *Nutrition and diet therapy.* Philadelphia: F. A. Davis Company.

Lutz, C., & Przytulski, K. (2004). *Nutri notes: Nutrition & diet therapy pocket guide.* Philadelphia: F. A. Davis Company.

Nutrition made incredibly easy. (2003). Philadelphia: Lippincott Williams & Wilkins.

Perry, A., & Potter, P. (2006). *Clinical nursing skills & technique.* St. Louis: Mosby Inc.

Taylor, C., Lillis, C., & LeMone, P. (2005). *Fundamentals of nursing.* Philadelphia: Lippincott, Williams & Wilkins.

Timby, B. K., & Smith, N. C. (2003). *Introductory medical-surgical nursing* (8th ed.). Philadelphia: J. B. Lippincott Williams & Wilkins.

20 Vegetarian Diet

■ Patient name: _____   Admission: _____

I.   The client/caregiver can define the types of vegetarian diets.

A. Ovolactovegetarian does not permit meat, fish, or poultry. They do eat dairy products and eggs.
B. Lactovegetarian does not permit meat, fish, poultry, or eggs. They do eat dairy products.
C. Ovovegetarian does not permit meat, fish, poultry, or dairy products. They do eat eggs.
D. Vegan does not permit meat, fish, poultry, dairy products, or eggs.

II. The client/caregiver can list measures to meet daily protein requirements when on a vegetarian diet.

A. Eat variety of foods from all food groups.
B. Use complementary plant proteins together to provide essential amino acids.
C. Consume enough calories to maintain your lifestyle and body's needs.
D. Use low-fat or nonfat products.
E. Use moderation in eating nuts and seeds to maintain a low-fat diet.
F. Use whole grains for fiber and iron content.
G. Include vitamin C at every meal to help with iron absorption.
H. Use vitamin supplements under physician's direction.

III. The client/caregiver can list plant sources of protein.

A. Plant sources of protein are
   • Bread, cereal, rice, pasta, oatmeal, and whole grain breads
   • Dark green and deep yellow vegetables (such as green beans and peas)
   • Soybeans, navy beans, kidney beans, black-eyed peas, and baby lima beans
   • Soybean sprouts and mung bean sprouts
   • Peanut butter, cashew nuts, English walnuts, almonds, and sesame seeds

B. Legumes are plants that have roots containing nitrogen-fixing bacteria to increase the nitrogen content. They are an excellent source of plant protein for the vegetarian. Examples of legumes are peas, beans, lentils, and peanuts.

IV. The client/caregiver can list the pros and cons of a vegetarian diet.

A. A vegetarian diet is healthy in that it is usually low in fat and cholesterol and high in fiber.
B. Special attention is needed to avoid deficiencies of calcium, vitamin B12, iron, and zinc. Vegetarian sources are
   1. Calcium—low-fat dairy foods, spinach, turnips, collard greens, kale, broccoli, tofu, and soy milk
   2. Vitamin B12—enriched cereals, fortified soy products, or supplements.
   3. Iron—dried beans and peas, lentils, enriched cereals, and whole-grain products. Mix them with foods high in vitamin C, such as strawberries, citrus fruits, tomatoes, cabbage, or broccoli to aid in the absorption of iron.
   4. Zinc—whole grains, soy products, nuts, and wheat germ.

REFERENCES

Lutz, C., & Przytulski, K. (2001). *Nutrition and diet therapy.* Philadelphia: F. A. Davis Company.

Lutz, C., & Przytulski, K. (2004). *Nutri notes: Nutrition & diet therapy pocket guide.* Philadelphia: F. A. Davis Company.

Nutrition made incredibly easy. (2003). Philadelphia: Lippincott Williams & Wilkins.

Perry, A., & Potter, P. (2006). *Clinical nursing skills & technique.* St. Louis: Mosby Inc.

Taylor, C., Lillis, C., & LeMone, P. (2005). *Fundamentals of nursing.* Philadelphia: Lippincott, Williams & Wilkins.

Timby, B. K., & Smith, N. C. (2003). *Introductory medical-surgical nursing* (8th ed.). Philadelphia: J. B. Lippincott Williams & Wilkins.

21 Diabetic Diet

Patient name: _____ Admission: _____

<table>
<tr><td>NRS
DATE INITIAL</td></tr>
</table>

I. The client/caregiver can explain nutrition therapy for treatment of diabetes.

A. The goal for nutrition therapy with diabetes is to control the blood glucose levels. This can be done by
1. Establishing a routine for eating meals and snacks at regular times every day
2. Choosing healthy foods in the correct amounts at each meal
3. Eating the same amount of carbohydrates at each meal or snack, thus keeping blood sugar from going too high or too low during the day
4. Having weight reduction if overweight
5. Complying with any ordered drug therapy

B. There are several methods to help develop an individual eating plan. The following suggestions are
1. The glycemic index is one method of counting carbohydrates or maintaining a consistent carbohydrate diet. Foods with a high glycemic index number will increase blood sugar levels more than a food with a lower number.
2. Food exchange system is when groups of foods are put into categories. One serving in any group is called an exchange. This means an exchange from one group can be traded for a serving in another group.
3. Consistent amounts of each macronutrient (carbohydrates, fats, and proteins) each day. Carbohydrates should consist of 45% to 65% of daily calories. Proteins should consist of 15% to 20% of daily calories. Fats should consist of 20% to 35% of daily calories.

<table>
<tr><td>NRS
DATE INITIAL</td></tr>
</table>

II. The client/caregiver can list general healthy diabetic eating habits.

A. Limit amount of sweets.
B. Eat often but in smaller amounts.
C. Watch when and how many carbohydrates are eaten.
D. Include lots of whole-grain foods and fruits and vegetables.
E. Eat less fat.
F. Limit the use of alcohol.

RESOURCES

Dietician

Diabetic Nurse Educator (American Association of Diabetes Educators)
http://members.aadenet.org/Scriptcontent/map.cfm

American Diabetes Association
www.diabetes.org

National Diabetes Information Clearinghouse
http://diabetes.niddk.nih.gov/

REFERENCES

Lutz, C., & Przytulski, K. (2001). *Nutrition and diet therapy.* Philadelphia: F. A. Davis Company.

Lutz, C., & Przytulski, K. (2004). *Nutri notes: Nutrition & diet therapy pocket guide.* Philadelphia: F. A. Davis Company.

Nutrition made incredibly easy. (2003). Philadelphia: Lippincott Williams & Wilkins.

Perry, A., & Potter, P. (2006). *Clinical nursing skills & technique.* St. Louis: Mosby Inc.

Taylor, C., Lillis, C., & LeMone, P. (2005). *Fundamentals of nursing.* Philadelphia: Lippincott, Williams & Wilkins.

Timby, B. K., & Smith, N. C. (2003). *Introductory medical-surgical nursing* (8th ed.). Philadelphia: J. B. Lippincott Williams & Wilkins.

Part VI

Medication Administration and Classification

Teaching Guides

1

Medication Administration
(Route of Administration)

Patient name: _____   **Admission:** _____

NRS
DATE INITIAL

I. **The client/caregiver can list measures used when administering medication to the eye (ophthalmic).**

A. Wash your hands. Read label.
B. Hold the bottle upside down.
C. Tilt your head back and look upward.
D. Hold the bottle in one hand, and place it as close as possible to the inner aspect of the eye.
E. With the other hand, pull down lower eyelid to form pocket.
F. Place correct number of drops into the pocket.
G. Avoid touching eye with tip of applicator.
H. If using more than one eyedrop medication, be sure to wait at least 5 minutes before second medication.
I. Close eye, or press lower lid lightly.
J. If applying ophthalmic ointment, apply thin line of ointment evenly along the inner edge of the lower lid (from inner to outer edge).

II. **The client/caregiver can list steps when administering ear drops.**

A. Wash hands. Read label.
B. Have client positioned with ear facing up. Stabilize head by placing hand on head.
C. Check for occlusion of outer ear canal with cerumen or drainage. Wipe outer canal with cotton-tipped applicator.
D. Check positioning of pinna before medication.
   1. For adults and children older than 3 years old, gently pull the pinna up and back.
   2. For children younger than 3 years old, gently pull down and back.
E. Hold the dropper 0.5 inch above ear canal, and instill ordered amount of drops.
F. Suggest that the client remains in same position for 5 to 10 minutes.

NRS
DATE INITIAL

G. If ordered, a cotton ball may be placed in the outer part of ear canal. Do not press into canal.

III. **The client/caregiver can explain steps to administer nasal drops or spray.**

A. Wash hands. Read label.
B. Ask client to blow nose to clear nasal passages.
C. Client should open and breathe through their mouth.
D. Hold tip above nostril (without touching), and direct medication toward the top of the nasal cavity.
E. Suggest client stay in position for 5 minutes.

IV. **The client/caregiver can list steps to apply transdermal medication.**

A. Read the manufacturer's instruction regarding application site and frequency of changing.
B. Apply gloves before handling medication to avoid absorption of medication.
C. Remove previous medication patch and cleanse area.
D. Press patch to clean, dry, and hairless skin.
E. Rotate sites to prevent skin irritation.
F. Label patch with date, time, and initials.
G. Discard old patch and gloves safely, keeping away from children.

V. **The client/caregiver can list steps to administer vaginal medication.**

A. Apply gloves, open suppository, or measure cream in provided syringe.
B. Lubricate rounded end of suppository.
C. Expose vaginal opening by separating the labia.
D. Insert rounded end of suppository along the posterior wall of vagina as far as it will pass.

(Continued)

NRS
DATE INITIAL

E. If using a cream, jelly, or foam, insert applicator along posterior wall and push plunger until empty.

VI.   **The client/caregiver can list steps to administer rectal suppositories.**

A. Lie on left side with knees pulled toward chest.
B. Apply gloves and open suppository. Lubricate the round end.
C. Gently insert the lubricated suppository into the rectum.
D. Remain in same position to prevent expulsion of the suppository.

VII.   **The client/caregiver can explain the method of Metered-Dose inhaler administration.**

A. Inhalers are hand-held pressurized devices that deliver a premeasured amount of medication to the respiratory system. It is delivered in a fine mist or spray.
B. Wash hands. Read medication label to check accurate medication and dose. Read any manufacturer's instructions.
C. Remove cover, and shake if indicated.
D. Hold inhaler in dominant hand and use inhaler in one of two ways:
   1. Place inhaler in mouth with opening toward back of throat, closing lips tightly around it or
   2. Position device 1 to 2 inches in front of widely opened mouth. Lips should not touch the inhaler.
E. Take deep breath and exhale. Depress medication canister with inhaler in place. Breathe in slowly, and hold breath for 10 seconds.
F. Remove inhaler, and exhale through nose or using pursed lips.
G. If using a spacer device with inhaler
   1. Remove mouthpiece cover from inhaler and spacer.
   2. Insert inhaler into the end of the spacer device.
   3. Continue as described previously.
H. Precautions when using inhaler are
   1. Use inhaler only as ordered by physician.
   2. If using bronchodilator with other medication, always use the bronchodilator first.
   3. Wait about 5 to 10 minutes between the two medications.

NRS
DATE INITIAL

VIII.   **The client/caregiver can list important points to remember when giving oral medications.**

A. Medications are most commonly given in tablet or capsule form.
B. Some medications are enteric coated and designed to dissolve in the small intestines. This is to avoid exposure to acids in the stomach. These medications should not be crushed.
C. Other medications have been designed to dissolve very slowly by creating a sustained-release tablet or capsule. They can be extended-release, long-acting, or slow-release tablets. They too should not be crushed or opened.
D. Client should be seated or in side-lying position to avoid aspiration.
E. Sublingual administered medications are placed under the tongue and allowed to dissolve.
F. Buccal-administered medications should be placed in mouth against the mucous membrane until dissolved.
G. Lozenges should not be chewed or swallowed.
H. Powdered medications mixed in liquid should be taken immediately after mixing.
I. Ensure that the client has safely swallowed medication.

IX.   **The client/caregiver can list measures to administer oral medications in tablet form.**

A. Wash hands. Read label.
B. Offer sips of liquid prior to medications for those people with a dry mouth.
C. If client has difficulty swallowing, (and there are no contraindications), pills may be crushed. Mix crushed medication in small amount of soft food (pudding, applesauce, etc.).
D. Rinse oral cavity, and offer or provide mouth care as needed.

X.   **The client/caregiver can list measures to administer liquid medication.**

A. Wash hands. Read label.
B. If medication is a suspension, shake well before using.
C. Do not use silverware spoons to measure or give medications.

(Continued)

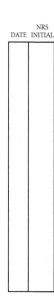

NRS
DATE INITIAL

D. Measuring spoons are accurate, but can spill easily.

E. Oral syringes or dosing cups can be used. Caution: The Food and Drug Administration has reports of young children choking on syringe caps. Caution: Do not use hypodermic syringe or syringe with a needle.

F. Measure into the dosing cup at eye level to be accurate.

G. Hold the bottle with label against palm of hand while pouring. This prevents future difficulty in reading label caused by spillage.

H. Flavorings can be added to liquid medications to improve taste.

RESOURCES

Health care provider

Pharmacist

Prepared information provided with medication by pharmacist and manufacturer

REFERENCES

Ackley, B. J., & Ladwig, G. B. (2006). *Nursing diagnosis handbook: A guide to planning care*. St. Louis: Mosby Elsevier.

Adams, M. P., Josephson, D. L., & Holland, L. N. Jr. (2005). *Pharmacology for nurses: A pathophysiologic approach*. Upper Saddle River, NJ: Pearson Education, Inc.

Deglin, J. F., & Vallerand, A. H. (2001). *Davis's drug guide for nurses*. Philadelphia: F. A. Davis Company.

Hunt, R. (2005). *Introduction to community based nursing*. Philadelphia: Lippincott Williams & Wilkins.

Nursing 2006 drug handbook. (2006). Philadelphia: Lippincott Williams and Wilkins.

Perry, A., & Potter, P. (2006). *Clinical nursing skills & technique*. St. Louis: Mosby Inc.

Rice, J. (1998). *Medications mathematics for the nurse*. Albany, NY: Delmar.

2 Medication Safety

Patient name: _____   Admission: _____

I. **The client/caregiver will list information to communicate with physician.**

A. Create a list of all medicines, vitamins, and herbal and/or dietary supplements that you are currently taking. Keep this list up to date. Make a copy of this list, and place it in safe place in an available location for emergencies.

B. Provide this list of medicines to all physicians and health care providers you visit. They need to have all this information before prescribing new medications or making changes.

C. Always check with physician before taking any nonprescription medication or over-the-counter products such as a laxative or aspirin.

D. Discuss the use of vitamins, minerals, and any dietary or herbal supplement before using.

E. Provide health care team with information regarding medicine allergies. Also, list any documented food (shellfish, etc.) or environmental allergies.

F. Learn the generic and brand name of your medications. They may look different; thus, check with pharmacist if in doubt.

G. Learn about any tests needed during use of medication.

H. Be aware of how many refills your physician has ordered.

I. Know the reason you are taking each medication.

J. Read the label each time you take medication.

K. Remember to take medications. Use a memory aid such as calendar and pill box.

II. **The client/caregiver can list information to discuss with pharmacist.**

A. Make sure that you can read and understand the prescription label.
    1. Ask for large print on the label if impaired vision is a problem.

2. Ask pharmacist to write the label in language (words) that you can understand.

B. Try to use the same pharmacy for all your medications.
    1. They will have a complete and up-to-date listing of your medications.
    2. They can monitor your medication for possible problems or interactions.

C. Read the attached information regarding your medications that come with each prescription.

D. Review the generic and brand name on your medications.

E. Clarify with the pharmacist information such as
    1. Interactions with foods, alcohol, or other medications
    2. Activity to avoid while taking medications
    3. Instructions about taking medication with food or on empty stomach

F. Ask for special lids on bottle if having problem opening medication.

III. **The client/caregiver can list general measures to promote safe and accurate medication administration.**

A. Read the label carefully in a well-lighted room. Check label for accurate information. Follow the "five rights" rule.
    1. Right medication
    2. Right dose
    3. Right person
    4. Right route
    5. Right time

B. Check label for expiration date.

C. Do not write over label prepared by pharmacist.

D. Do not combine different medications in same prescription bottles.

E. Do not store medication near heat or humidity. Avoid areas in bathroom or near sink or stove.

(Continued)

NRS
DATE INITIAL

F. Do not share prescribed medication with other people.

G. Store medications out of the reach of children.

H. Plan ahead to reorder so no doses are missed.

I. Take all medications as ordered (complete antibiotic prescriptions).

J. Report any side effects or problems to physician.

K. Read the label each time you take medication.

L. Remember to take medications. Use a memory aid such as a calendar, chart, or medication box that can be prefilled for a week's supply.

M. Ask pharmacist or physician what to do if doses are missed.

IV. **The client/caregiver states adequate knowledge of each medication.**

A. Side effects of medication and what side effects should be reported to physician.

B. Recommendations for when to take medication in relation to meals or appropriate time of day.

C. Generic and brand names.

D. Any special safety precautions (i.e., decreased alertness makes certain activities dangerous and avoid taking with aspirin).

RESOURCES
Health care provider

Pharmacist

REFERENCES

Ackley, B. J., & Ladwig, G. B. (2006). *Nursing diagnosis handbook: A guide to planning care.* St. Louis: Mosby Elsevier.

Adams, M. P., Josephson, D. L., & Holland, L. N. Jr. (2005). *Pharmacology for nurses: A pathophysiologic approach.* Upper Saddle River, NJ: Pearson Education, Inc.

Deglin, J. F., & Vallerand, A. H. (2001). *Davis's drug guide for nurses.* Philadelphia: F. A. Davis Company.

Hunt, R. (2005). *Introduction to community based nursing.* Philadelphia: Lippincott Williams & Wilkins.

Nursing 2006 drug handbook. (2006). Philadelphia: Lippincott Williams and Wilkins.

Perry, A., & Potter, P. (2006). *Clinical nursing skills & technique.* St. Louis: Mosby Inc.

Rice, J. (1998). *Medications mathematics for the nurse.* Albany, NY: Delmar.

Your medicine: Play it safe. Patient Guide. AHRQ Publication No. 03-0019 (February 2003). Available from: *www.ahrq .gov/consumer/safemeds/safemeds.htm.* Bethesda, MD: Agency for Healthcare Research and Quality and Rockville, MD: National Council on Patient Information and Education.

Circulatory and Cardiac Medications

Patient name: _____   **Admission:** _____

<small>NRS
DATE INITIAL</small>

I. The client/caregiver can define the classifications of cardiac and circulatory medications.

  A. Antihypertensive drugs are used to lower blood pressure to a normal level.
  B. Antianginal drugs are used to treat and prevent attacks of chest pain (angina).
  C. Antiarrhythmic drugs are used to correct cardiac arrhythmias (irregular heart beats).

II. The client/caregiver can describe the desired results of each type of medication.

  A. The effective use of antihypertensives will result in decreased blood pressure to normal levels.
  B. Antianginal agents should decrease the frequency and severity of any chest pain. The client should be able to increase their level of activity without chest pain.
  C. Antiarrhythmic drug therapy should resolve the arrhythmia without untoward side effects from medication.

III. The client/caregiver can list important assessments and evaluations for cardiac medications.

  A. Monitor blood pressure and pulse at regular times. Blood pressure and pulse should be taken weekly, and any significant changes should be reported to the physician.
  B. Teach client/caregiver how to take pulse to monitor rate and rhythm. Report any pulse

<small>NRS
DATE INITIAL</small>

  rate below 50 or above 120 to physician, and ask for directions in whether to take medication.
  C. Instruct the client to take medication as prescribed.
  D. Advise client to report to physician before taking any supplements or over-the-counter medications.
  E. Caution client/caregiver to monitor for any signs of dizziness or lightheadedness when moving to a standing position.
  F. Monitor supply, and refill medications as needed.
  G. Encourage other recommendations for control of heart disease such as increased exercise, required diet restrictions, and maintenance of healthy weight.
  H. Monitor any episodes of chest pain, shortness of breath, or dizziness. Report any changes to physician.
  I. Maintain follow-up visits to physician.
  J. Advise client to carry identification to include the disease and medications used.

REFERENCES

Ackley, B. J., & Ladwig, G. B. (2006). *Nursing diagnosis handbook: A guide to planning care*. St. Louis: Mosby Elsevier.

Deglin, J. H., & Vallerand, A. H. (2001). *Davis's drug guide for nurses*. Philadelphia: F. A. Davis Company.

Nursing 2006 drug handbook. (2006). Philadelphia: Lippincott Williams and Wilkins.

Rice, J. (1998). *Medications mathematics for the nurse*. Albany, NY: Delmar.

2

Anticoagulant and Antiplatelet Agents

Patient name: _____

Admission: _____

NRS
DATE INITIAL

I. **The client/caregiver can define the purpose and action of oral anticoagulant and antiplatelet agents.**

A. The anticoagulant and antiplatelet medication is used to treat or prevent a blood clot that could result in a heart attack, stroke, and other life-threatening problems.

B. The medications discussed here are to be taken as oral medication.

II. **The client/caregiver can list important assessments and evaluations used when taking oral anticoagulants.**

A. Report any signs of bleeding (nosebleeds, bleeding gums, or blood in urine) or bruising promptly.

B. Avoid taking drugs that may increase the risk of bleeding, such as aspirin or nonsteroidal antiinflammatory drugs without approval of physician.

C. Instruct client to avoid activities with high risk of injury.

NRS
DATE INITIAL

D. Male clients should use electric razor.

E. Take medication exactly as prescribed.

F. Have blood work done at times specified by physician.

G. Keep all follow-up visits with physician.

H. Keep record of any medication changes your physician may give over the phone as a result of recent laboratory tests.

I. Read food labels. Any foods or supplements that contain vitamin K may impair the effectiveness of anticoagulant medication.

REFERENCES

Ackley, B. J., & Ladwig, G. B. (2006). *Nursing diagnosis handbook: A guide to planning care*. St. Louis: Mosby Elsevier.

Deglin, J. H., & Vallerand, A. H. (2001). *Davis's drug guide for nurses*. Philadelphia: F. A. Davis Company.

Nursing 2006 drug handbook. (2006). Philadelphia: Lippincott Williams and Wilkins.

Rice, J. (1998). *Medications mathematics for the nurse*. Albany, NY: Delmar.

3 Anticonvulsants

Patient name: _____   Admission: _____

NRS
DATE INITIAL

I. **The client/caregiver can define purpose and action of anticonvulsant medications.**

A. Anticonvulsants work with the central nervous system.
B. They depress any abnormal neuronal activity in the central nervous system that can produce seizure activity.

II. **The client/caregiver can describe the desired outcome when using these medications.**

A. Seizure activity will be eliminated without having adverse reactions.
B. Do not stop medications abruptly. Call your physician immediately if having problems.
C. Be aware of type or types of seizure prior to starting medication. Keep record of any seizure activity during use of medication.

III. **The client/caregiver can list important teaching tips and possible adverse reactions.**

A. Advise patient to avoid driving and other activities that require mental alertness until the effect of the specific drug is known.
B. Keep track of medication supply so as not to interrupt use. Do not stop abruptly.

NRS
DATE INITIAL

C. Watch for behavior changes, especially in children and older persons.
D. Report to physician if pregnancy is suspected.
E. Check medication label and discuss with pharmacist for any specific instructions in taking this type of medication, such as storage or if to be taken with food.
F. Acute or chronic alcohol abuse will interfere with this type of drug.
G. Wear a Medic Alert identification.
H. Avoid over-the-counter medications without consulting with physician.
I. Monitor for vitamin D, vitamin K, folic acid, and vitamin B deficiencies.

REFERENCES

Ackley, B. J., & Ladwig, G. B. (2006). *Nursing diagnosis handbook: A guide to planning care*. St. Louis: Mosby Elsevier.

Adams, M. P., Josephson, D. L., & Holland, L. N. Jr. (2005). *Pharmacology for nurses: A pathophysiologic approach*. Upper Saddle River, NJ: Pearson Education, Inc.

Deglin, J. H., & Vallerand, A. H. (2001). *Davis's drug guide for nurses*. Philadelphia: F. A. Davis Company.

Nursing 2006 drug handbook. (2006). Philadelphia: Lippincott Williams and Wilkins.

Rice, J. (1998). *Medications mathematics for the nurse*. Albany, NY: Delmar.

Antidepressants and Antianxiety Agents

4

NRS
DATE INITIAL

I. **The client/caregiver can define purpose and action of antidepressant medication.**

A. These drugs prevent or relieve the symptoms of depression.

B. Many of these drugs also are used to treat social anxiety disorders, obsessive compulsive disorders, panic disorders, chronic pain, some eating disorders, premenstrual dysphoric disorder, and posttraumatic stress disorders.

C. Antidepressants work by two methods. One method is to inhibit the uptake of serotonin. Another method is the tricyclic which increases the amount of norepinephrine and serotonin by blocking their reuptake.

D. Tricyclic antidepressants should not be given with monoamine oxidase inhibitor.

E. Antidepressants can be prescribed for short-term or continual use.

II. **The client/caregiver can describe the desired outcome when using these medications.**

A. Relief of symptoms of depression and decrease in anxiety levels without adverse effects.

NRS
DATE INITIAL

III. **The client/caregiver can list important teaching tips and possible adverse reactions.**

A. These drugs may impair mental and/or physical abilities such as driving or using heavy equipment.

B. Advise client not to use alcohol or over-the-counter medications without checking with physician first.

C. Advise physician if client becomes pregnant or is planning a pregnancy.

D. These medications should be kept out of the reach of children.

E. Encourage client/caregiver to contact physician if symptoms do not improve.

F. Report any suspicion or thoughts of suicide at once.

G. Side effects can range from dry mouth, hives, and constipation to urinary retention and dizziness or drowsiness.

REFERENCES

Ackley, B. J., & Ladwig, G. B. (2006). *Nursing diagnosis handbook: A guide to planning care.* St. Louis: Mosby Elsevier.

Adams, M. P., Josephson, D. L., & Holland, L. N. Jr. (2005). *Pharmacology for nurses: A pathophysiologic approach.* Upper Saddle River, NJ: Pearson Education, Inc.

Deglin, J. H., & Vallerand, A. H. (2001). *Davis's drug guide for nurses.* Philadelphia: F. A. Davis Company.

Nursing 2006 drug handbook. (2006). Philadelphia: Lippincott Williams and Wilkins.

Rice, J. (1998). *Medications mathematics for the nurse.* Albany, NY: Delmar.

5 Analgesics—Nonsteroidal Antiinflammatory, Nonopioid Analgesics, and Antipyretics

Patient name: _____ Admission: _____

NRS
DATE INITIAL

I. **The client/caregiver can define purpose of nonopioid analgesic medication.**

   A. Nonopioid analgesic medications include nonsteroidal antiinflammatory drugs and another group, including acetaminophen, aspirin, and ibuprofen.
   B. Nonsteroidal antiinflammatory drugs (NSAIDs) are used for mild to moderate pain, especially when pain is from condition having inflammation.
   C. Acetaminophen, aspirin, and ibuprofen are also used for the relief of mild to moderate pain. They also are very effective for reducing fevers.

II. **The client/caregiver can list the advantages of the use of nonopioid analgesic medications.**

   A. Acetaminophen, aspirin, and ibuprofen are available over the counter and are relatively inexpensive.
   B. These can be taken orally and can be given in liquid form for children or others who are have difficulty swallowing.

III. **The client/caregiver can list cautions when using these medications.**

   A. Use extreme caution in giving aspirin to children or adolescents.
   B. Use with caution for clients having long history of alcohol use.
   C. Acetaminophen can appear in breast milk.
   D. NSAIDs should be used with caution for clients with a history of bleeding disorders, gastric ulcers, and severe liver or kidney disease or during pregnancy.

NRS
DATE INITIAL

IV. **The client/caregiver can list possible side effects when taking these medications.**

   A. If taking high doses of these medications, monitor for symptoms of toxicity kidneys, such as frequent or painful urination. Also, bloody urine should be reported.
   B. Allergic reactions to these drugs may produce a rash or itch.
   C. Other undesired side effects would be nausea, abdominal pain, loss of appetite, dizziness, or drowsiness.

V. **The client/caregiver can list important teaching facts when taking this class of drugs.**

   A. Goals of the pain relief medication and how to classify level of pain.
   B. Obtaining routine laboratory tests to monitor for liver or kidney damage.
   C. Enteric-coated medication should not be crushed.
   D. To decrease gastrointestinal symptoms, medication should be taken with food and plenty of fluids.

REFERENCES

Ackley, B. J., & Ladwig, G. B. (2006). *Nursing diagnosis handbook: A guide to planning care.* St. Louis: Mosby Elsevier.

Adams, M. P., Josephson, D. L., & Holland, L. N. Jr. (2005). *Pharmacology for nurses: A pathophysiologic approach.* Upper Saddle River, NJ: Pearson Education, Inc.

Deglin, J. H., & Vallerand, A. H. (2001). *Davis's drug guide for nurses.* Philadelphia: F. A. Davis Company.

Nursing 2006 drug handbook. (2006). Philadelphia: Lippincott Williams and Wilkins.

Rice, J. (1998). *Medications mathematics for the nurse.* Albany, NY: Delmar.

6 Oral Antidiabetic Agents

Patient name: _____ Admission: _____

NRS
DATE INITIAL

I. **The client/caregiver can define purpose and action of antidiabetic medication.**

   A. These oral medications help to lower the glucose levels in type 2 diabetes.
   B. They may be also used with insulin for the treatment of type 1 diabetes.

II. **The client/caregiver can describe the desired outcome when using these medications.**

   A. Along with proper dietary and lifestyle changes (i.e., exercise and healthy weight), these medications help lower the serum glucose levels to normal levels. With diabetic teaching, the desired glucose levels will be discussed.
   B. These medications treat but do not cure diabetes.
   C. The client/caregiver should be aware that changes in medications and/or use of insulin may be necessary to maintain desired glucose levels.

NRS
DATE INITIAL

III. **The client/caregiver can list important teaching tips and possible adverse reactions.**

   A. Advise client to wear a medical alert identification.
   B. Take medication exactly as prescribed.
   C. Instruct client/caregiver in proper diet as listed in nutritional section.
   D. The client/caregiver will learn how and when to monitor blood glucose levels.
   E. The client/caregiver will be able to recognize signs and symptoms of hypoglycemia.
   F. Review with client/caregiver the general diabetic teaching regimen.

REFERENCES

Ackley, B. J., & Ladwig, G. B. (2006). *Nursing diagnosis handbook: A guide to planning care.* St. Louis: Mosby Elsevier.

Adams, M. P., Josephson, D. L., & Holland, L. N. Jr. (2005). *Pharmacology for nurses: A pathophysiologic approach.* Upper Saddle River, NJ: Pearson Education, Inc.

Deglin, J. H., & Vallerand, A. H. (2001). *Davis's drug guide for nurses.* Philadelphia: F. A. Davis Company.

Nursing 2006 drug handbook. (2006). Philadelphia: Lippincott Williams and Wilkins.

7   Lipid-Lowering Medications

Patient name: _____   Admission: _____

<table>
<tr><td>NRS
DATE INITIAL</td></tr>
</table>

I. **The client/caregiver can describe indications for this class of medication.**

   A. They are used in addition to dietary and lifestyle changes to reduce total cholesterol and triglyceride levels.

II. **The client/caregiver can list important medication teaching and concerns.**

   A. Knowledge and evaluation of client's understanding of dietary management.

   B. Avoid alcohol. Use this medication with caution if documented history of alcohol abuse.

   C. Notify physician if pregnancy is planned or suspected.

   D. Monitor cholesterol and triglyceride levels as prescribed. Physician may also want to monitor liver function during therapy.

   E. Monitor for deficiencies of fat-soluble vitamins (vitamins A, D, E, and K).

   F. Report unexplained muscle pain, weakness, fever, or unexplained numbness or tingling in feet and hands.

   G. Ask pharmacist for specific instruction on how to take medication (with or without food, time of day, etc.).

   H. Monitor bowel habits for constipation or diarrhea. A high-fiber diet and fluids can be used for constipation.

REFERENCES

Ackley, B. J., & Ladwig, G. B. (2006). *Nursing diagnosis handbook: A guide to planning care*. St. Louis: Mosby Elsevier.

Adams, M. P., Josephson, D. L., & Holland, L. N. Jr. (2005). *Pharmacology for nurses: A pathophysiologic approach*. Upper Saddle River, NJ: Pearson Education, Inc.

Deglin, J. H., & Vallerand, A. H. (2001). *Davis's drug guide for nurses*. Philadelphia: F. A. Davis Company.

Nursing 2006 drug handbook. (2006). Philadelphia: Lippincott Williams and Wilkins.

8 Diuretics

Patient name: _____

Admission: _____

NRS
DATE INITIAL

I. **The client/caregiver can define indications for the use of diuretics.**

A. Diuretics increase the volume of urine production and excretion.

B. Along with antihypertensive medications, they are used in the treatment of hypertension and heart failure and sometimes with kidney disease.

C. Because this type of medication affects electrolytes, it is important to maintain electrolyte balance.

II. **The client/caregiver can list concerns and needed actions/considerations when taking diuretics.**

A. Client will understand signs of dehydration or electrolyte imbalance.
   - Low potassium levels may be evidenced by generalized weakness and muscle cramps.
   - Dehydration may present as decreased urine output and thirst.

B. Use a weight schedule to monitor for changes.

C. Clients with kidney disease should be monitored more closely.

D. A balanced diet and proper amounts of fluids are encouraged.

E. Diuretics should be taken during the day, preferably in the morning.

F. Ambulation ability or self-care issues should be addressed because of increased urinary output.

NRS
DATE INITIAL

G. Have routine laboratory tests to evaluate electrolyte levels and liver and kidney function.

H. Glucose and uric acids levels may increase with diuretic use. Clients with diabetes and/or gout should be monitored.

I. Monitor blood pressure, and report any unusual changes.

J. Avoid herbal or dietary supplements unless approved by physician.

K. Discuss high-potassium diets (included teaching guide) or potassium supplements if prescribed by physician.

L. Discuss low-sodium diets (included teaching guide) if prescribed by physician.

M. If needed, instruct how to measure intake and output.

N. Limit exposure to sunlight due to possible side effect of photosensitivity.

O. Consult physician for instruction if experiencing an acute illness with fever, vomiting, or diarrhea.

P. Restrict use of alcohol and caffeine.

REFERENCES

Ackley, B. J., & Ladwig, G. B. (2006). *Nursing diagnosis handbook: A guide to planning care.* St. Louis: Mosby Elsevier.

Adams, M. P., Josephson, D. L., & Holland, L. N. Jr. (2005). *Pharmacology for nurses: A pathophysiologic approach.* Upper Saddle River, NJ: Pearson Education, Inc.

Deglin, J. H., & Vallerand, A. H. (2001). *Davis's drug guide for nurses.* Philadelphia: F. A. Davis Company.

Nursing 2006 drug handbook. (2006). Philadelphia: Lippincott Williams and Wilkins.

9 Antiparkinson Medications

Patient name: _____   Admission: _____

NRS
DATE INITIAL

I. The client/caregiver can define indications of this type of medication.

A. These drugs relieve some of the symptoms of Parkinson's disease by restoring the balance of dopamine and acetylcholine in the brain.

II. The client/caregiver can list important teaching concerns.

A. Medication should be taken with meals.
B. Nutritional concerns are
1. Increase fiber and fluids to prevent constipation.
2. Avoid foods high in pyridoxine (vitamin B6) because they decrease the effectiveness of medication. Foods such as beef, liver, ham and pork, egg yolks, and oatmeal are to be avoided or limited.
3. High-protein foods also may decrease the effects of this medication.
4. Eating and swallowing difficulties are discussed in dysphagia teaching guide.
C. Possible dizziness when standing quickly can be avoided by changing position slowly.

NRS
DATE INITIAL

D. Central nervous system adverse reactions can range from agitation and anxiety to fatigue and lethargy.
E. There may be dry mouth, changes in taste, loss of appetite, abdominal discomfort, and changes ranging from constipation to diarrhea.
F. Observe for any changes in disease symptoms. They can cause symptoms to worsen.
G. Observe for hallucinations, confusion, and so forth.
H. Periodic evaluation and laboratory test to evaluate effectiveness of medication and for any indication of liver or kidney damage.
I. Take medication exactly as ordered. Do not change doses or stop medication without direction from physician.

REFERENCES

Ackley, B. J., & Ladwig, G. B. (2006). *Nursing diagnosis handbook: A guide to planning care.* St. Louis: Mosby Elsevier.

Adams, M. P., Josephson, D. L., & Holland, L. N. Jr. (2005). *Pharmacology for nurses: A pathophysiologic approach.* Upper Saddle River, NJ: Pearson Education, Inc.

Deglin, J. H., & Vallerand, A. H. (2001). *Davis's drug guide for nurses.* Philadelphia: F. A. Davis Company.

Nursing 2006 drug handbook. (2006). Philadelphia: Lippincott Williams and Wilkins.

10 Gastrointestinal Drugs—Antiulcer

Patient name: _____   Admission: _____

NRS
DATE INITIAL

I. **The client/caregiver can describe purpose of antiulcer medication.**

  A. Used to treat duodenal ulcers
  B. Used to help heal damage created in esophagitis
  C. Used to relieve symptoms of gastroesophageal reflux disease and heartburn
  D. Used to reduce the gastric irritation caused by other medications, such as the NSAIDs

II. **The client/caregiver can list considerations and/or concerns when using antiulcer medications.**

  A. Monitor for abdominal pain or blood in vomit or stool.
  B. Avoid the use of alcohol, caffeine, and tobacco.
  C. Follow specific instructions related to individual medication.
    1. Do not chew or crush medication if alert on prescription label.

NRS
DATE INITIAL

  2. Take with foods or empty stomach as directed on label.
  3. Take medication at specific time of day as ordered.
  4. Continue follow-up and evaluation with physician during treatment.
  5. Talk with physician regarding taking any other over-the-counter antacids.
  6. Alert physician if pregnant or planning pregnancy.
  7. Observe for adverse symptoms of drowsiness or dizziness.

REFERENCES

Ackley, B. J., & Ladwig, G. B. (2006). *Nursing diagnosis handbook: A guide to planning care.* St. Louis: Mosby Elsevier.

Adams, M. P., Josephson, D. L., & Holland, L. N. Jr. (2005). *Pharmacology for nurses: A pathophysiologic approach.* Upper Saddle River, NJ: Pearson Education, Inc.

Deglin, J. H., & Vallerand, A. H. (2001). *Davis's drug guide for nurses.* Philadelphia: F. A. Davis Company.

Nursing 2006 drug handbook. (2006). Philadelphia: Lippincott Williams and Wilkins.

Part VII

Disease Prevention and Health Promotion

Teaching Guides

1 | Basic Nutrition

Patient name: _____ **Admission:** _____

NRS
DATE INITIAL

I. **The client/caregiver can list reasons to eat a well-balanced diet.**

A. It provides energy, builds and repairs body tissues, and regulates body processes.
B. It is essential for preventing disease and for healing of disease.
C. It is essential for emotional and physical well-being.

II. **The client/caregiver can explain the MyPyramid program.**

A. The U.S. Department of Agriculture introduced this program in 2006.
B. It offers a personal eating plan with suggested foods and amount of food intake.
C. They are not therapeutic diets for specific health conditions (see therapeutic diets teaching guides for specific health conditions).
D. The program can track your food intake and physical activity level.
E. They offer some basic advice when starting the program:
1. Make wise choices from every food group.
2. Find a balance between food and physical activity.
3. Get the most nutrition out of your calories. Avoid empty calories.
4. Stay within your daily calorie needs.
5. Make half your grains whole.
6. Vary your vegetables.
7. Focus on fruit selections.
8. Use calcium-rich foods.
9. Use lean proteins.
10. Find a balance between food intake and physical activity.

III. **The client/caregiver can list methods to evaluate healthy weight.**

A. Body mass index was created to provide a measurement of weight that is not related to height.

NRS
DATE INITIAL

B. It is often used as an indicator of obesity.
1. BMI of 25 to 29.5 is considered overweight.
2. BMI over 30 is considered obese.
C. Another method to evaluate a healthy weight is to use one of the height–weight tables. Adults and older children are measured standing. Infants and small children are measured lying on a flat surface.

IV. **The client/caregiver can list the Dietary Guidelines presented by the Surgeon General of the United States, the U.S. Department of Agriculture, and the U.S. Department of Human Resources (2005).**

A. Eat a variety of foods.
B. Balance the food you eat with physical activity. Maintain or improve your weight.
  • Engage in 30 minutes of moderate-intensity activity most days of the week.
C. Choose a diet with plenty of grain products, vegetables, and fruits. Daily suggested amounts per a 2000 calorie diet are
  • 2 cups of fruit
  • 2.5 cups of vegetables
  • 3 or more servings of whole-grain products
  • 3 cups of fat-free or low-fat milk or milk products
D. Choose a diet low in fat, saturated fat, and cholesterol.
1. Consume less than 10% of calories from saturated fatty acids.
2. Consume less than 300 mg/day of cholesterol.
3. Limit intake of fats and oils high in saturated or trans fatty acids.
E. Choose a diet moderate in sugars.
1. Choose and prepare foods/beverages with little added sugars.
F. Choose a diet moderate in salt and sugars.
1. Consume less than 2300 mg (approximately 1 teaspoon of salt) of sodium per day.

(Continued)

NRS
DATE INITIAL

2. Choose and prepare foods with little salt.

G. If you drink alcoholic beverages, do so in moderation. Moderate consumption is considered
   1. One drink per day for women
   2. Up to two drinks per day for men

H. Avoid foods that are contaminated with bacteria, viruses, parasites, toxins, and chemical or physical contaminants.

V. **The client/caregiver can list general nutritional tips for different ages thru the lifespan.**

A. Recommendations for children are
   1. Engage in 60 minutes of physical activity most days of the week.
   2. At least half of grains consumed should be whole grains.
   3. Children 2 to 8 years old should consume 2 cups of fat-free or low-fat milk products. Children over 9 years old should consume 3 cups of milk or milk products daily.
   4. Consume most fats coming from polyunsaturated and monounsaturated fatty acids, such as fish, nuts, and vegetable oils.
   5. Obtain sufficient amounts of fiber, but avoid excessive amounts of added sugars.
   6. Do not eat or drink raw milk or raw milk products, raw eggs, raw or undercooked meats, poultry or fish, unpasteurized juice, or raw sprouts.

B. Women of childbearing age who may become pregnant or are pregnant and breastfeeding women should
   1. Eat foods high in heme iron, iron-rich plant foods, or iron-fortified foods.
   2. Include vitamin C-rich foods to aid in iron absorption.
   3. Consume adequate amounts of folic acid from fortified foods or supplements.

NRS
DATE INITIAL

4. Eat only certain deli meats and frankfurters that have been reheated to steaming hot.
5. Avoid raw milk or raw milk products.

C. Older adults should
   1. Consume extra vitamin D from fortified foods.
   2. Increase dietary fiber to prevent constipation.
   3. Limit intake of sodium per day to no more than 1500 mg.
   4. Eat foods with potassium recommendations of 4700 mg/day.

RESOURCES

National Institutes of Health/National Heart, Lung and Blood Institute
www.nhlbi.nih.gov/health/public/heart/obesity/lose_wt/

U.S. Department of Agriculture. MyPyramid/Steps to a Better Healthier You
www.mypyramid.gov/

USDA Dietary Guidelines for Americans 2005
www.health.gov/dietaryguidelines

Nutritionist

Dietician

REFERENCES

Ackley, B. J., & Ladwig, G. B. (2006). *Nursing diagnosis handbook: A guide to planning care.* St. Louis: Mosby Inc.

Canobbio, M. M. (2006). *Mosby's handbook of patient teaching.* St. Louis: Mosby Inc.

Hitchcock, J. E., Schubert, P. E., & Thomas, S. A. (2003). *Community health nursing: Caring in action.* Clifton Park, NY: Thomson Delmar Learning.

Lutz, C., & Przytulski, K. (2001). *Nutrition and diet therapy.* Philadelphia: F. A. Davis Company.

Nutrition made incredibly easy. (2003). Philadelphia: Lippincott Williams & Wilkins.

Timby, B. K. (2005). *Fundamental nursing skills and concepts.* Philadelphia: J. B. Lippincott Williams & Wilkins.

2   Exercise Teaching Guides

Patient name: _____   Admission: _____

NRS
DATE INITIAL

I. **The client/caregiver will state benefits of exercise.**

 A. Strengthens your cardiovascular and respiratory systems
 B. Promotes feeling of emotional well-being and improved self-esteem
 C. Keeps bones and muscles strong
 D. Manages weight
 E. Prevents and manages diabetes
 F. Eases depression and manages pain and stress
 G. Lowers the risk of colon, prostate, uterus, and breast cancer
 H. Improves sleep habits and increases energy

II. **The client/caregiver can list recommended types of exercise.**

 A. There are four basic fitness components.
  1. Cardiorespiratory endurance. Examples are long runs and swims.
  2. Muscular strength. Weight-lifting exercises are an example.
  3. Muscular endurance. Pushups are a common example.
  4. Flexibility. Using muscles to complete a full range of motion is an example.
 B. Each workout should begin with a warmup.

III. **The client/caregiver can state general rules for exercise.**

 A. Get a physician's approval before beginning exercise program if over 35 years old and sedentary or has a cardiovascular problem.
 B. Stop exercise, and notify a physician if chest pain, dizziness, or fainting occurs.
 C. Drink plenty of water before, during, and after the workout.
 D. Dress in loose-fitting clothing to permit freedom of movement. Wear supportive shoes.
 E. Wait 90 minutes after a meal to exercise.

NRS
DATE INITIAL

 F. Avoid exercising in very hot or humid weather.
 G. Decrease the intensity of exercise if unable to hold a conversation during exercise.
 H. Have fun while exercising.
 I. Exercise with someone or with a group.
 J. Set realistic goals.
 K. Give yourself rewards for meeting those goals.

IV. **The client/caregiver can describe an aerobic exercise plan.**

 A. Warm up before exercise.
  1. Start slowly, gradually increasing the pace.
  2. Allow at least 5 minutes for the warm up.
  3. The warm-up period prepares the body by gradually increasing heart rate and warming the muscles. It protects the body from injury.
 B. Take pulse several times during exercise and adjust intensity of exercise to maintain the target heart rate.
  1. Target heart rate is the heart rate you should reach and maintain for 20 minutes.
  2. One way to determine what your target heart rate is
   • Maximum heart rate (220 − age) times 70%
 C. Cool down after exercise.
  1. Gradually decrease the pace of the exercise.
  2. Allow at least 5 minutes for the cool-down period.
  3. It returns blood to the heart, preventing a buildup of lactic acid in the muscles.
  4. It allows for gradual recovery of the body.
  5. Perform a stretching routine at the end of the exercise.
 D. The exercise should be performed at least three times per week for at least a 20-minute duration to improve cardiovascular status.

(Continued)

RESOURCES

The President's Council on Physical Fitness and Sports
www.fitness.gov/

Health and fitness clubs

YMCA

REFERENCES

Ackley, B. J., & Ladwig, G. B. (2006). *Nursing diagnosis handbook: A guide to planning care.* St. Louis: Mosby Inc.

Canobbio, M. M. (2006). *Mosby's handbook of patient teaching.* St. Louis: Mosby Inc.

Hitchcock, J. E., Schubert, P. E., & Thomas, S. A. (2003). *Community health nursing: Caring in action.* Clifton Park, NY: Thomson Delmar Learning.

Lutz, C., & Przytulski, K. (2001). *Nutrition and diet therapy.* Philadelphia: F. A. Davis Company.

Nutrition made incredibly easy. (2003). Philadelphia: Lippincott Williams & Wilkins.

Timby, B. K. (2005). *Fundamental nursing skills and concepts.* Philadelphia: J. B. Lippincott Williams & Wilkins.

3 Stress Management and Relaxation Techniques

Patient name: _____   Admission: _____

<table>
<tr><td>NRS
DATE INITIAL</td><td></td></tr>
</table>

I. The client/caregiver can define stress.

A. It is a pressure or a strain caused by a real or perceived threat.
B. It can cause mental, physical, intellectual, emotional, and/or spiritual consequences.
C. It creates a physical reaction in which hormones are released, causing symptoms such as tense muscles, pounding heart, increase in blood pressure, cold clammy hands, and tense stomach.
D. Prolonged or chronic stress can be particularly harmful.

II. The client/caregiver can list benefits of stress.

A. Increases concentration
B. Increases alertness
C. Improves performance
D. Increases strength
E. Provides incentive for accomplishment

III. The client/caregiver can list bad effects of stress.

A. Chronic fatigue and sleep disturbances
B. Increased pulse, blood pressure, and respirations
C. Constipation, diarrhea, or ulcers
D. Chronic back pain, headache, and stiff neck
E. Increased susceptibility to disease
F. Loss of appetite, nausea, and weight loss

IV. The client/caregiver can list methods to cope with stress.

A. Identify stressors.
B. Attend support groups.
C. Have psychotherapy.
D. Simplify life.
E. Do not self-medicate with alcohol or drugs.
F. Promote better organizational skills.
    1. Delegate jobs to others.
    2. Use time management.

3. Establish priorities.
4. Learn to say "no."
G. Take care of the body.
    1. Eat a well-balanced diet.
    2. Avoid caffeine, alcohol, and tobacco.
    3. Take vitamin and mineral supplements.
    4. Obtain adequate rest.
    5. Exercise regularly.
H. Develop positive thinking.
    1. Learn and practice assertiveness.
    2. Use good posture.
I. Keep your expectations realistic.
J. Keep a sense of humor.

V. The client/caregiver can list techniques and activities that may decrease stress.

A. Mental imagery/visualization
B. Progressive muscle relaxation
C. Meditation
D. Biofeedback
E. Aromatherapy
F. Deep breathing exercises
G. Massage
H. Therapeutic touch
I. Stretching
J. Walking
K. Gardening
L. Spending time with pet
M. Hot baths
N. Listening to music
O. Reading
P. Physical activities such as swimming

VI. The client/caregiver can list stress management techniques that have been used in other countries many years ago and are now becoming popular in our society.

A. Acupuncture uses needles at certain points on the body to promote the flow of energy.
B. Acupressure uses application of pressure on certain points on the body to promote flow of energy.

(Continued)

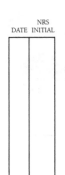

C. Reflexology is the use of pressure on specific areas of the foot or hand that corresponds to body organs.

D. Shiatsu is a form of manipulation to correct internal malfunctioning.

E. Aroma therapy is the use of essential oils to promote healing.

F. Massage has been used in many countries to reduce stress and pain.

RESOURCES

National Center for Complementary and Alternative Medicine
http://nccam.nih.gov/

Counseling/clergy

Support groups

Health clubs

YMCA

REFERENCES

Ackley, B. J., & Ladwig, G. B. (2006). *Nursing diagnosis handbook: A guide to planning care.* St. Louis: Mosby Inc.

Canobbio, M. M. (2006). *Mosby's handbook of patient teaching.* St. Louis: Mosby Inc.

Hitchcock, J. E., Schubert, P. E., & Thomas, S. A. (2003). *Community health nursing: Caring in action.* Clifton Park, NY: Thomson Delmar Learning.

Lutz, C., & Przytulski, K. (2001). *Nutrition and diet therapy.* Philadelphia: F. A. Davis Company.

Nutrition made incredibly easy. (2003). Philadelphia: Lippincott Williams & Wilkins.

Timby, B. K. (2005). *Fundamental nursing skills and concepts.* Philadelphia: J. B. Lippincott Williams & Wilkins.

4 Preventive Dental Care

Patient name: _____   Admission: _____

I. The client/caregiver can state purpose of good oral hygiene.

A. To provide comfort
B. To decrease unpleasant tastes and odors
C. To decrease the possibility of irritation, infection, or disease in mouth
D. To prevent cavities and gum disease

II. The client/caregiver can list measures to assure good dental/oral health.

A. Brush teeth at least twice a day with fluoride toothpaste.
B. Floss teeth daily.
C. Eat snack smart—limit sugary or sticky snacks.
D. Get enough calcium in diet to support the health of teeth.
E. Do not smoke or use tobacco products.
F. Have regular dental exams.

III. The client/caregiver can demonstrate the correct method for brushing teeth.

A. Use a soft-bristled toothbrush.
B. Hold toothbrush at slight angle against teeth, and use short back and forth motions.
C. Brush inside and chewing surfaces of teeth.
D. Brush your tongue.
E. Brush your teeth for about 2 minutes each time.
F. Rinse mouth well.

IV. The client/caregiver can demonstrate proper method for flossing.

A. After brushing teeth, wrap approximately 18 inches of floss around your middle fingers.

B. Slide floss between teeth until it reaches the gum.
C. Pull floss against tooth and gum to remove plaque.
D. Floss each tooth several times using fresh floss as needed.
E. If there is a problem handling the floss, try a manufactured floss holder.
F. Rinse mouth well.

V. The client/caregiver can demonstrate care of dentures.

A. Remove dentures, and place in a denture container.
B. Place a washcloth over the sink to prevent breaking if they are dropped.
C. Use tepid water because hot water may change the shape of some dentures.
D. If removing dentures during the night, place in covered denture container with water.
E. Have dentures adjusted as needed for proper fit.

RESOURCES

American Dental Association
www.ada.org/

Local dentist

REFERENCES

Lutz, C., & Przytulski, K. (2001). *Nutrition and diet therapy.* Philadelphia: F. A. Davis Company.
Perry, A., & Potter, P. (2006). *Clinical nursing skills & technique.* St. Louis: Mosby Inc.
Timby, B. K. (2005). *Fundamental nursing skills and concepts.* Philadelphia: J. B. Lippincott Williams & Wilkins.

5   Preventive Health Care

Patient name: _____   Admission: _____

NRS
DATE INITIAL

I. **The client/caregiver can define health.**

A. It is mental, physical, emotional, and spiritual well-being.
B. Each aspect is interdependent on the others.

II. **The client/caregiver can list measures suggested by Healthy People 2010.**

A. Be physically active.
B. Eat a nutritious diet.
C. Get preventive screenings.
D. Make healthy choices.

III. **The client/caregiver can list screening measures for early detection of various types of cancer.**

A. Breast cancer
   1. Breast self-exams monthly
   2. Women 40 years old and older should have yearly mammograms.
   3. Clinical breast exams should be a part of regular physical exams (preferably before mammograms).
B. Colorectal cancer screening guidelines. Beginning at the age of 50 years, both men and women (with average risk) should have one of the following screening tests:
   1. Yearly stool blood test (FOBT) or fecal immunochemical test (FIT). Often the physician will give supplies to collect sample at home and return for analysis.
   2. Flexible sigmoidoscopy should be done every 5 years.
   3. Yearly stool blood test plus sigmoidoscopy should be done every 5 years. This is the preferred plan.
   4. Digital rectal exams should be done as part of a regular physical exam.
C. Skin cancer
   1. Monthly exam of full-body skin surface. Use mirror to view hard to see areas, or have spouse or partner help with exam. Include palms and soles of feet.

NRS
DATE INITIAL

D. Oral cavity or oropharyngeal cancer
   1. Routine dental exams
E. Cervical, ovarian, and uterine cancer
   1. Pelvic exam with pap smear yearly
F. Prostate cancer
   1. Digital exam and prostate-specific antigen (PSA) blood test yearly after the age of 50 years.
   2. Men at higher risk can begin testing at the age of 40 years.
G. Testicular cancer
   1. Testicular exam as part of regular physical exam
   2. Self-exam schedule as recommended by physician

IV. **The client/caregiver can list warning signs of cancer.**

A. Unusual bleeding or discharge
B. Thickening or lump in breast or elsewhere
C. Changing wart or mole
D. Chronic hoarseness or cough
E. Indigestion or difficulty swallowing
F. Change in bladder or bowel habits
G. Sore that does not heal

RESOURCES

Healthy People 2010
www.healthypeople.gov/About/whatis.htm

American Cancer Society
www.cancer.org

U.S. Public Health Service Office of Disease Prevention and Health Promotion
http://odphp.osophs.dhhs.gov/

REFERENCES

Hunt, R. (2005). *Introduction to community based nursing.* Philadelphia: Lippincott Williams & Wilkins.
Perry, A., & Potter, P. (2006). *Clinical nursing skills & technique.* St. Louis, Missouri: Mosby Inc.
Timby, B. K. (2005). *Fundamental nursing skills and concepts.* Philadelphia: J. B. Lippincott Williams & Wilkins.

6 Immunization

Patient name: _____   Admission: _____

NRS
DATE INITIAL

I. **The client/caregiver can give important facts about immunizations.**

   A. Immunization for both children and adults is one of the best examples of primary prevention. They prevent the initial occurrence of a specific disease.
   B. Vaccines contain a killed or weakened form or derivative of specific infectious germs.
   C. This vaccine given to a healthy person will trigger an immune response without exposure to the actual disease-producing germ.
   D. Later, if exposed to the real disease, the body will produce antibodies to destroy the disease.

II. **The client/caregiver can list any possible reactions to childhood immunizations.**

   A. The most common reactions include
      • Redness or swelling at the site of injection
      • Rash
      • Fever

III. **The client/caregiver can list measures to manage common reactions to immunizations.**

   A. Pain at injection site
      1. Apply ice or cold compress to the area for 20 minutes.
      2. Give acetaminophen or ibuprofen per physician's recommendation.
   B. Fever
      1. For a fever over 102°F, give acetaminophen or ibuprofen per physician's recommendation.
   C. General reactions for children that do not need treatment unless they have not resolved in 24 to 48 hours are
      • Mild fussiness, irritability, or restless sleep
      • Decreased appetite or activity level

NRS
DATE INITIAL

IV. **The client/caregiver can describe symptoms that need the prompt attention of a physician.**

   A. Fever that lasts more than 3 days
   B. Pain that lasts more than 3 days
   C. An injection site that shows signs of infection

V. **The client/caregiver can list one treatment/medication to avoid with children.**

   A. Never give aspirin for fever or pain to a child.
   B. Reye's syndrome is a rare but serious brain disease that can result from use of aspirin in children.

VI. **The client/caregiver can list the recommended immunizations for children and adults (2007 schedule).**

   A. Childhood immunizations should include
      • Hepatitis B
      • Rotavirus
      • Diphtheria/pertussis/tetanus
      • Haemophilus influenzae type b
      • Pneumococcal
      • Inactivated poliovirus
      • Influenza
      • Measles, mumps, and rubella
      • Varicella
      • Hepatitis A
      • Meningococcal
   B. Adult immunizations should include
      • Tetanus/diphtheria/acellular pertussis (Td/Tdap)
      • Human papillomavirus (HPV2) for females
      • Measles, mumps, and rubella
      • Varicella
      • Influenza
      • Pneumococcal
      • Hepatitis A
      • Hepatitis B
      • Meningococcal

(Continued)

NRS
DATE INITIAL

C. Contact health care provider or the
    Centers for Disease Control and
    Prevention for more information on
    immunization schedules, requirements,
    and any updates.

RESOURCES

American Academy of Family Physicians
www.aafp.org/

American Academy of Pediatrics
www.cispimmunize.org

National Immunization Program
www.cdc.gov/Nip/recs/child-schedule

Women, Infants, and Children
www.fns.usda.gov/wic

Community health clinics

REFERENCES

Hitchcock, J. E., Schubert, P. E., & Thomas, S. A. (2003).
    Community health nursing: Caring in action. Clifton Park, NY:
    Thomson Delmar Learning.
Hunt, R. (2005). *Introduction to community based nursing.*
    Philadelphia: Lippincott Williams & Wilkins.
Muscari, M. E. (2005). *Pediatric nursing.* Philadelphia:
    Lippincott Williams & Wilkins.
Perry, A., & Potter, P. (2006). *Clinical nursing skills & technique.*
    St. Louis, Missouri: Mosby Inc.
Timby, B. K., & Smith, N. C. (2003). *Introductory medical-
    surgical nursing* (8th ed.). Philadelphia: J. B. Lippincott
    Williams & Wilkins.

1 Older Adult Safety

Patient name: _____   **Admission:** _____

I. **The client/caregiver can discuss the importance of safety and fall prevention for the older adult.**

   A. Falls are the leading cause of injury death for Americans 65 years old and older. Each year, between 35% and 40% of adults 65 years old and older will fall at least once.

   B. The Centers for Disease Control and Prevention has four suggestions to improve safety and prevent injuries.
      1. Begin a regular exercise program.
      2. Have your health care provider review you medicines (especially any that would increase risk of falls).
      3. Have your vision checked.
      4. Make your home safer.

   C. In 2002, more than 12,800 people over the age of 65 years died as a result of a fall and injury.

   D. In the same year, 1.6 million people over the age of 65 years were treated in emergency departments because of falls.

   E. For many older adults, being able to drive their automobile is a very large symbol of independence. The decision of whether to continue driving is a difficult problem for individuals and their families. The American Association of Retired Persons (AARP) and other organizations offer testing and refresher courses for the older adult to help improve safety, and they even serve as an evaluation tool for driving ability.

II. **The client/caregiver can list general measures to promote safety and prevent falls.**

   A. Display emergency numbers and home address near all phones.

   B. Install smoke alarms near all bedrooms and in the kitchen.

   C. Make sure handrails are installed on both sides of stairways.

   D. Keep hallways and stairwells clear of all clutter. Do not use these areas for storage.

   E. Install nightlights for late-night trips to the kitchen or bathroom.

   F. Do not use throw rugs.

   G. Avoid clutter. Keep walking areas free of clutter and furniture.

   H. Wear shoes with nonskid soles.

   I. Keep all cords, phones, extension cords, and so forth safely out of flow of traffic.

   J. Make sure that electrical cords are in good condition, with no fraying or cracking.

   K. Provide adequate lighting. Change light bulbs as needed. Use the appropriate size and type of light bulk for each fixture.

   L. Do not rush or run—allow plenty of time to get things done. Change positions slowly.

   M. Maintain an adequate fluid intake.

   N. Eat a well-balanced diet.

   O. Wear visual aids (i.e., glasses) and hearing aids.

   P. Place a contrasting color along the edge of the tread to help differentiate the steps.

III. **The client/caregiver can list measures to promote safety and prevent falls in the bathroom and kitchen.**

   A. Adjust the temperature of the water heater to 120°F to avoid burns.

   B. Consider dismantling the garbage disposal.

   C. Keep good, clean lighting over the stove, sink, and countertop work areas, especially where food is sliced and cut.

   D. Keep towels, curtains, and other flammable items away from the range.

   E. Wear clothes with short or close-fitting sleeves when cooking.

   F. Make sure that kitchen ventilation systems or range exhaust is functioning.

   G. Install smoke detectors, and check batteries routinely.

   H. In the bathroom, use grab bars on the walls and nonskid mats or strips in the bathtub and shower.

(Continued)

I. If needed, use extended toilet seat with handrails.

J. Use shower stool/chair and hand-held showerhead for bathing.

K. Keep ash trays, smoking materials, and other fire sources (heaters, hot plates, etc.) away from beds and bedding.

L. Keep a telephone close to the bed, and have lamps and light switches in reach.

M. Clean any spills immediately.

N. Store frequently used items in easy-to-reach locations.

IV. **The client/caregiver can list measures to promote safety and prevent falls outside of the home and entryways.**

A. Make sure outdoor steps and walkways are kept in good repair.

B. Spread sand or salt on icy walkways.

C. Consider using a ramp with handrail as needed.

D. Avoid clutter on walkways such as toys, gardening tools, hoses, and so forth.

E. Eliminate uneven surfaces or walkways.

F. Place a small bench or table by entry to hold packages while unlocking doors.

G. Check entryways and walk for adequate lighting.

H. Keep shrubbery and foliage away from pathway and doorway.

V. **The client/caregiver can list precautions regarding the telephone.**

A. Place an enlarged or lighted dial on the phone to aid with impaired vision.

B. Place adaptive devices on the phone to help with the hearing impaired.

C. Keep phone within easy reach day or night. Make sure the phone is properly charged.

D. Keep emergency numbers, including doctor, police, fire department, ambulance, nearest neighbor, and relative, near the phone.

E. Consider a medical alert and alarm system that client can wear to signal for help.

RESOURCES

Senior centers

Adult day care centers

Office of the aging in local county

American Association of Retired Persons (AARP)
www.aarp.org/

AARP—Driver Safety Classes
www.aarp.org/families/driver_safety/driver_ed/

Gerontological Society of America
www.geron.org/

Home Safety Counsel
www.homesafetycouncil.org

National Safety Counsel
www.nsc.org/

The U.S. Administration on Aging
www.aoa.dhhs.gov/

REFERENCES

Hitchcock, J. E., Schubert, P. E., & Thomas, S. A. (2003). *Community health nursing: Caring in action.* Clifton Park, NY: Thomson Delmar Learning.

National Center for Injury Prevention and Control. (2006). *What you can do to prevent falls.* Available from: *www.cdc.gov/ncipc/pub-res/toolkit/WhatYouCanDoToPreventFalls.htm.* Washington, DC: Centers for Disease Control and Prevention.

National Center for Injury Prevention and Control. (2007). *Older adult drivers: Fact sheet.* Available at: *www.cdc.gov/ncipc/factsheets/older.htm.* Washington, DC: Centers for Disease Control and Prevention.

Perry, A., & Potter, P. (2006). *Clinical nursing skills & technique.* St. Louis: Mosby Inc.

The Older Adult Driver (*American Family Physician*). (January 1, 2000). Available at *www.aafp.org/afp/20000101/141.html.*

Timby, B. K., & Smith, N. C. (2003). *Introductory medical-surgical nursing* (8th ed.). Philadelphia: J. B. Lippincott Williams & Wilkins.

2 Child and Adolescent Safety

Patient name: _____   **Admission:** _____

I.   **The client/caregiver can discuss child safety.**

A. Safety for infants and toddlers
1. Things to keep away from children this age are
- Knives and sharp objects
- Medicine
- Cleaning supplies
- Houseplants
- Plastic bags
- Balloons (especially burst balloons)
2. Keep crib away from electric cords, curtains, or blind cords that could get around the child's neck, thus preventing choking or strangulation.
3. The room should be painted with a nontoxic paint.
4. Crib features should be checked for safety.
- Bars should be no more than $2\frac{3}{8}$ inches apart.
- Railing should be at least 26 inches higher than the lowest level of the mattress support.
- Mattress should fit snugly into crib.
- Surfaces should all be smooth.
- Bumper guards should be used to protect infant from the hard railing.
- Crib should be placed away from hot radiators or cold drafts.
- No pillows should be used in the crib.
- Drop-side latches should not be easily released by infant.
5. Changing table safety tips are
- It should be sturdy, with a strap to prevent falls.
- It should have drawers or shelves that are easily accessible to prevent turning away from the infant.

II.   **The client/caregiver can discuss general safety measures for children.**

A. Measures to prevent poisoning
1. Remove any houseplants in the home that are poisonous.
2. Give medications as a drug, and stress that they are not candy.
3. Apply hooks to cupboards that contain dangerous chemicals, such as may be in kitchen, laundry, or bathroom.
4. Have emergency numbers and numbers for the regional poison center posted.
B. Measures to prevent falls
1. Keep children away from windows. Lock windows when possible, as screens will not prevent falls.
2. Keep chairs and furniture away from windows so that children cannot climb up. Open windows from the top whenever possible.
3. Do not let children play alone on fire escapes, balconies, and so forth.
4. Install safety gates to block stairs.
5. Secure area rugs.
6. Avoid use of extension cords.
7. Fasten safety belts on highchairs, strollers, and shopping carts.
8. Never leave child unattended.
C. Measures to prevent burns
1. Avoid hot spills from food or drinks. Turn handles of pots and pans away from front of stove.
2. Avoid use of tablecloths with toddlers. They could pull heavy or hot items down on themselves.
3. Establish a "no zone" area, such as in front of your stove/oven.
4. Unplug irons (curling and clothes) when not in use. Keep out of children's reach.
5. Test food and beverage temperature. Microwave can heat unevenly.

(Continued)

6. Childproof electrical outlets.
7. Never leave a grill unattended.
8. Secure matches and lighters away from children.
9. Be careful with cigarettes.
10. Use space heaters with care.
11. Place candles away from reach of children, and never leave unattended.
12. Place "totfinder" symbol in child's bedroom window.
13. Have smoke alarms and fire extinguisher in the home.

D. Measures for yard and water safety
1. Home playground equipment should be age appropriate.
2. Equipment should be surrounded 6 feet in all direction by loose material such as shredded rubber or wood chips.
3. Install four-sided isolation fencing with self-closing and self-latching gates around pools and spas. Wading pools should be emptied after each use. Always supervise children when around water.
4. Keep ignition keys out of riding movers, vehicles, and so forth.
5. Look before going backwards in a motor vehicle.
6. Remove poisonous plants, pesticides, pool chemical, and so forth from the reach of children.
7. Use sunscreen and insect repellent carefully after reading directions for use.

E. Safety measures for children when using computer at home or school
1. Never give personal information such as your name, address, school or phone number. Never send a picture.
2. Do not write to someone who has made you feel uncomfortable or scared.
3. Do not meet someone or have them visit without the permission of your parents.
4. Tell your parents or teacher if you read or view anything on the Internet that makes you feel uncomfortable.

F. Safety tips from the National Center for Missing and Exploited Children
1. Teach children to run away from danger and to yell loudly and make efforts to get away by kicking, screaming, and resisting.
2. Never let your children go places alone. Make sure older children always take a friend with them.
3. Know where your children are and whom they are with at all times.
4. Remind children never to accept anything or respond to anyone they do not know.
5. Talk openly to children about safety and talking to you or a trusted adult regarding anything that makes them scared or uncomfortable.
6. Have a list of family members who could be contacted in case of an emergency.
7. Report any suspicious persons or activities to law enforcement.
8. Maintain a recent photograph of child. The photograph should be in color. Often local law enforcement agencies will offer a free program to fingerprint children. Both pictures and fingerprints should be stored in an easily accessible place.
9. Teach child home address and phone number.
10. Get references for baby sitters.

G. General wellness care should include the following:
1. Have routine exams to monitor growth and development.
2. Vision and dental exam are recommended before beginning school.
3. Keep immunizations up to date.

H. Car safety measures
1. An appropriate car seat is required for all children less than 40 pounds.
2. Seatbelts should be worn for all children over 40 pounds.
3. Children under the age of 12 years should be placed in the back seat.

NRS
DATE INITIAL

(Continued)

RESOURCES

Child Safety Publications. U.S. Consumer Product Safety Commission
www.cpsc.gov/cpscpub/pubs/chld_sfy.html

American Academy of Pediatrics

Consumer Product Safety Commission

National Center for Missing and Exploited Children
www.missingkids.com/missingkids/

Federal Bureau of Investigation
www.fbi.gov/kids/k5th/safety1.htm

REFERENCES

Canobbio, M. M. (2006). *Mosby's handbook of patient teaching.* St. Louis: Mosby Inc.

Muscari, M. E. (2005). *Pediatric nursing.* Philadelphia: Lippincott Williams & Wilkins.

Novak, J. C., & Broom, B. L. (1999). *Maternal and child health nursing.* St. Louis: Mosby, Inc.

3   Fire Safety

Patient name: _____   Admission: _____

<table>
<tr><td>NRS
DATE INITIAL</td><td></td><td>NRS
DATE INITIAL</td><td></td></tr>
</table>

I. The client/caregiver can list measures to promote fire safety.

A. Measures to protect home from fires
1. Keep electrical appliances and cords in good condition.
2. Do not overload outlets or extension cords.
3. Keep the correct wattage light bulbs in light fixtures.
4. Avoid smoking in bed or when sleepy.
5. Have chimneys cleaned and inspected yearly.
6. Install a smoke detector on each floor, and check batteries.
7. Make sure that lamps and night lights are not touching bedspreads, drapes, or other fabrics.
8. Use electric blankets with caution.
9. Never leave candles burning unattended.
10. Put doors and screens on fireplaces.
11. Use precautions with wood-burning stoves.
12. Never place space heater too close to a bed, especially a child's bed.
13. Keep newspapers, magazines, curtains, and bedding away from space heaters, radiators, and fireplaces. Heaters should be at least 3 feet from anything flammable.
14. Keep lighters and matches away from children.
15. Turn off appliances before leaving the home (i.e., iron, oven, and curling iron).
16. Store flammable substances in a well-ventilated area.

II. The client/caregiver can explain the use of a fire extinguisher.

A. The National Fire Protection Agency suggests the following instruction called PASS:
1. Pull the pin. Release the lock with the nozzle pointing away from you.
2. Aim low. Point the extinguisher at the base of the fire.
3. Squeeze the lever slowly and evenly.
4. Sweep the nozzle from side to side.
B. Check the fire extinguisher regularly to make sure that it is functioning.

III. The client/caregiver can list measures to plan an escape route in case of fire.

A. Plan for two escape routes in case one is blocked by fire.
B. Make sure that windows in all rooms are easy to open.
C. If living in an apartment, know where stairways and escape routes are.
D. If living in a two-story house or apartment, have a fire-safe approved ladder to use in case of fire.
E. Provide baby-sitters, cleaning personnel, and so forth know the escape routes and plans.

IV. The client/caregiver can list measures to perform in case of a fire emergency.

A. Evacuate. Call 911 if possible.
B. Feel a door (not the doorknob) before opening it.
C. Keep low to the floor if smoke is in the building.

(Continued)

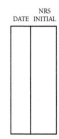

D. Use stairs—never elevators.
E. Cover mouth and nose with moist towel or clothing to keep out fumes.
F. Never stop to take personal items. Never go back into a burning building.
G. Stop, drop, and roll to extinguish flames if an article of clothing catches on fire.

RESOURCES

Local fire company

United States Fire Administration
www.usfa.dhs.gov/

National Fire Protection Agency
www.nfpa.org

REFERENCES

Perry, A., & Potter, P. (2006). *Clinical nursing skills & technique.* St. Louis: Mosby Inc.

Taylor, C., Lillis, C., & LeMone, P. (2005). *Fundamentals of nursing.* Philadelphia: Lippincott, Williams & Wilkins.

Timby, B. K., & Smith, N. C. (2003). *Introductory medical-surgical nursing* (8th ed.). Philadelphia: J. B. Lippincott Williams & Wilkins.

4 | Food Safety

Patient name: _____   **Admission:** _____

<table>
<tr><td>NRS
DATE INITIAL</td><td>I.</td><td>The client/caregiver can list measures to promote food safety.</td></tr>
</table>

I.   **The client/caregiver can list measures to promote food safety.**

   A.   Major things to remember when working with food
1. Wash hands and surfaces often.
2. Do not cross-contaminate foods.
3. Cook foods to proper temperature.
4. Refrigerate foods promptly.

   B.   Specific measures to prevent food-borne illness
1. Wash hands with warm water and soap before and after handling food and after using the bathroom, changing diapers, or handling pets.
2. Wash cutting boards, dishes, utensils, and countertops with hot, soapy water after preparing each food item.
3. Rinse fresh fruits and vegetables under tap water.
4. Separate raw meat, poultry, seafood, and eggs from other foods in your grocery cart and in the refrigerator.
5. Never place cooked food on a plate that had held raw meat, poultry, seafood, and eggs.
6. Refrigerate or freeze perishables as soon as you get home.
7. Never defrost food at room temperature.

II.   **The client/caregiver can list complications of food-borne illness.**

   A.   The Centers for Disease Control and Prevention reports that 76 million Americans suffer from food-borne illness.

   B.   They also report that as many as 5000 people die from this illness.

RESOURCES

U.S. National Food Safety Programs
www.foodsafety.gov/~dms/fs-toc.html

Food and Drug Administration

U.S. Department of Agriculture

U.S. Environmental Protection Agency

Centers for Disease Control and Prevention
www.cdc.gov/foodsafety/disease.htm

USDA National Agricultural Library
http://foodsafety.nal.usda.gov/nal_web/fsic/Contact_Us.php

REFERENCES

Lutz, C., & Przytulski, K. (2001). *Nutrition and diet therapy.* Philadelphia: F. A. Davis Company.
Nutrition made incredibly easy. (2003). Philadelphia: Lippincott Williams & Wilkins.

5 Handwashing

Patient name: _____   **Admission:** _____

NRS
DATE INITIAL

I. **The client/caregiver can list reasons for using good handwashing.**

   A. Prevention of spread of infections such as colds, flu, gastrointestinal disorders
   B. Prevention of the spread of food-borne illness

II. **The client/caregiver can list when it is important to wash hands.**

   A. After using the bathroom
   B. After changing a diaper—wash baby's hands, too.
   C. After touching animals or animal waste
   D. Before and after preparing food (especially when handling raw meat)
   E. Before eating
   F. After blowing your nose
   G. After coughing or sneezing into your hands
   H. Before and after treating wounds or cuts
   I. Before and after touching a sick or injured person
   J. After handling garbage
   K. Before inserting or removing contact lenses
   L. When using public restrooms

III. **The client/caregiver can describe good handwashing techniques.**

   A. Instructions for washing with soap and water
      1. Wet hands with warm, running water and apply soap. Lather well.
      2. Rub hands together vigorously for at least 15 seconds.

NRS
DATE INITIAL

   3. Scrub the backs of your hands and wrists and between your fingers and under fingernails.
   4. Rinse well.
   5. Dry hands with clean or disposable towel.
   6. Use towel to turn off the faucet.

   B. Instructions for the use of alcohol-based hand sanitizer.
      1. Use only alcohol-based products.
      2. If your hands are visibly dirty, use soap and water.
      3. Apply about 1/2 teaspoon of product to hands.
      4. Rub hands together, covering all surfaces, until hands are dry.

RESOURCE
Centers for Disease Control and Prevention
www.cdc.gov/cleanhands/

REFERENCES
Perry, A., & Potter, P. (2006). *Clinical nursing skills & technique.* St. Louis: Mosby Inc.

Taylor, C., Lillis, C., & LeMone, P. (2005). *Fundamentals of nursing.* Philadelphia: Lippincott, Williams & Wilkins.

Timby, B. K., & Smith, N. C. (2003). *Introductory medical-surgical nursing* (8th ed.). Philadelphia: J. B. Lippincott Williams & Wilkins.

1 Alcohol Abuse

Patient name: _____ Admission: _____

NRS
DATE INITIAL

I. **The client/caregiver can list general facts about alcohol and alcohol abuse.**

A. Alcohol is a drug that causes central nervous system depression.
B. It contains 200 calories per ounce and has no nutritional value. It is absorbed easily and can reach all areas of the body.
C. Alcohol abuse or alcoholism is a disease with four main features.
   1. Craving or a strong need to drink
   2. Loss of control and not being able to stop drinking once you have begun
   3. Physical dependence and withdrawal symptoms, such as nausea, sweating, or shakiness after drinking has stopped
   4. Tolerance for alcohol and need to drink greater amounts of alcohol to get "high" or desired effect
D. The signs and symptoms of alcohol intoxication will vary with the amount of alcohol ingested. The blood alcohol level is one method of measuring alcohol intake. A person with a blood alcohol level between .08 and .10 is considered legally intoxicated in most states.
E. Some studies indicate that between 25% and 50% of people seen in medical situations have physical and emotional problems related to alcoholism. That number increases when people are seen in the mental health setting.
F. The use of alcohol is growing in adolescents and underage drinkers. Often they will participate in binge drinking.

II. **The client/caregiver can list the effects of alcohol (directly and indirectly) on the body.**

A. Specific brain and nervous system changes can be
   • Slower reaction time
   • Decreased inhibitions
   • Impaired concentration and memory

NRS
DATE INITIAL

   • Impaired judgment and decision-making skills
   • Decreased physical control, such as loss of balance, slurred speech, or blurred vision
B. Blood vessels may dilate, and hypertension can result.
C. Irritation of the gastrointestinal tract can result in the following:
   • Bleeding
   • Diarrhea
   • Inability to absorb required nutrition
D. Alcohol poisoning or an overdose of alcohol can lead to respiratory depression and even death.
E. There is an increased risk of certain cancers (liver, esophagus, nasopharynx, and larynx).
F. Permanent damage can occur to liver, brain, and other organs.

III. **The client/caregiver can describe results and complications of alcohol abuse.**

A. Depression
B. Drinking during pregnancy can result in birth defects.
C. There is an increased risk of death from automobile accidents.
D. There is an increased risk of injuries from falls and accidents.
   1. Alcoholics are 16 times more likely than other to die in falls.
   2. Alcoholics are 10 times more likely to become fire or burn victims.
   3. Alcohol is associated with between 47% and 65% of adult drownings.
   4. Forty percent of industrial fatalities and 47% of industrial injuries can be linked to alcohol consumption and alcoholism.
E. There is an increased risk of suicide and involvement in homicide.
   1. Twenty percent of suicide victims are alcoholics.

(Continued)

NRS
DATE INITIAL

F. Family dysfunction, marital problems, and possible abuse can occur.

IV.   **The client/caregiver can explain the CAGE test as one example of screening for alcoholism.**

A. The test consists of four questions for the person to answer. More than one positive response is a good indication that a problem exists.

B. The questions are as follows:
   1. Have you ever felt the need to cut down on your drinking?
   2. Have you ever felt annoyed at criticism of your drinking?
   3. Have you ever felt guilty about something that's happened while drinking?
   4. Have you ever felt the need for an eye opener?

V.   **The client/caregiver can list signs and symptoms of alcohol withdrawal.**

A. Anxiety
B. Agitation
C. Irritability
D. Tremors
E. Sweating
F. Seizures
G. Delirium tremens

VI.   **The client/caregiver can list treatments available.**

A. Alcohol abuse treatment programs such as Alcoholics Anonymous
B. Inpatient programs
C. Residential treatment
D. Outpatient treatment
E. Halfway houses
F. Community-based treatment
G. Employee assistance programs and referrals

RESOURCES

Alcoholics Anonymous
212-870-3400
www.aa.org

Al-Anon Family Group Headquarters
800-356-9996
www.al-anon.alateen.org

National Institute on Alcohol Abuse and Alcoholism
www.niaaa.nih.gov

Substance Abuse and Mental Health Services Administration
www.samhsa.gov/

National Council on Alcoholism and Drug Dependence
www.ncadd.org

Department of Health and Human Services Surgeon General's Call to Action for the Prevention of Underage Drinking
www.surgeongeneral.gov

Employee assistance program

State or local mental health agencies

REFERENCES

Ackley, B. J., & Ladwig, G. B. (2006). *Nursing diagnosis handbook: A guide to planning care.* St. Louis: Mosby Inc.

Hitchcock, J. E., Schubert, P. E., & Thomas, S. A. (2003). *Community health nursing: Caring in action.* Clifton Park, NY: Thomson Delmar Learning.

Lutz, C., & Przytulski, K. (2001). *Nutrition and diet therapy.* Philadelphia: F. A. Davis Company.

Varcarolis, E. M. (2006). *Manual of psychiatric nursing care plans.* St. Louis: Saunders Elsevier.

2 Substance (Drug) Abuse

Patient name: _____   Admission: _____

NRS
DATE INITIAL

I. **The client/caregiver can define substance abuse.**

A. Substance abuse is the abuse of tobacco, alcohol, and other drugs (legal and illegal).

B. According to the National Institute on Drug Abuse, addiction is defined as a chronic, relapsing brain disease that is characterized by compulsive drug seeking and use despite harmful consequences.

C. The National Institute on Drug Abuse fact sheets from 1999 report
   - 14.8 million Americans used illicit drugs.
   - 3.5 million Americans were dependent on drugs.
   - 8.2 million Americans were dependent on alcohol.

D. Drug abuse can change the structure of the brain and how it works. These changes can be permanent.

E. Addiction is a developmental disease. It usually begins in childhood or adolescence.

F. Substances frequently abused include (but are not limited to) the following:
   - Marijuana
   - Hallucinogens (such as LSD)
   - Cocaine (stimulant that is snorted or injected)
   - Amphetamines (methamphetamine, a stimulant that is growing in popularity)
   - Opiates, such as heroin
   - Anabolic steroids (used to build muscle strength)
   - Prescription drugs (oxycodone is the most abused prescription drug in the United States)
   - Sedatives, hypnotics, and antianxiety medication
   - Inhalants
   - Designer or party drugs

II. **The client/caregiver can list indicators of substance abuse.**

A. Behavioral changes such as
   - Secretiveness
   - Change in friends

NRS
DATE INITIAL

   - Missed work or school
   - Poor performance at job or school
   - Frequent job changes
   - Legal difficulties
   - Increase in accidents and injuries

B. Physical signs such as
   - Unsteady gait
   - Slurred speech
   - Odor of alcohol or inhalant on breath or clothes
   - Constricted or dilated pupils
   - Needle marks
   - Runny nose or constant sniffling
   - Twitchiness or tremors
   - Seizures
   - Sores from picking or scratching skin
   - Weight loss
   - Red eyes

C. Emotional symptoms such as
   - Personality changes
   - Moodiness
   - Irritability
   - Anxiety
   - Poor attention or concentration
   - Restlessness
   - Euphoria
   - Depression
   - Agitation
   - Paranoia

D. Environmental factors such as
   - Poor living facilities or frequent moves
   - Poor personal hygiene of self or dependent children
   - Unkempt house
   - Presence of empty bottles or drug paraphernalia
   - Cigarette burns on furniture, rugs, or clothes

III. **The client/caregiver can list results of drug abuse.**

A. Violence
B. Car accidents
C. Financial difficulties
D. Addiction

(Continued)

NRS
DATE INITIAL

E. Crimes, including homicide, theft, and assault
F. Mental illness
G. Family and child abuse
H. Birth defects
I. AIDS
J. Death

IV. **The client/caregiver can list some community settings/activities for all three levels of prevention and health promotion.**

A. School
   1. Education of the students, parents, and educators
   2. Health fairs, presentations by positive role models, and so forth
   3. Training for peer counselors
B. Workplace
   1. Seminars, presentations, discussion groups
   2. Referrals
C. Community in general
   1. Health fairs, educational presentations at various centers (senior centers, neighborhood meetings, child and teen organizations such as scouts, homeless centers, etc.)
D. Home and neighborhood
   1. Talk openly with family members.
   2. Have accountability for any prescription drugs or alcohol used in the home.
   3. Supervise children's activities, and know the people they interact with.
   4. Form discussion and/or support groups.
E. Church
   1. Offer facilities for support groups such as Narcotics Anonymous or AA to meet.
   2. Have social activities without use of drugs and alcohol.
   3. Make health screenings for blood pressure and other things available.
   4. A parish nurse can assist in education and support.

V. **The client/caregiver can list treatments available.**

A. Substance-abuse treatment program
B. Inpatient programs
C. Residential treatment

NRS
DATE INITIAL

D. Outpatient treatment
E. Halfway houses
F. Community-based treatment
G. Employee assistance programs
H. Holistic treatments
   1. Massage
   2. Nutrition therapy
   3. Acupuncture or acupressure
   4. Hypnosis, meditation, or guided imagery
   5. Aromatherapy
   6. Energy medicine such as Reiki or Therapeutic Touch

RESOURCES

National Institute on Drug Abuse
www.nida.nih.gov/

U.S. Department of Health/SAMSHA Clearinghouse for alcohol and drug information
http://ncadi.samhsa.gov/

Narcotics Anonymous World Service
www.na.org/

National Center for Complementary and Alternative Medicine/National Institutes of Health
http://nccam.nih.gov/

National Center for Health Statistics
www.cdc.gov/nchs/fastats/druguse.htm

Drug testing

Counseling

Support groups

REFERENCES

Ackley, B. J., & Ladwig, G. B. (2006). *Nursing diagnosis handbook: A guide to planning care.* St. Louis: Mosby Inc.

Canobbio, M. M. (2006). *Mosby's handbook of patient teaching.* St. Louis: Mosby Inc.

Hitchcock, J. E., Schubert, P. E., & Thomas, S. A. (2003). *Community health nursing: Caring in action.* Clifton Park, NY: Thomson Delmar Learning.

Hunt, R. (2005). *Introduction to community based nursing.* Philadelphia: Lippincott Williams & Wilkins.

Varcarolis, E. M. (2006). *Manual of psychiatric nursing care plans.* St. Louis: Saunders Elsevier.

Tobacco Abuse

3

Patient name: _____ Admission: _____

NRS
DATE INITIAL

I. **The client/caregiver can describe physical changes caused by tobacco.**

A. Tobacco products include cigarettes, cigars, pipe tobacco, and chewing tobacco.
B. All tobacco products contain tar, carbon monoxide, and nicotine.
C. Tar in the tobacco increases the risk of lung cancer, emphysema, and other bronchial problems.
D. The carbon monoxide in tobacco smoke increases the chance of cardiovascular diseases. The Environmental Protection Agency has done studies that indicate second-hand smoke can cause lung cancer in adults and greatly increases the risk of respiratory illnesses in children and sudden infant death.
E. Nicotine is the drug in tobacco that causes addiction. Nicotine restricts blood vessels, causing increased blood pressure and circulatory problems. Nicotine can reach the brain within 8 seconds after inhalation.
F. The Centers for Disease Control and Prevention states this:
   1. The use of tobacco products is the leading preventable cause of death in the United States.
   2. More than $75 billion dollars have been used for direct medical costs related to smoking in 1 year.

II. **The client/caregiver can list ill effects of tobacco abuse.**

A. Coughing, shortness of breath, bad breath, and stained teeth
B. Financial problems (heavy smokers can spend $1,000 per year on cigarettes).
C. Addiction
D. Disease
   1. Cancer (all tobacco contains tar, a cancer-causing substance)
   2. Vascular diseases (nicotine causes blood vessels to constrict)
   3. Heart disease

4. Stroke
5. A constant oxygen deficiency in body
6. Chronic bronchitis
7. Gum disease
8. Stomach ulcers

E. Women who smoke increase the risk of
   • Earlier menopause
   • Stillborn or premature infants
   • Having low birth weight infants
F. Nutritional problems. Smokers use vitamin C twice as fast as nonsmokers. Vitamin C is one of the useful antioxidants.

III. **The client/caregiver can list signs and symptoms of withdrawal.**

A. Anxiety
B. Nervousness and possibly anger
C. A loss of concentration
D. Headaches
E. An intense craving for nicotine
F. A rise in blood pressure
G. Stomach pain

IV. **The client/caregiver can list methods to stop smoking.**

A. Counseling or behavioral training. Do not exchange one addiction for another, such as eating.
B. Nicotine-replacement products
   • Gum
   • Inhaler
   • Patch
C. Nonnicotine medications as prescribed by physician
D. Realistic goals because repeated attempts to stop smoking may be needed.
E. Many community programs that assist in smoking cessation. They offer group and personal support.
F. Keep busy. Find new things to do. Avoid situations or activities that can tempt you to smoke.
G. The Centers for Disease Control and Prevention has an online program (*www.smokefree.gov*) to help. It has a

(Continued)

NRS
DATE INITIAL

five-step plan to use when you decide to quit smoking.

- S = Set a quit date.
- T = Tell family, friends, and co-workers that you plan to quit.
- A = Anticipate and plan for the challenges you will face while quitting.
- R = Remove cigarettes and other tobacco products from your home, car, and work.
- T = Talk to your doctor about getting help to quit.

H. Explore complementary treatments such as
- Acupuncture or acupressure
- Hypnosis, meditation, or guided imagery
- Aromatherapy

V. **The client/caregiver can list methods to avoid weight gain.**

A. Eat low-calorie foods, including plenty of fresh fruits and vegetables.

B. Increase exercise. Take a walk. Seek activities that interest you, such as gardening.

RESOURCES

Health care professionals

American Cancer Society
www.cancer.org

American Lung Association
www.lungusa.org

American Heart Association
www.americanheart.org

Government Internet sites
www.surgeongeneral.gov/tobacco
www.cdc.gov/tobacco/how2quit.htm
www.smokefree.gov/
wsw.nlm.nih.gov/medlineplus/smokingcessation

REFERENCES

Ackley, B. J., & Ladwig, G. B. (2006). *Nursing diagnosis handbook: A guide to planning care.* St. Louis: Mosby Inc.

Canobbio, M. M. (2006). *Mosby's handbook of patient teaching.* St. Louis: Mosby Inc.

Hitchcock, J. E., Schubert, P. E., & Thomas, S. A. (2003). *Community health nursing: Caring in action.* Clifton Park, NY: Thomson Delmar Learning.

Hunt, R. (2005). *Introduction to community based nursing.* Philadelphia: Lippincott Williams & Wilkins.

Varcarolis, E. M. (2006). *Manual of psychiatric nursing care plans.* St. Louis: Saunders Elsevier.

You can quit smoking. (2007). Available from: *www.cdc.gov/tobacco/quit_smoking/you_can_quit/index.htm.* Washington, DC: Centers for Disease Control and Prevention.

4   Inhalant Abuse

Patient name: _____   Admission: _____

I.   **The client/caregiver can define inhalant abuse or "huffing."**

   A. Deliberately sniffing, inhaling, or huffing concentrated amounts of household products to produce a quick "high." They also depress the central nervous system.

   B. This form of substance abuse is usually seen in late childhood and early adolescence. Studies show that one in five students have used inhalants by the time they reach 8th grade.

   C. Inhalant abuse is growing in popularity because
      1. They are inexpensive.
      2. They are available in the home, the grocery store, the hardware store, pharmacies, and even school.
      3. They can be easily concealed in outer clothing, backpacks, closets, lockers, and so forth.
      4. They offer a very quick "high."

II. **The client/caregiver can list signs and symptoms of inhalant abuse.**

   A. Strong link between inhalant abuse and problems in school
   B. Paint or stains on body or clothing
   C. Red or runny eyes or nose
   D. Chemical breathe odor
   E. Drunk, dazed, or dizzy appearance
   F. Nausea and loss of appetite
   G. Anxiety, excitability, and irritability

III. **The client/caregiver can list products that can be used as inhalants.**

   A. Model airplane glue, rubber cement, and household glue
   B. Spray paint, aerosol hairspray, air freshener, deodorant, fabric protector, computer keyboard cleaner, and video head cleaners
   C. Nail polish remover, paint thinner, correction fluid, toxic markers, lighter fluid, gasoline, and carburetor cleaner

   D. Vegetable cooking spray, dessert topping spray (whipped cream), and whippets
   E. Nitrous oxide, butane, propane, and helium

IV. **The client/caregiver can list possible complications or results of inhalant abuse.**

   A. "Sudden sniffing death syndrome" can occur with use of any inhalant and even the first time it is used.
   B. Brain damage
      • Cell death of the brain
      • Permanent personality changes
      • Memory impairment
      • Hallucinations
      • Learning disabilities
   C. Muscle damage
      • Loss of coordination
      • Tremors and uncontrollable shaking
      • Muscle wasting
      • Reduced muscle tone and strength
   D. Peripheral nervous system
      • Numbness
      • Tingling sensation or total paralysis
   E. Bone marrow
      • Leukemia
   F. Liver, lung, and kidney damage
   G. Vision and hearing impairment

V.   **The client/caregiver can discuss measures to use when someone is "huffing."**

   A. Remain calm and do not panic.
   B. If the person is unconscious or not breathing, call for help and start CPR.
   C. If the person is conscious, keep him or her calm and in a well-ventilated room.
   D. Do not argue with or excite the abuser when he or she is under the influence.
   E. Excitement or stimulation can cause hallucinations or violence.
   F. Activity or stress may cause heart problems leading to "sudden sniffing death."
   G. Check the area for clues to what was used.

(Continued)

H. Seek professional help for the abuser from the school nurse, counselor, physician, and so forth.

VI. **The client/caregiver can discuss measures to prevent inhalant abuse.**

A. Start talking. Talk about the products that could be used, and emphasize the dangerous results.

B. Be educated regarding the products and methods of use. Learn the signs and symptoms of inhalant abuse.

C. Encourage your child to bring questions and concerns to you for discussion.

D. Set limits, and state that you will not tolerate use of inhalants.

E. Be involved with your child's friends and activities. Know where they are and what they are doing.

F. Promote an awareness of inhalant abuse to others, such as teachers or coaches.

RESOURCES

Substance Abuse and Mental Health Services Administration

National Inhalant Prevention Coalition
www.inhalants.org

National Institute on Alcohol Abuse and Alcoholism
www.niaaa.nih.gov/

REFERENCES

Hitchcock, J. E., Schubert, P. E., & Thomas, S. A. (2003). *Community health nursing: Caring in action.* Clifton Park, NY: Thomson Delmar Learning.

Varcarolis, E. M. (2006). *Manual of psychiatric nursing care plans.* St. Louis: Saunders Elsevier.

1 Energy Conservation

Patient name: _____ Admission: _____

NRS
DATE INITIAL

I. **The client/caregiver can state reasons for energy conservation.**

A. It decreases the physical stress on the body and promotes healing.
B. It decreases consumption of oxygen in the body.
C. It is needed for those with respiratory diseases and with physical limitations.

II. **The client/caregiver can state methods to promote energy conservation.**

A. Perform stretching and relaxation exercises before getting out of bed.
B. Use a tub seat and handheld showerhead when bathing.
C. Rest before difficult tasks.
D. Take frequent rest periods during the activity.
E. Pace activities, and do not rush.
F. Plan trips before going up and down stairs.
G. Roll, push, or pull instead of lifting. Use a cart to carry things.
H. Organize work area, and keep frequently used items within reach.

NRS
DATE INITIAL

I. Avoid having a work area that is too high or too low.
J. Delegate work to others.
K. Avoid extreme heat and cold.
L. Schedule activity when most able to tolerate it (i.e., after rest periods, after pain medication, and at least 1 hour after meals).
M. Sit to perform an activity instead of standing, when possible.
N. Hold objects close to you instead of away from your body.
O. Use arm supports to perform an activity (i.e., resting elbows on table while shaving, brushing teeth, and eating).
P. Limit activity on days of high air pollution.

REFERENCES

Canobbio, M. M. (2006). *Mosby's handbook of patient teaching.* St. Louis: Mosby Inc.

Perry, A., & Potter, P. (2006). *Clinical nursing skills & technique.* St. Louis: Mosby Inc.

Timby, B. K. (2005). *Fundamental nursing skills and concepts.* Philadelphia: J. B. Lippincott Williams & Wilkins.

2

Body Mechanics

Patient name: _____

Admission: _____

DATE | NRS INITIAL

DATE | NRS INITIAL

I. **The client/caregiver can list advantages of good body mechanics.**

A. Decreases possibility of back injury.
B. Decreases possibility of falls.
C. Increases work force with decreased energy.

II. **The client/caregiver can list good body mechanics in various positions and activities.**

A. Standing
1. Use good posture when standing. Check your posture by standing with heels, shoulders, and head against the wall.
2. Stand with feet slightly apart and toes pointed straight ahead.
B. Sitting
1. Sit with your back completely against the back of the chair.
2. Change position frequently if sitting for a long time.
C. Walking
1. Walk with feet parallel and close together.
2. Take a step by pushing off with the back foot.
3. Swing arms easily as you walk.
D. Sleeping
1. Sleep on a firm mattress.
2. Lying flat provides the least pressure on the back.
E. Lifting or carrying objects
1. Lift objects by flexing knees and hips, placing one foot in front of the other one and keeping the back straight.
2. Spread feet for a broad base of support to decrease the possibility of falling.

3. Prepare muscles by taking a deep breath and setting muscles before lifting.
4. Ask for assistance to lift or carry anything.
5. Use mechanical lifting aids whenever possible, such as a lever, hydraulic lift, and so forth.
6. Roll, push, pull, or slide if possible instead of lifting.
7. Keep load of weight close to the body to decrease workload.
8. Use wheels to move objects instead of carrying.
F. Pivoting
1. Place one foot in front of the other.
2. Raise heels slightly, placing weight on the balls of the feet to turn 90 degrees.
3. Face the direction of movement to prevent twisting of the spine.

III. **The client/caregiver can list other general measures for good body mechanics.**

A. Plan movements to avoid using poor body mechanics.
B. Move muscles in a smooth coordinated manner, avoiding any jerking.
C. Keep work material at appropriate level to avoid bending or stretching.

REFERENCES

Canobbio, M. M. (2006). *Mosby's handbook of patient teaching.* St. Louis: Mosby Inc.

Perry, A., & Potter, P. (2006). *Clinical nursing skills & technique.* St. Louis: Mosby Inc.

Timby, B. K. (2005). *Fundamental nursing skills and concepts.* Philadelphia: J. B. Lippincott Williams & Wilkins.

3 Joint Protection

Patient name: _____ **Admission:** _____

NRS
DATE INITIAL

I. **Definition: Joint protection is a means of using your joints wisely. Joint protection does not mean eliminating use of that joint.**

A. Principle 1: Use the strongest or largest joint possible to accomplish a task. Example: A doorknob extender allows you to open the door with the palm of the hand instead of with fingers.

B. Principle 2: Distribute the load over several joints. Example: Carry an object by using two hands instead of one.

C. Principle 3: Use each joint in its most stable and functional position. Example: To pick up an object, make sure that you face it directly to avoid twisting the trunk.

D. Principle 4: Use good body mechanics. Example: To lift objects from the ground, bend your legs instead of your back: pick up the object, holding it as close to your body as possible and rise, letting your leg muscles do the work.

E. Principle 5: Reduce the effort required to do the job. Example: Use wheels to transport. Utility carts, tea tables, and shopping carts are just a few examples.

F. Principle 6: Avoid prolonged periods of maintaining the same joint position. Example: Alternate between sitting and standing positions.

G. Principle 7: Encourage full and complete motions during daily activities. Example: Reach as high as possible when washing windows.

H. Principle 8: Avoid positions and activities leading to possible joint deformities. Example: Sleeping with pillows under the knees should be avoided unless otherwise advised.

1. Principle 8a: Avoid excessive pressure against the back of the fingers, the pads

of the thumb, and the tip of each finger. Example: When using spray cans or bottles, push down with the palm of the hand instead of the thumb tip.

2. Principle 8b: Avoid tight grasps on objects and keep hand open whenever possible. Example: Foam padding added to such articles as a toothbrush, pen, razor, fork, or comb will increase the size of the handle. The larger the grip, the less tension required to maintain your hold on these objects.

I. Principle 9: Organize your work. Example: Combine several errands in one trip whenever possible, especially if climbing stairs is involved.

J. Principle 10: Balance work with rest. Example: Schedule frequent rest periods during the day. Alternate heavy and light work tasks.

K. Principle 11: Use efficient storage. Example: Determine the easy way to reach areas and use them for the most frequently used supplies.

L. Principle 12: Eliminate unnecessary tasks. Example: Use convenience foods or prepare food in the easiest manner possible. For example, bake potatoes instead of mashing them.

Source: K. Lorig and J. Fries, *The Arthritis Helpbook* (pp. 69–92), ©1980 Addison-Wesley Publishing Company Inc. Reprinted by permission of Addison-Wesley Longman, Inc.

RESOURCE

Arthritis Foundation
www.arthritis.org

4   Walking with a Cane

Patient name: _____   **Admission:** _____

NRS DATE	INITIAL	

I. **The client/caregiver can list types of canes available.**

   A. A tripod cane has three legs.
   B. A quad cane has four legs.
   C. A standard straight cane has one leg.

II. **The client/caregiver can list general guidelines for use of a cane.**

   A. Choose a cane that has proper support and proper height.
   B. Canes should have rubber tips to improve traction and prevent slipping.
   C. Always wear sturdy, nonskid shoes to prevent falls.

III. **The client can demonstrate walking with a cane.**

   A. Hold cane on the strongest side of the body.
   B. Place cane about 4 inches in front of body and slightly to the side.
   C. Move the cane forward with the weaker leg bearing weight on the strong leg.
   D. Then move the strong leg forward while bearing weight on the cane and weaker leg.
   E. Look ahead, not at the floor, when walking.

IV. **The client can demonstrate walking the stairs with a cane.**

   A. Walking up the steps
      1. Place strong leg up first.
      2. Then move cane and affected leg up.
      3. Continue one step at a time.
   B. Walking down the steps
      1. Place cane and affected leg down first.
      2. Then move strong leg down.
      3. Continue one step at a time.

V. **The client can demonstrate getting into and out of a chair.**

   A. Sitting down in a chair
      1. Stand with backs of legs against a chair.
      2. Reach back with both hands to grasp armrests.
   B. Getting out of a chair
      1. Hold cane on stronger side as you grasp armrests.
      2. Lean forward and push up using armrests.

REFERENCES

Canobbio, M. M. (2006). *Mosby's handbook of patient teaching.* St. Louis: Mosby Inc.

Perry, A., & Potter, P. (2006). *Clinical nursing skills & technique.* St. Louis: Mosby Inc.

Timby, B. K. (2005). *Fundamental nursing skills and concepts.* Philadelphia: J. B. Lippincott Williams & Wilkins.

5   Walking with Crutches

Patient name: _____   **Admission:** _____

NRS
DATE INITIAL

I. **The client can demonstrate type of crutch walking as instructed.**

  A. Four-point gait
    1. Move the right crutch forward 4 to 6 inches.
    2. Move the left foot forward to level of right crutch.
    3. Move the left crutch forward 4 to 6 inches.
    4. Move the right foot forward to level of left crutch.
  B. Three-point gait
    1. Balance weight on crutches.
    2. Move both crutches and affected leg forward while body weight is supported on unaffected leg.
    3. Move unaffected leg forward.
  C. Two-point gait
    1. Advance right foot and left crutch together.
    2. Advance left foot and right crutch together.
  D. Swing-to gait
    1. Move both crutches ahead together.
    2. Lift body weight and swing to the crutches.
  E. Swing-through gait
    1. Move both crutches ahead together.
    2. Lift body weight and swing through and beyond the crutches.

II. **The client can demonstrate rising from a sitting position.**

  A. Slide forward in chair and place unaffected leg slightly under or at edge of chair.
  B. Hold both crutches by the hand bars in one hand on affected side.
  C. Use the hand on the unaffected side to grasp the arm of the chair and push up to a standing position.

NRS
DATE INITIAL

III. **The client can demonstrate getting into a chair.**

  A. Stand close to chair with chair touching back of legs.
  B. Hold both crutches in one hand.
  C. Use the free hand to hold the arm of the chair.
  D. Bear weight on the crutches and lower self into the chair.

IV. **The client can state precautions when using crutches.**

  A. Only use crutches that have a proper fit:
    1. The top of crutch should be about 1.5 inches below armpits.
    2. Elbows should be flexed 15 to 30 degrees.
  B. Do not lean or walk with weight on armpits because this may cause damage to nerves.
  C. Report any numbness or tingling down arms.
  D. Clear pathways by removing any objects that could cause falls.
  E. Avoid walking on slick or wet floor surfaces.
  F. Use only crutches in good condition.
    1. The underarms should be well padded for comfort.
    2. The ends should have rubber tips to prevent sliding.
  G. Keep crutch tips clean.
  H. Avoid walking on wet or slippery floors.

REFERENCES

Canobbio, M. M. (2006). *Mosby's handbook of patient teaching.* St. Louis: Mosby Inc.

Perry, A., & Potter, P. (2006). *Clinical nursing skills & technique.* St. Louis: Mosby Inc.

Timby, B. K. (2005). *Fundamental nursing skills and concepts.* Philadelphia: J. B. Lippincott Williams & Wilkins.

6 Cast Care

Patient name: _____ Admission: _____

NRS
DATE INITIAL

I. **The client/caregiver can list types of casts.**

   A. Plaster of Paris
   B. Fiberglass
   C. Plastic

II. **The client/caregiver can describe the care of a newly applied cast.**

   A. Handle it carefully by using palms of hands instead of fingers to prevent indentations in the cast.
   B. Allow air to circulate around it.
   C. Turn cast every 2 hours to ensure even drying.
   D. Support cast on a pillow, and place an absorbent material over the pillow to aid in drying.
   E. Do not bear weight on new cast for at least 48 hours.
   F. Apply ice to cast for the first 24 hours if prescribed by physician to decrease pain and swelling of tissue.
   G. Expect cast to feel warm as it dries.

III. **The client/caregiver can describe skin care with a cast.**

   A. Inspect skin regularly for irritation.
   B. Petal edges of cast with adhesive tape or mole skin to decrease irritation.
   C. Avoid inserting any objects into the cast. (If itchiness occurs, cool air can be blown into the cast or ice can be applied.)
   D. Report any breakage of the cast to the physician.
   E. Avoid getting cast wet.
   F. Avoid covering the cast tightly.
   G. Keep follow-up appointments.

IV. **The client/caregiver can list measures to prevent possible complications.**

   A. Edema
      1. Exercise joints above and below the cast.
      2. Elevate extremity above heart to prevent edema.
      3. Apply ice if swelling occurs.

NRS
DATE INITIAL

   B. Constipation
      1. Eat a diet high in bulk and roughage.
      2. Take stool softeners as needed.
   C. Renal calculi
      1. Increase fluids to 2000 to 3000 ml per day.
   D. Pressure sores and skin irritation
      1. Petal edges of cast with small strips of tape.
      2. Change positions frequently.

V. **The client/caregiver can list signs and symptoms of complications to report immediately.**

   A. Impaired blood supply
      1. Lack of pulse
      2. Skin pale and cool
      3. Pain and swelling
      4. Numbness, tingling, and prickling
   B. Nerve damage
      1. Increasing localized pain
      2. Numbness, tingling, and prickling
      3. Feelings of deep pressure
      4. Weakness or paralysis not noticed before
   C. Infection
      1. Musty odor over cast
      2. Hot spot or warmth felt on cast
      3. Pain
      4. Drainage
   D. Cast syndrome
      1. Prolonged nausea and vomiting
      2. Abdominal distention

REFERENCES

Canobbio, M. M. (2006). *Mosby's handbook of patient teaching.* St. Louis: Mosby Inc.

Perry, A., & Potter, P. (2006). *Clinical nursing skills & technique.* St. Louis: Mosby Inc.

Timby, B. K. (2005). *Fundamental nursing skills and concepts.* Philadelphia: J. B. Lippincott Williams & Wilkins.

7 Effective Breathing

Patient name: _____ **Admission:** _____

I. **The client/caregiver can list goals of effective breathing.**

   A. To increase expiration of air
   B. To decrease air trapping
   C. To increase lung expansion
   D. To decrease shortness of breath

II. **The client/caregiver can describe procedure for diaphragmatic or abdominal breathing.**

   A. Lie on your back with a pillow under your head and with knees slightly bent over a pillow.
   B. Clear airway passages first with coughing.
   C. Press one hand lightly on abdomen, and rest the other hand on the chest.
   D. Breathe in slowly through your nose, letting abdomen protrude.
   E. The hand on the stomach should rise during inspiration and fall during expiration while the hand on the chest should be almost still.

III. **The client/caregiver can demonstrate procedure for pursed lip breathing.**

   A. Breathe in slowly through the nose, counting to three while keeping mouth shut.
   B. Exhale through pursed lips (as if blowing out a candle), counting to seven.
   C. Breathing out should take at least twice as long as breathing in.

   D. When doing pursed lip breathing during an activity, breathe in before exertion and breathe out doing the activity.
   E. The client/caregiver can list methods to practice.
      1. Blow through a straw into a glass of water to form bubbles.
      2. Blow at a candle to bend the flame without blowing it out.
      3. Blow a tennis ball across a table at a steady pace.

IV. **The client/caregiver can demonstrate procedure for counted breathing.**

   A. Assess usual pattern of breathing by counting seconds required for inspiration and seconds required for expiration.
   B. Breathe out slowly, attempting to increase expiration time.
   C. Then breathing should be coordinated with walking by counting steps taken with inspiration and counting steps taken for each expiration.

REFERENCES

Canobbio, M. M. (2006). *Mosby's handbook of patient teaching.* St. Louis: Mosby Inc.

Perry, A., & Potter, P. (2006). *Clinical nursing skills & technique.* St. Louis: Mosby Inc.

Timby, B. K. (2005). *Fundamental nursing skills and concepts.* Philadelphia: J. B. Lippincott Williams & Wilkins.

8 Effective Coughing

Patient name: _____   **Admission:** _____

NRS
DATE INITIAL

I. **The client/caregiver can list benefits of controlled, effective coughing.**

   A. To conserve energy and decrease fatigue
   B. To remove mucus from airways
   C. To prevent respiratory complications

II. **The client/caregiver can demonstrate positioning methods for effective coughing.**

   A. Sit upright on chair or edge of bed with feet firmly on the floor, leaning forward slightly.
   B. If unable to sit upright, elevate head of bed and flex knees, or lie on the side keeping upper body flexed forward and knees bent toward body.

III. **The client/caregiver can demonstrate controlled coughing.**

   A. Take a deep breath, placing your hands on your stomach while allowing stomach to expand.
   B. Hold breath for 2 seconds.
   C. Cough twice with mouth open. The first cough loosens mucus and the second cough helps to remove it.
   D. Cough the mucus into a tissue and dispose of it.
   E. Breath in slowly through nose. Fast mouth breathing can drive mucus back into lungs.

IV. **The client/caregiver can demonstrate cascade coughing, another version of controlled coughing.**

   A. Take a slow deep breath and contract abdominal muscles.

NRS
DATE INITIAL

   B. Hold breath for 2 seconds.
   C. Open mouth and perform a series of coughs from the beginning to the end of the expiration. This clears large and small airways.
   D. Then breathe slowly through the nose and rest.

V. **The client/caregiver can list other general measures to promote effective coughing and clearing of airways.**

   A. Take pain medication as needed.
   B. Support incision with a pillow to decrease pain when coughing.
   C. Increase fluids to 2000 ml per day, unless contraindicated, to thin mucus.
   D. Use medications as ordered.

VI. **The client/caregiver can list possible complications of ineffective coughing.**

   A. Collapse of airways
   B. Rupture of alveoli
   C. Pneumothorax

REFERENCES

Canobbio, M. M. (2006). *Mosby's handbook of patient teaching.* St. Louis: Mosby Inc.

Perry, A., & Potter, P. (2006). *Clinical nursing skills & technique.* St. Louis: Mosby Inc.

Timby, B. K. (2005). *Fundamental nursing skills and concepts.* Philadelphia: J. B. Lippincott Williams & Wilkins.

9 Reality Orientation

Patient name: _____   **Admission:** _____

NRS
DATE INITIAL

I.   **The client/caregiver can list benefits of reality orientation.**

   A. Keeps the client in touch with reality
   B. Decreases confusion and disorientation
   C. Decreases fear and anxiety
   D. Improves quality of interactions with others

II. **The client/caregiver can list measures for orientation.**

   A. Use devices to improve memory.
       1. Simple clocks
       2. Calendars
       3. Label cabinets, doors, and drawers with words or pictures.
   B. Do not reinforce hallucinations or delusions.
   C. Give information slowly and simply.
   D. Allow time for response.
   E. Praise client for appropriate behavior.
   F. Encourage independence.
   G. Be sure client has glasses and/or hearing aid and that they are adequate for the client.
   H. Maintain good eye contact.

NRS
DATE INITIAL

   I. Treat client with respect, patience, and acceptance.
   J. Encourage socialization with family and friends.
   K. Encourage verbalization, and allow client to talk about past events.
   L. Encourage activities as tolerated.
   M. Maintain familiar routines.
   N. Tell client frequently what day and what time it is.
   O. Discuss current events.
   P. Give client only one instruction at a time.
   Q. Do not argue with client over inaccurate information.
   R. Provide good lighting.
   S. All caretakers and family should be included in promoting reality orientation.

REFERENCES

Canobbio, M. M. (2006). *Mosby's handbook of patient teaching.* St. Louis: Mosby Inc.

Perry, A., & Potter, P. (2006). *Clinical nursing skills & technique.* St. Louis: Mosby Inc.

Timby, B. K. (2005). *Fundamental nursing skills and concepts.* Philadelphia: J. B. Lippincott Williams & Wilkins.

10   Relaxation Techniques

Patient name: _____ Admission: _____

I.   **The client/caregiver can demonstrate quiet breathing technique.**

 A. Assume a comfortable sitting position.
 B. Take a deep, slow breath.
 C. As you exhale, envision all your tensions and anxieties flowing outward with each breath.
 D. Repeat as needed.

II. **The client/caregiver can demonstrate progressive relaxation.**

 A. Assume a comfortable sitting position; close your eyes.
 B. Take slow deep breaths, with the exhalation taking longer than the inhalation.
 C. Continue slow breathing, feeling the tension leaving your body and its becoming heavy.
 D. Perform progressive relaxation of muscles by tightening muscles during inspiration and relaxing muscles during expiration.
 E. Begin with muscles in feet and progress upward through the body muscles through every muscle group.

III. **The client/caregiver can demonstrate use of mental imagery.**

 A. Assume a comfortable sitting position.
 B. Use your imagination to experience a pleasant place or event.
 C. Using all your senses, smell the pleasant smells. Feel the warmth or softness. Taste something pleasant. See the pleasant surroundings, and hear the pleasant sounds.

IV. **The client/caregiver can demonstrate autogenic training.**

 A. Assume a comfortable sitting position.
 B. Take several slow, deep breaths.

 C. Have someone say these phrases in a slow monotonous tone three times, and then you say them silently and begin to relax.
  1. My right arm is heavy and warm.
  2. My left arm is heavy and warm.
  3. My forehead is cool and my face is relaxed.
  4. My neck and shoulders are warm and heavy.
  5. My breathing is slow and steady.
  6. My heartbeat is slow and steady.
  7. My entire body is warm and relaxed.

V.   **The client/caregiver can describe the thought-stopping technique.**

 A. Identify a few very pleasant experiences.
 B. Whenever an unpleasant thought enters your mind, say "stop."
 C. Begin thinking about a pleasant experience.
 D. As this process is repeated, it will become habit forming.

VI. **The client/caregiver can demonstrate massage therapy.**

 A. Use warm lotion with massage to relax muscles.
 B. Use a gliding light stroke to relax muscles.
 C. Use strong, circular movements to loosen tight muscles and to improve circulation.
 D. Use a kneading-type motion to relax tight muscles.

REFERENCES

Canobbio, M. M. (2006). *Mosby's handbook of patient teaching.* St. Louis: Mosby Inc.

Dossey, B. M., Keegan, L., Guzzetta, C. E., & Kolmeier, L. G. (1995). *Holistic nursing: A handbook for practice.* Gaithersburg, MD: Aspen Publishers.

Perry, A., & Potter, P. (2006). *Clinical nursing skills & technique.* St. Louis: Mosby Inc.

Timby, B. K. (2005). *Fundamental nursing skills and concepts.* Philadelphia: J. B. Lippincott Williams & Wilkins.

11 Bladder Retraining

Patient name: _____   **Admission:** _____

NRS
DATE INITIAL

I. **The client/caregiver can list goals of bladder retraining.**

  A. To re-establish bladder control
  B. To increase self-esteem of client
  C. To promote skin integrity

II. **The client/caregiver can list general measures to promote bladder retraining.**

  A. Keep a record for several days before training begins.
    1. Record amount of fluid intake.
    2. Record times that client voids.
    3. Record amount voided.
  B. Encourage large fluid intake (approximately 3,000 ml if not contraindicated) during the day.
  C. Restrict fluid in the evening.
  D. Avoid drinks with diuretic effect (coffee, tea, etc.).
  E. Give diuretic medication early in the day to avoid nighttime incontinence.
  F. Strengthen perineal muscles with Kegel exercises. Tighten buttocks together, and hold several times a day.
  G. Notify physician of signs of infection (i.e., frequency, burning, fever, and foul odor).

III. **The client/caregiver can describe the procedure for bladder training procedure.**

  A. Drink a glass of water about 30 minutes before voiding.

NRS
DATE INITIAL

  B. Begin by taking client to bathroom every 1 to 2 hours and then gradually increasing time between voiding to no more than every 3 to 4 hours.
  C. Several methods can be used to encourage voiding.
    1. Running water from the faucet
    2. Drinking water
    3. Pouring warm water over the perineum
    4. Tightening and relaxing pelvic muscles
    5. Massaging bladder
  D. Client should be taken to bathroom if possible, or provide a bedside commode so that the client can assume position used to void.
  E. Establish a strict schedule of voiding, usually before and after meals and on rising and before bedtime.
  F. Keep accurate records of when client voids in the commode and when incontinence occurs.

REFERENCES

Canobbio, M. M. (2006). *Mosby's handbook of patient teaching.* St. Louis: Mosby Inc.

Perry, A., & Potter, P. (2006). *Clinical nursing skills & technique.* St. Louis: Mosby Inc.

Timby, B. K. (2005). *Fundamental nursing skills and concepts.* Philadelphia: J. B. Lippincott Williams & Wilkins.

12 Bowel Retraining

Patient name: _____ **Admission:** _____

I. **The client/caregiver can list goals of bowel retraining.**

    A. Regularity of bowel function
    B. Prevention of fecal incontinence and impaction
    C. Prevention of skin breakdown
    D. Improvement of client's self-esteem

II. **The client/caregiver can list preparatory measures to promote bowel retraining.**

    A. Assess and record client's usual pattern of elimination.
       1. Record times of elimination.
       2. Record usual stimulus for elimination.
    B. Establish a specific time for elimination, usually after a meal consistent with client's history.
    C. Eat diet high in fiber to prevent constipation, but avoid foods that may cause diarrhea.
    D. Drink 3000 to 4000 ml of fluid per day unless contraindicated.
    E. Exercise regularly.
    F. Attain as normal a position as possible for defecation, such as sitting on a bedside commode or toilet and leaning forward.

III. **The client/caregiver can describe the procedure for bowel retraining.**

    A. Drink 4 ounces of prune juice each evening.
    B. Drink warm fluids just before evacuation to promote peristalsis.
    C. Insert rectal glycerin suppository (Dulcolax if glycerin is not effective) 30 minutes before scheduled time for defecation.
    D. Have client sit on toilet with feet placed on a stool, if possible, for defecation.
    E. Instruct client to bear down and contract abdominal muscles.
    F. Massaging abdomen from right to left may be helpful.
    G. Rectal stimulation may also be required to promote defecation.
    H. Allow adequate time for defecation.
    I. Record daily the stool amount, consistency, and so forth.

REFERENCES

Canobbio, M. M. (2006). *Mosby's handbook of patient teaching.* St. Louis: Mosby Inc.

Perry, A., & Potter, P. (2006). *Clinical nursing skills & technique.* St. Louis: Mosby Inc.

Timby, B. K. (2005). *Fundamental nursing skills and concepts.* Philadelphia: J. B. Lippincott Williams & Wilkins.

Part VIII

Resources

Advance directives (American Medical Association)
www.medem.com/index.cfm

AIDS Info
PO Box 6303
Rockville, MD 20849
800-448-0440
www.aidsinfo.nih.gov

Alcoholics Anonymous World Services
Grand Central Station
PO Box 459
New York, NY 10163
212-870-3400
www.alcoholics-anonymous.org

Alexander Graham Bell Association for the Deaf and Hard of
   Hearing
3417 Volta Place, NW
Washington, DC 20007
202-337-5220 (V); 202-337-5221 (TTY)
E-mail: info@agbell.org
www.agbell.org

ALS (Amyotrophic Lateral Sclerosis Association)
27001 Agoura Road Suite 150
Calabasas Hills, CA 91301-5104
800-782-4747
www.alsa.org

Alzheimer's Association
225 N Michigan Ave. Floor 17
Chicago, IL 60601
800-272-3900
www.alz.org

American Academy of Allergy, Asthma and Immunology
555 East Wells Street, Suite 1100
Milwaukee, WI 53202-3823
800-822-2762
www.aaaai.org

American Academy of Dermatology
1350 I Street, NW, Suite 870
Washington, DC 20005-4355
202-842-3555
www.aad.org

American Academy of Ophthalmology
PO Box 7424
San Francisco, CA 94120-7424
415-561-8500
www.eyenet.org

American Cancer Society
National Center
1599 Clifton Road NE
Atlanta, GA 30329
800-227-2345
www.cancer.org

American Chronic Pain Association (ACPA)
PO Box 850
Rocklin, CA 95677-0850
800-533-3231
www.theacpa.org

American College of Rheumatology
Association of Rheumatology Health Professionals
1800 Century Place, Suite 250
Atlanta, GA 30345
404-633-3777
www.rheumatology.org

American Council of the Blind
1155 15th St. NW, Suite 1004
Washington, D.C. 20005
800-424-8666
E-mail: info@acb.org
www.acb.org

American Diabetes Association
National Call Center
1701 N. Beauregard St.
Alexandria, VA 22311
800-DIABETES
www.diabetes.org

American Dietetic Association
120 South Riverside Plaza, Suite 2000
Chicago, IL 60606-6995
800-877-1600
E-mail: hotline@eatright.org
www.eatright.org

American Foundation for the Blind
11 Penn Plaza, Suite 300
New York, NY 10001
800-232-5463 (Hotline)
For publications: 800-232-3044
E-mail: afbinfo@afb.net
www.afb.org

American Heart Association
National Center
7272 Greenville Ave.
Dallas, TX 75231
800-242-1793
www.americanheart.org

American Kidney Fund
6110 Executive Boulevard, Suite 1010
Rockville, MD 20852
800-638-8299
E-mail: helpline@kidneyfund.org
www.kidneyfund.org

American Lung Association, National Headquarters
61 Broadway, Sixth Floor
New York, NY 10006
800-548-8252
www.lungusa.org

American Parkinson Disease Association
1250 Hylan Blvd., Suite 4B
Staten Island, NY 10305-1943
800-223-2732
www.apdaparkinson.com

American Speech-Language-Hearing Association (ASHA)
10801 Rockville Pike
Rockville, MD 20852
Voice: 301-897-5700
Toll-free voice: 800-638-8255
TTY: 301-897-0157
E-mail: actioncenter@asha.org
www.asha.org

American Stroke Connection, National Center
7272 Greenville Ave.
Dallas, TX 75231
888-STROKE
www.strokeassociation.org

American Thyroid Association
6066 Leesburg Pike, Suite 550
Falls Church, Virginia 22041
703-998-8890
www.thyroid.org/

Anxiety Disorders Association of America
8730 Georgia Avenue, Suite 600
Silver Springs, MD 20910
240-485-1001
www.adaa.org

Arthritis Foundation
1330 W. Peachtree St.
Atlanta, GA 30309
800-283-7800
www.arthritis.org

Attention Deficit Disorder Association (ADDA)
PO Box 543
Pottstown, PA 19464
484-945-2101
E-mail: mail@add.org
www.add.org

Back to Sleep
31 Center Drive, Building 31, Room 2A32
Bethesda, MD 20892
800-505-CRIB
E-mail: NICHDIRC@mail.nih.gov

Brain Injury Association of America
8201 Greenboro Dr., Suite 611
McLean, VA 22102
800-444-6443
www.biausa.org

Celiac Disease Foundation
13251 Ventura Boulevard, #1
Studio City, CA 91604
818-990-2354
E-mail: cdf@celiac.org
www.celiac.org

Centers for Disease Control and Prevention
1600 Clifton Road, N.E.
Atlanta, GA 30333 USA
800-311-3435
www.cdc.gov/

CHADD—Children and Adults with Attention-
    Deficit/Hyperactivity Disorder
8181 Professional Place, Suite 150
Landover, MD 20785
800-233-4050
www.chadd.org

Children's Safety Network
Washington office:
Education Development Center, Inc.
1000 Potomac St., Suite 350
Washington, DC 20007
202-572-3734
E-mail: eschmidt@edc.org
www.childrenssafetynetwork.org/

Crohn's and Colitis Foundation of America
386 Park Avenue S. Seventeen Floor
New York, NY 10016-7374
800-932-2423
www.ccfa.org

Cystic Fibrosis Foundation
6931 Arlington Rd.
Bethesda MD 20814
800-344-4823
www.cff.org/

Epilepsy Foundation
4351 Garden City Dr.
Landover, MD 20785
800-EFA-1000
www.epilepsyfoundation.org

The Glaucoma Foundation
116 John St., Suite 1605
New York, NY 10038
800-GLAUCOMA
www.glaucomafoundation.org

Healthy People 2010
www.health.gov/healthypeople

Hospice Association of America
228 Seventh St. SE
Washington, DC 20003
202-546-4759
www.nahc.org/

International Association of Infant Massage
PO Box 6370
Ventura, CA 93006
805-644-8524
E-mail: IAIM4US@aol.com

La Leche League International
www.lalecheleague.org/

Learning Disabilities Association of America
4156 Library Road, Suite 1
Pittsburgh, PA 15234-1349
E-mail: info@ldaamerica.org
www.ldaamerica.org

Leukemia and Lymphoma Society
Home Office
1311 Mamaroneck Ave.
White Plains, NY 10605
800-955-4572
www.leukemia.org

Lupus Foundation of America
National Office
2000 L Street NW, Suite 710
Washington, DC 20036
800-558-0121
www.lupus.org

March of Dimes Birth Defects Foundation
1275 Mamaroneck Avenue
White Plains, NY 10605
888-MODIMES (663-4637)
E-mail: askus@marchofdimes.com
www.marchofdimes.com

MedicAlert
2323 Colorado Ave.
Turlock, CA 95382
888-633-4298
www.medicalert.org

Medline Plus, National Library of Medicine
Patient Education material
http://medlineplus.gov/

Multiple Sclerosis Association of America, National
  Headquarters
706 Haddonfield Road
Cherry Hill, NJ 08002
800-LEARN-MS
www.msaa.com

My Pyramid-United State Department of Agriculture
www.mypyramid.gov

Narcotics Anonymous World Service
www.na.org/

National Association for Continence
PO Box 1019
Charleston, SC 29402-1019
800-BLADDER (252-3337)
E-mail: memberservices@nafc.org
www.nafc.org

National Association for Visually Handicapped
22 West 21st Street, 6th Floor
New York, NY 10010
212-889-3141
E-mail: staff@navh.org
www.navh.org

National Braille Association, Inc. (NBA)
3 Townline Circle
Rochester, NY 14623-2513
585-427-8260
E-mail: nbaoffice@nationalbraille.org
www.nationalbraille.org

National Cancer Institute (NCI)
NCI Public Inquiries Office
6116 Executive Boulevard, Room 3036A
Bethesda, MD 20892-8322
www.cancer.gov/

National Council on Alcoholism and Drug Dependence
   (NCADD)
22 Cortlandt Street, Suite 801
New York, NY 10007-3128
212-269-7797; Fax: 212-269-7510
HOPELINE: 800-NCA-CALL (24-hour affiliate referral)
E-mail: national@ncadd.org
www.ncadd.org

National Center for Complementary and Alternative
   Medicine/National Institutes of Health
http://nccam.nih.gov/

National Diabetes Information Clearinghouse
1 Information Way
Bethesda, MD 20892-3560
800-860-8747
http://diabetes.niddk.nih.gov

National Eye Institute
National Institutes of Health
2020 Vision Place
Bethesda, MD 20892-3655
301-496-5248
E-mail: 2020@nei.nih.gov
www.nei.nih.gov

National Foundation for the Treatment of Pain
PO Box 70045
Houston, TX 77270
713-862-9332
E-mail: NFTPain@cwo.com
www.paincare.org

National Heart, Lung, and Blood Institute
Health Information Center
PO Box 30105
Bethesda, MD 20824-0105
www.nhlbi.nih.gov

National Hemophilia Foundation
116 W. 32nd St., 11th Floor
New York, NY 10001
800-42-HANDI
www.hemophilia.org

National Hospice and Palliative Care Organization
1700 Diagonal Rd., Suite 625
Alexandria, VA 22314
703-837-1500
www.nho.org

National Inhalant Prevention Coalition
322-A Thompson Street
Chattanooga, TN 37405
800-269-4237
E-mail: nipc@io.com
www.inhalants.org

National Institute on Alcohol Abuse and Alcoholism (NIAAA)
5635 Fishers Lane, MSC 9304
Bethesda, MD 20892-9304
301-443-3860; Fax: 301-480-1726
www.niaaa.nih.gov

National Institute of Aging
Building 31, Room 5C27
31 Center Drive, MSC 2292
Bethesda, MD 20892
www.nihseniorhealth.gov

National Institute of Allergy and Infectious Diseases
6610 Rockledge Dr. MSC 6612
Bethesda, MD 200892-6612
301-496-5717
www.niaid.nih.gov

National Institute of Arthritis and Musculoskeletal and Skin
   Diseases
National Institutes of Health
31 Center Dr. MSC 2350, Building 31, Room 4C02
Bethesda, MD 20892-2350
301-496-8190
www.niams.nih.gov

National Institute on Deafness and Other Communication
   Disorders
31 Center Dr. MSC 2320
Bethesda, MD 20892-2320
301-496-7243
301-402-0252 (TTY)
www.nidcd.nih.gov/

National Institute of Dental and Craniofacial Research
   (NIDCR)
National Institutes of Health, DHHS
31 Center Drive, Room 5B-55
Bethesda, MD 20892
E-mail: nidcrinfo@mail.nih.gov

National Institute on Drug Abuse/National Institutes of Health
6001 Executive Boulevard, Room 5213
Bethesda, MD 20892-9561
www.nida.nih.gov/

National Institute of Mental Health (NIMH)
National Institutes of Health, DHHS
6001 Executive Blvd., Rm. 8184, MSC 9663
Bethesda, MD 20892-9663
E-mail: nimhinfo@nih.gov
www.nimh.nih.gov

National Kidney Foundation
30 E. 33rd St., 11th Floor
New York, NY 10016
800-622-9010
www.kidney.org

National Kidney and Urologic Diseases Information
    Clearinghouse
3 Information Way
Bethesda, MD 20892-3580
E-mail: nkudic@info.niddk.nih.gov

National Library Service for the Blind and Physically
    Handicapped, Library of Congress
1291 Taylor Street, N.W.
Washington, D. C. 20011
800-424-8567
www.loc.gov/nls

National Maternal and Child Health Clearinghouse (NMCHC)
Health Resources and Services Administration (HRSA)
U.S. Department of Health and Human Resources
Parklawn Building
5600 Fishers Lane
Rockville, Maryland 20857
888-ASK-HRSA (275-4772)
www.ask.hrsa.gov/MCH.cfm

National Organization on Fetal Alcohol Syndrome (NOFAS)
900 17th Street, NW, Suite 910
Washington, DC 20006
800-66-NOFAS
www.nofas.org

National Osteoporosis Foundation, National Headquarters
1232 22nd St., NW
Washington, DC 20037-1292
202-223-2226
www.nof.org

National Parkinson Foundation, Inc.
1501 N.W. Ninth Ave./Bob Hope Rd.
Miami, FL 33136-1494
800-327-4545
www.parkinson.org

National PKU News
www.pkunews.org/

National Scoliosis Foundation (NSF)
5 Cabot Place
Stoughton, MA 02072
781-341-6333
E-mail: scoliosis@aol.com
www.scoliosis.org

National Spinal Cord Injury Association
6701 Democracy Blvd., Suite 202
Bethesda, MD 20817
800-962-9629
www.spinalcord.org

National Stroke Association
9707 E. Easter La.
Englewood, CO 80112-5341
800-STROKES
www.stroke.org

The National Women's Health Information Center
U.S. Department of Health and Human Services
Office on Women's Health
www.4woman.gov/

The Office of the Surgeon General (OSG)
www.surgeongeneral.gov/sgoffice

Smoking Cessation
www.surgeongeneral.gov/tobacco/index.html
www.smokefree.gov/

Obsessive-Compulsive Foundation, Inc.
337 Notch Hill Road
North Branford, CT 06471
203-315-2190
www.ocfoundation.org

Organ Donor Programs
www.organdonor.gov/

Ovarian Cancer National Alliance
910 17th Street, N.W., Suite 1190
Washington, D.C. 20006
866-399-6262
E-mail: ocna@ovariancancer.org
www.ovariancancer.org/

Prostate Cancer Foundation
1250 Fourth Street
Santa Monica, CA 90401
www.prostatecancerfoundation.org/

Sickle Cell Disease Association of America
231 East Baltimore Street, STE 800
Baltimore, MD 21202
800-421-8453
E-mail: scdaa@sicklecelldisease.org

Sjogren's Syndrome Foundation
8120 Woodmont Ave., Suite 530
Bethesda, MD 20814-1437
800-4-SJOGREN (475-6473)
www.sjogrens.org

Spina Bifida Association of America
4590 MacArthur Blvd. NW, Suite 250
Washington, DC 20007-4266
800-621-3141
www.sbaa.org

Substance Abuse and Mental Health Services Administration
    (SAMHSA) Treatment Facility Locator
800-662-HELP
www.findtreatment.samhsa.gov

United Cerebral Palsy Associations, Inc.
1660 L Street NW, Suite 700
Washington, DC 20036
202-776-0406; 202-973-7197 (TT)
800-872-5827 (V/TT)
E-mail: ucpanatl@ucpa.org
www.ucpa.org

U.S. Food and Drug Administration
www.fda.gov/

United Ostomy Association
19772 MacArthur Blvd., Suite 200
Irvine, CA 92612-2405
800-826-0826
www.uoa.org

Women, Infants, Children (WIC) Program
www.fns.usda.gov/wic/

World Health Organization
Avenue Appia 20
1211 Geneva 27, Switzerland
E-mail: info@who.int
www.who.int

Wound, Ostomy, Continence Nurses
1550 S. Coast Highway, Suite 201
Laguna Beach, CA 92651
888-224-9626
www.wocn.org

Index

Index

Index